Creationist Diet

Second Edition

A Comprehensive Guide to Bible and Science Based Nutrition

By Gary F. Zeolla

Table of Contents

Introductory Pages – 5

Section One
Plant Foods – 27

Section Two
Animal Foods – 149

Section Three
Miscellaneous – 379

Appendixes – 533

Notes:

The First Edition of this book contained two chapters on supplements. But I have plans to write a full book on that subject, so I will forgo comments in that regard until then (see Appendix Two).

The First Edition of this book also contained two chapters on exercise. But my fitness website contains much information in that regard, as does my book *Starting and Progressing in Powerlifting*, so I will refer the reader to those resources (see Appendixes Two and Three).

Other chapters were renamed and reconfigured, with information from different chapters being combined into one, and a couple of new chapters were added.

Introductory Pages

Creationist Diet

Preface

What did God give to human beings for food? What does the Bible teach about diet and nutrition? How do the Biblical teachings on foods compare to scientific research on nutrition and the relationship of diet to degenerative disease like heart disease, cancer, stroke, diabetes, and osteoporosis? These and other questions are addressed in this book.

Starting with God's decrees about foods at Creation, in the Garden of Eden, after the Fall, and after the Flood, and gleaning nutrition information from the rest of the Bible, this book proposes four different possible Creationist Diets, presenting the pros and cons of each. These different possible diets are also correlated with scientific research. In this way, information is given to help the reader to decide on what type of diet would be best for you personally.

In addition, foods are divided into "God-given foods" and "not God-given foods." These lists are compared to what foods scientific research has shown to increase or decrease the risk of heart disease, cancer, and stroke. Thus the reader can know what foods to include in your own diet and what foods to avoid.

This Second Edition is 2-1/2 times as long as the First Edition. Along with being much longer, this Second Edition presents a different perspective on diet. The First Edition mostly advocated a vegan diet, while this Second Edition also advocates for a diet that includes animal foods. But, and this is very important, those animal foods are to be what are called "old-fashioned" meats, dairy, and eggs, not the "factory farm" products that most people eat. What is meant by these two terms and the incredible difference between them is explained in this book.

In addition, this book covers a wide range of diet related topics to help the reader to understand how to live a healthier lifestyle according to God's design. It is truly a comprehensive to diet and nutrition for Christians and others, as it covers every subject imaginable in regard to sound nutritional practices that would be helpful for the average person.

About the Author:

The author has a B.S. in Nutrition Science (Penn State; 1983) and attended Denver Seminary from 1988-1990. He is the translator of the *Analytical-Literal Translation of the Bible* and the author of numerous Christian and fitness books. He is also a powerlifter, being listed on the Top 20 All-time open (all ages) ranking lists and holds All-time masters (50-59 age) American and world records.

Zeolla is the director, webmaster, and primary writer for his four websites: his personal website (www.Zeolla.org), Darkness to Light Christian Ministry (www.Zeolla.org/Christian), Fitness for One and All (www.Zeolla.org/Fitness), and Biblical and Constitutional Politics (www.Zeolla.org/Politics). A detailed autobiography is available on the personal website.

Disclaimers:

The material presented in this book is intended for educational purposes only. The author is not offering medical or legal advice. Accuracy of information is attempted but not guaranteed. Before undertaking any diet plan, making any dietary changes, or beginning an exercise program, consult your doctor. The author is in no way responsible or liable for any harm (physical, mental, emotional, or financial) that results from following any of the advice in this book.

All brand names are trademarks or registered trademarks of their respective companies. The author is not being paid to endorse any of the products, companies, or websites mentioned in this book.

Scripture Verses:

Unless otherwise indicated, all Scripture verses are from the author's *Analytical-Literal Translation of the Bible* (ALT). Copyright © 1999-2016 by Gary F. Zeolla (www.Zeolla.org).

Scripture verses marked NKJV are from: *The New King James Version*. Nashville: Thomas Nelson Publisher, 1982. Word counts from the Bible are based on the NKJV.

Terminology

The words: creation, creationism, and creationist are being used in this book to refer to a belief in divine creation as opposed to atheistic evolution. There are various forms of creationist theories, but the view being used in this book would more specifically be called "young-earth creationism." This is contrasted with old-earth creationism, intelligent design, and other theistic theories of origins. For more in this regard, see Chapter One of Volume One of the author's three volume set, *Why Are These Books in the Bible and Not Others?*

The "Fall" refers to when Adam and Eve sinned against God by eating of the forbidden fruit (Gen 3:1ff).

"Antediluvian" refers to "of or belonging to the time before the Biblical Flood" (Oxford). It refers to the 1,500 years or so between the sin of Adam and Eve and the Flood of Noah.

In this book, the word "meats" refers to red meat (beef), poultry (chicken and turkey), fish, and other flesh foods, though sometimes fish is considered separately. The term "processed meats" refers to sausage, bacon, ham, kielbasa, pepperoni, and lunch meats (bologna, salami, and the like).

The term "animal foods" refers to all foodstuff attained from animals, which is to say, meats, dairy, eggs, and honey.

The term "plant foods" refers to fruits, vegetables, nuts, seeds, grains, legumes, and other edible plant stuff.

The term "produce" refers to "products of agriculture, particularly fruits and vegetables" (YourDictionary)

The term "vegan" refers to an eating plan in which only plant foods are consumed; no animal foods of any kind are consumed, no meat, no dairy, no eggs, not even honey.

The term "ovo-lacto-vegetarian" refers to an eating plan in which no meat is consumed, but in which dairy, eggs, and usually honey is consumed. But for simplicity's sake, such a diet will be referred to in this book simply as "vegetarian."

The term "omnivore" refers to an eating plan in which both plant foods and animal foods are consumed. The term "carnivore" would refer to an eating plan in which only animal foods are consumed, usually only meats.

"Vitamins" are "any of a group of organic compounds that are essential for normal growth and nutrition and are required in small quantities in the diet because they cannot be synthesized by the body" (Oxford)

Creationist Diet

"Minerals" are "a solid inorganic substance of natural occurrence" (Oxford). Nutritionally essential minerals are like vitamins in that they are essential for normal growth but cannot be synthesized by the body.

The three macronutrients are: fats, carbohydrates (carbs), and protein. These provide calories, which is energy for the body. Fats provide nine calories per gram, while carbs and protein provide four calories per gram. Alcohol also provides calories (seven per gram), but it will not be discussed in this book.

Amino acids are the building blocks of protein, which in addition to providing energy, is essential for many body processes, most notably the building of muscle. There are eight essential amino acids, meaning they cannot be created by the body and thus must be attained through the diet. A food that contains all eight essential amino acids is said to be a complete protein, while one that is lacking in one or more is said to be an incomplete protein.

Fatty acids are the components of fat. There arc three types of fatty acids: saturated fatty acids (SFA), monounsaturated fatty acids (MUFA), and polyunsaturated fatty acids (PUFA). Essential fatty acids cannot be created by the body and thus must be attained through the diet. The essential fatty acids are omega 3s, 6s, and 9s.

The term "phytonutrients" or "phytochemicals" refers to "chemical compounds that occur naturally in plants. Some are responsible for color and other organoleptic properties." They are not vitamins or minerals, but are important for our study, as they are "a substance found in certain plants which is believed to be beneficial to human health and help prevent various diseases" (Meriam).

Similar to phytonutrients are flavonoids. These are, "any of a large class of plant pigments having a structure based on or similar to that of flavone" (Oxford). The important point for this book is, "This nutrient group is most famous for its antioxidant and anti-inflammatory health benefits, as well as its contribution of vibrant color to the foods we eat" (World's).

Bibliography:

Merriam Webster – www.merriam-webster.com

Oxford Dictionary. As found on Microsoft *Word 365*.

World's Healthiest Foods. Flavonoids. http://www.whfoods.com/genpage.php?tname=nutrient&dbid=119

YourDictionary. http://www.yourdictionary.com

Creation Theory

A popular diet plan being promoted today is the "Paleolithic Diet." The idea of the diet is to eat like a "Paleo-man" i.e., a caveman. The theory behind the diet is that the healthiest way to eat is the way our ancestors ate from when we first starting evolving into *Homo sapiens* about two million years ago, until our diets changed a few thousand years ago. Such a diet would be how evolution "intended" for us to eat.

Such a diet does have plausibility, if one believes in the theory of evolution. I for one do not. But this "Paleolithic Diet" got me thinking as to what a diet based on the theory of creation would look like. But before looking at what a "Creationist Diet" would involve, some of the basic points of the creationist position need to be summarized.

Summary of Creation Theory

According to the young-earth theory of creation, God "made the heaven and the earth" (Gen 1:1) about 6,000 years ago. This creation was accomplished in six, 24-hour days. On day six, God created the man (Adam) and the woman (Eve) and placed them in the Garden of Eden.

At the time of their creation, Adam and Eve and their descendants had the same if not greater intellectual capabilities as we do today. They each also had a greater genetic diversity than we do today.

After an unspecified amount of time, Adam and Eve sinned against God and were cast out of the Garden of Eden (Gen 3:1ff). It was at that time that suffering and death entered the world (Rom 5:12). Adam and Eve proceeded to have "sons and daughters" (Gen 5:4). These children populated the world.

But over the next 1,500 years or so, humanity became increasing wicked, and God punished the world with a worldwide flood (Gen 6-9). But first He told righteous Noah to build an ark for himself, his family, and sets of animals. This Flood destroyed all humans and animals, except for those kept safely on the ark. After the Flood, the world was repopulated by Noah and his family and the animals from the ark.

However, rather than scattering over the earth as they were supposed to, these humans built a tower "whose top will be as far as the heaven" (Gen 11:4). God judged this project by confusing the languages of the people. Then "the LORD scattered them abroad over the face of the earth" (Gen 11:7-9). This scattering of people and the inbreeding that followed was the origin of the different human races. As a result, the genetic diversity of each race would become more limited.

11

Then a few hundred years after the Flood, God chose one man, Abram/ Abraham, and through him and his descendants, God would continue to give revelations that would be for him, his descendants, and ultimately for all peoples. These revelations are the Books of the Old Testament.

Then "in these last days He spoke to us by [His] Son" (Heb 1:1). Thus the words and actions of Jesus and of His disciples are the words of God and also contain revelations for us today. These revelations became the New Testament.

Implications of Creation Scenario

This creation scenario has several implications that will bear on the subject of diet. First off, all human beings are descendants of Adam and Eve. As such, any dietary directives God gave to Adam and Eve would be the earliest directives and would apply to and have been passed on to all human beings directly. Furthermore, these were the only God-given dietary directives for human beings during the entire antediluvian (before the Flood) era.

Second, all human beings alive today are descendants of Noah and his family. Thus again, any dietary directives God gave to Noah would apply to and have been passed on directly to all human beings. These directives would be later but still as important as the previous ones, as they would have been directly given by God to all peoples.

Third, the Tower of Babel is a turning point in human history. With the scattering of humans over the planet and the division into races, no longer could dietary directives be given directly to the entire human race. Over time, each people group would begin to develop and adapt to their own unique dietary habits.

But the directives given to one race, the Hebrews, the descendants of Abram/ Abraham, would still be the Word of God. Therefore, any dietary directives given through them would be important for all peoples. Though these directives would be later and not known by most people, unless they came in contact with the Hebrews or their writings.

Finally, the example and teachings of Jesus and of His disciples would also be God-given revelations, though still later and known only to those to whom the Gospel would be preached.

The import of these points is this: any dietary directives given to Adam and Eve would constitute the original diet for all humans and be known by all. Dietary directives given to Noah and his family would be later but just as important and for all peoples. Information about diet in the Bible after the time of the Tower of Babel would be still important, but later and not known by all people.

Consequently, the thesis of the Creationist Diet is that the earlier a dietary directive is given, the more basic and applicable it is to all peoples. Or to put it another way, the earlier a food entered into the human diet, the more likely it is that it is a healthy food for all peoples. Whereas, the later a food entered into the human diet, the less likely it is to be a healthy food for all people. But what the Bible says about it is still important as the entirety of the Bible is the Word of God.

Also important is the form of the food. If eaten in the form in which it was created by God and thus found in nature, it would definitely be a God-given food, as it would contain all of the naturally occurring nutrients. If a food undergoes a form of processing that would have been possible in Biblical times, it would still be considered to be a God-given food, as it would still most likely contain the naturally occurring nutrients.

However, if a food is processed in such a way that was not possible in Biblical times and which removes a significant amount of nutrients, then that food would no longer be considered to be a God-given food. The same would be true if elements are added to the food that did not exist in Bible times. The difference between Biblical and more modern day food processing methods will be explained further at the appropriate places.

With that background, this book will try to ascertain from Scripture when different kinds of foods and processing thereof entered into the human diet. And most of all, this book will try to discern what are "God-given foods" based on dietary directives given in the Bible.

What this means is, Genesis chapters 1-11 will receive the most emphasis in developing a Creationist Diet, which is appropriate as it is from these chapters that the creation theory is developed. However, since "All Scripture [is] God-breathed and [is] beneficial" (2Tim 3:16), other parts of Scripture will be taken into account at appropriate points.

In addition, throughout this book, numerous quotes and scientific studies will be cited which demonstrate modern-day knowledge is finally catching up with the Biblical teachings on diet and nutrition.

Creationist Diet

Background to Second Edition

The first edition of this book was published in September 2000. For many years prior to that time, this writer had been following a mostly plant-based diet. I would eat meats, dairy, and eggs, but only in limited amounts. But then about the time I started work on the first edition of this book, I eliminated dairy from my diet. The type of reasons for doing so will be mentioned in this book. I also rarely ate eggs, but I was eating one serving of meat a day. My health was not good at that time; that was the reason for the dietary changes, an effort to improve my health.

I was following that mostly-plant based diet for most of the time I was working on this book. My preference for such a diet affected my interpretation of Scripture and the tone of the first edition of this book. It did not advocate a vegan diet *per se*, but it did recommend only eating animal foods in very limited amounts.

Then just before the First Edition was published, I eliminated even the small amount of animal food I had been eating from my diet. I was thus following a full vegan diet. I updated the final chapter of the book at the last minute prior to publication to reflect that dietary change.

I followed that full vegan diet for a few months, and I did feel better initially. But then after a few months, my health completely fell apart, and I struggled greatly health-wise for the next few years. I thus re-investigated the reasons I had been following a near-vegetarian or full vegan diet, and I came to believe most of the reasons were faulty. I also restudied the Scriptures and realized I had been mistaken in thinking the Scriptures advocated a vegan, vegetarian, or even near-vegetarian diet.

As a result, I began eating meats, dairy, and eggs again. I still have health struggles, but I am doing much better than when I was following the near vegetarian diet and especially the vegan diet. I even started competing in powerlifting again for the first time in two decades. Therefore, in 2008, rather than updating this book, I published a new book on nutrition and the Bible. It is titled *God-given Foods Eating Plan* and was published through a new publisher.

That book addresses the subject of nutrition and the Bible in a rather different manner than this one. It goes into great detail exegeting the Scriptures as to what God's eating plan is for us, while refuting vegetarian claims in this regard. It is also packed with scientific studies supporting the eating plan advocated in it. It is thus similar to this book, but there is very little redundant material between the two books.

Now to be clear, the eating plan advocated in that book is not that different from what was promoted in the First Edition of this book. In both, I advocate eating copious amounts of unprocessed plant foods.

15

And even in regards to animal foods, some of what I said in the First Edition of this book did not change. However, I changed the rather negative attitude towards animal foods from the First Edition to that book. As such, I only regretted somewhat that the First Edition of this book was still in circulation.

But I especially regretted the last-minute change that reflected my change to a full vegan diet. But it was not possible to alter the First Edition given the policies of that publisher without great expense or to pull it from circulation. Although a year later, I was able to correct the last part in the Kindle version. But even at that time, I was still only consuming limited amounts of meats and no dairy and eggs.

But with my new publisher, it is less expensive to publish books and it is possible to alter previously published ones. Thus after publishing a couple of dozen books over the next 16 years, at the end of 2016, I decided to go back over all of my books and to update them. But most of these were to be minor not full updates; more like an Edition 1.1.

These updates also included republishing this book with my new publisher. But since it was published in 2000 and is also out of date in other respects, it required a full update and is labeled "Second Edition." Most though not all of the quotes and cited scientific studies have been updated, with much new material added. In fact, this Second Edition is two and a half times the size of the First Edition.

In some cases, I have kept original information that is no longer accurate but have added new correcting information after it. I have done so as despite being out of date, very often that older information is still being circulated. In this way, the reader will know that when you see that information elsewhere, it is out of date and no longer accurate.

I also changed the Scripture quotes from the *New King James Version* (NKJV) to my own *Analytical Literal Translation of the Bible* (ALT). But the counts of word occurrences in the Bible are still based on the NKJV. I also corrected typos and made many other changes.

Lastly, I changed the subtitle. The original was *Nutrition and God-given Foods According to the Bible*. But I incorporated the phrase "God-given Foods" into the title of my other book. As indicated, that book addresses the same issues as this book but in a different manner, but both books look at what the Bible and science have to say about healthy eating. To make those two points clear for this book, and given its depth of coverage, I changed the subtitle to *A Comprehensive Guide to Bible and Science Based Nutrition*.

It is my hope and prayer that this Second Edition of this book will encourage the reader to follow a healthier way of eating. May the LORD use this book to lead His people into a healthier lifestyle, enabling them to better serve Him.

Analytical-Literal Translation

Unless otherwise indicated, all Bible verses in this book are quoted from the author's *Analytical-Literal Translation* (ALT; see Appendixes One and Two). The ALT is published in seven volumes.

Volumes I – IV are the Old Testament (OT). One unique feature of the ALT: OT is it is translated from the Septuagint (LXX) rather than the Hebrew text. The LXX is a third century BC Greek translation of the Hebrew Bible. The name and abbreviation comes from the tradition that 70 (or 72) Jewish scholars worked on its translation, six from each of the twelve tribes of Israel.

As such, the wording of some OT verses quoted in this book might differ from Bible versions based upon the Hebrew text, which most versions are. In cases where there is a difference between texts affecting the subject of this book, the verses will also be quoted from the author's own translation of the Hebrew text or from the *New King James Version* (NKJV), which is based on the Hebrew text.

Volume V of the ALT contains the Apocryphal/ Deuterocanonical (A/D) Books. These are the "extra" books found in Roman Catholic and Eastern Orthodox Bibles as compared to Jewish and Protestant Bibles. Since there is debate as to whether these A/D books should be included in the Bible, they will not be quoted as authoritative in this book.

Volume VI of the ALT is the New Testament (NT). It is translated from the Majority Text. This Greek text differs slightly from the other two Greek texts used in Bible translation: the *Textus Receptus* (used by the KJV and NKJV) and the "Critical Text" (used by the ESV, NASB, NIV, and most other modern-day versions). Thus again, the wording of some NT verses quoted in this book might differ from the wording in other Bibles. If a textual variant affects the interpretation of a verse, then that point is mentioned.

However, more often than these textual reasons, the wording of the ALT differs from other versions due to the ALT being a literal translation while many Bible versions use a less than literal translation method. These textual and translation differences are addressed in this writer's book *Differences Between Bible Versions* (see Appendix One).

Volume VII of the ALT is the Apostolic Fathers (APF). These are the writings of the Church leaders of the late first through mid-second centuries, some of which were considered for inclusion in the NT. These writings will not be quoted as authoritative in this book, since they are not included in the Bible proper and are only included in the ALT as an appendix to the NT.

For a discussion of the canonicity (authoritative nature) of all of these books, see the author's three volume set, *Why Are These Books in the Bible and Not Others* (see Appendix One).

Copyright Information for the Individual Volumes of the ALT:

Analytical-Literal Translation of the Old Testament: Volume I: The Torah. Copyright © 2012 by Gary F. Zeolla (www.Zeolla.org).

Analytical-Literal Translation of the Old Testament: Volume II: The Historical Books. Copyright © 2013 by Gary F. Zeolla (www.Zeolla.org).

Analytical-Literal Translation of the Old Testament: Volume III: The Poetic Books. Copyright © 2013 by Gary F. Zeolla (www.Zeolla.org).

Analytical-Literal Translation of the Old Testament: Volume IV: The Prophetic Books. Copyright © 2014 by Gary F. Zeolla (www.Zeolla.org).

Analytical-Literal Translation of the Apocryphal/ Deuterocanonical Books: Volume V of the ALT: Copyright © 2014 by Gary F. Zeolla (www.Zeolla.org).

Analytical-Literal Translation of the New Testament: Third Edition. Copyright © 2012 by Gary F. Zeolla (www.Zeolla.org). Previously copyrighted © 1999, 2001, 2005, 2007 by Gary F. Zeolla.

Analytical-Literal Translation of the Apostolic Fathers: Volume VII of the ALT: Copyright © 2016 by Gary F. Zeolla (www.Zeolla.org).

Where referring to all seven volumes collectively, the copyright information is: *Analytical-Literal Translation of the Bible* (ALT). Copyright © 1999-2016 by Gary F. Zeolla (www.Zeolla.org).

Note: There are some differences between the text of the ALT as quoted in this book versus the texts in the published volumes. That is because this writer/ translator has been making changes and corrections to the texts in my own files in preparation for new editions of all seven of these volumes (see Appendix Three).

Abbreviations Used in this Book

General

a – Only the first half of the verse is being quoted or referred to (e.g., Exodus 15:25a, only the first half of verse 25 is quoted or referred to).

b – Only the second half of the verse is being quoted or referred to (e.g., Exodus 15:25b, only the second half of verse 25 is quoted or referred to).

c – Circa. About. Used with approximate dates.

cf. – confer

cp. – compare

ct. – contrast

e.g. – Latin *exempli gratia*, meaning "for example"

i.e. – Latin *id est*, meaning "that is" or "in explanation"

f – And the following verse (e.g. Psalm 22:9f means verses 9 and 10 are quoted or referred to).

ff – And the following verses (e.g., 22:9ff means verse 9 and several following verses are quoted or referred to).

Gr. – Greek

Heb. – Hebrew

LXX – Septuagint: A third-century BC, Greek translation of the Hebrew OT.

NT – New Testament

OT – Old Testament

v. – verse

vv. – verses

Bible Versions

ALT – *Analytical–Literal Translation of the Holy Bible*. Copyright © 1999-2016 by Gary F. Zeolla (www.Zeolla.org). Unless otherwise indicated, all Scripture verses are from the ALT.

ESV – *English Standard Version*. Copyright © July 2001 by Crossway Books/Good News Publishers, Wheaton, IL.

KJV – *King James Version*. Public domain.

NASB – *New American Standard Bible*. Copyright 1977, 1995 by the Lockman Foundation. All rights reserved.

NIV – *New International Version*. Copyright © 1973, 1984, 1987 by the International Bible Society.

NKJV – *New King James Version*. Nashville, TN: Thomas Nelson Publishers, 1982. All Bible word counts are based on the NKJV.

Abbreviations and Notations in the ALT

Following are the meanings of abbreviations and notations seen in the *Analytical Literal Translation*.

[wife] – Words added for clarity are bracketed (e.g., Matt 1:6). Within bracketed alternative translations, bracketed words indicate words added for clarity, i.e. "[or, the kingdom [of Satan]]" (Matt 8:12) indicates the words "of Satan" are added.

[Isaiah 7:14] – Reference for the preceding OT quote. The quote itself is in italics (e.g., Matt 1:23).

"Yahweh is Salvation" – Meaning of a proper name, placed in quotation marks (e.g., Matt 1:21).

About – Modern–day equivalent for measurements and monetary units (e.g., Matt 13:33).

A.D. – *Anno Domini*. In the year of the Lord. Used in dates (e.g., Matt 3:1).

and elsewhere in – The bracketed information applies to other occurrences of the preceding word or phrase in the given range, but not necessarily to all occurrences (e.g., Rom 8:1).

and throughout/ and in – The bracketed information applies to all occurrences of the preceding word or phrase throughout the given range (e.g., Matt 1:20).

B.C. – Before Christ. Used in dates (e.g., Matt 2:1).

cp. – Compare. A cross reference (e.g., Matt 1:1).

fig. – Figurative. Possible figurative meaning or paraphrase of preceding literal translation (e.g., Matt 1:18).

Gr. – Greek. The Greek word previously translated, with the Greek letters transliterated (changed) into English letters (e.g., Matt 3:6).

Heb. – Hebrew. The OT quote is taken from the Hebrew text of the OT and not the LXX since the quote matches the Hebrew but differs from the LXX (e.g., Matt 2:15).

i.e. – Explanatory note ("that is" or "in explanation") (e.g., Matt 2:11).

LXX – Septuagint, a third century B.C., Greek translation of the Hebrew OT. The notation means the OT quote is taken from the LXX rather than from the Hebrew text since the quote matches the LXX but differs from the Hebrew (e.g., Matt 3:2). When there is no notation, it means the source could be either the Hebrew or the LXX (e.g., Matt 2:6).

NT – New Testament (e.g., Matt 6:13).

OT – Old Testament (e.g., Matt 3:23).

or – Alternative, traditional, or slightly less literal translation (e.g., Matt 1:2).

see – Cross reference (e.g., John 18:32).

Miscellaneous Abbreviations and Notations

But – Indicates the use of the Greek strong adversative (*alla* – e.g., Matt 4:4) instead of the weak adversative (*de*, translated as "but" when used in an adversative sense – e.g., Matt 3:7).

LORD – Lord – The former indicates the OT verse from which the quote is taken has *Yahweh* (the Hebrew proper name for God – Matt 4:7). The latter indicates the OT has *adonai* (the general word for "lord" – e.g., Matt 22:44).

you – Indicates the pronoun is emphasized in the Greek text (also, <u>he</u>, <u>she</u>, etc. – e.g., Matt 3:11,14).

you* – Indicates the original is plural (also, your* – e.g., Matt 2:8). With no asterisk the second person pronoun is singular (e.g., Matt 1:20).

Quotations Notes

Much of this book consists of extended Scripture quotations. These have not been put in block quotes (indented) as is normally done for extended quotes due to the length and number of them, as to do so would have made this book even longer than it already is in hardcopy formats and difficult to read in electronic formats. But the superscript verse numbers are retained, so Scripture quotes are easily identified.

However, extended quotes from sources other than the Bible are indented for easy identification. The sources are cited after the quote in parentheses by the first word or two of the main title of the source, followed by part of an article title if applicable. The full biographical data is then given at the end of each chapter.

All bolding in Biblical and other quotes is added for emphasis, unless otherwise indicated.

The LORD

Throughout the ALT, I use "LORD" (written in all capital letters) to indicate when the Greek word *kurios* is a translation of the Hebrew Divine Name (*YHWH*; traditionally pronounced "Jehovah" but more likely pronounced "Yahweh"). As a result, I have gotten in the habit of using "LORD" in all my writings. That is why "LORD" is used throughout this book. But whether LORD, Lord, or God, the reference is to the one true God, the God of the Bible.

Bible Book Names

The Old Testament

Gen – Genesis
Ex, Exod – Exodus
Lev – Leviticus
Num, Numb – Numbers
Dt, Deut – Deuteronomy
Josh – Joshua
Jud, Judg – Judges
Ruth – Ruth
1Sam – 1Samuel
2Sam – 2Samuel
1Ki – 1Kings
2Ki – 2Kings
1Chr, 1Chron – 1Chronicles
2Chr, 2Chron – 2Chronicles
Ez – Ezra
Neh – Nehemiah
Est – Esther
Job – Job
Ps – Psalms
Pr, Prov – Proverbs
Eccl – Ecclesiastes
Song – Song of Solomon
Isa – Isaiah
Jer – Jeremiah
Lam – Lamentations
Ez, Ezek – Ezekiel
Dan – Daniel
Hos – Hosea
Joel – Joel
Amos – Amos
Ob, Obad – Obadiah
Jon – Jonah
Mic – Micah
Nah – Nahum
Hab – Habakkuk
Zeph – Zephaniah
Hag – Haggai
Zech – Zechariah
Mal – Malachi

The New Testament
Mt, Matt – Matthew
Mk – Mark
Lk – Luke
Jn – John
Ac – Acts
Rom – Romans
1Cor – 1Corinthians
2Cor – 2Corinthians
Gal – Galatians
Eph – Ephesians
Phil – Philippians
Col – Colossians
1Th, 1Thes – 1Thessalonians
2Th, 2Thes – 2Thessalonians
1Tim – 1Timothy
2Tim – 2Timothy
Tit – Titus
Phlm – Philemon
Heb – Hebrews
Jam – James
1Pet – 1Peter
2Pet – 2Peter
1Jn – 1John
2Jn – 2John
3Jn – 3John
Jd – Jude
Rev – Revelation

Dedication/ Memorial to my Mom

This book is dedicated to my mom (Marcella Rose Zeolla), who went to be with the LORD on my birthday while I was working on this book, on Monday, March 27, 2017 at 10:15 am. She was 81 years old.

She had struggled with many health problems for most of her life and spent the last year of her life in a nursing home. But her love for her family was unquestioned. She always was there for me and the rest of her family, and she always kept each one of us in her prayers.

She was a very faithful and dedicated mother, grandmother, great-grandmother, and wife. In fact, my parents missed by just a few weeks being married for 60 years.

Along with me and my dad (Nicholas "Nick" Zeolla), she is survived by her older son, Allen "Al" Zeolla (and his wife Kim), her three grandchildren though them: April Barnes (and her husband Pat), Daniel Zeolla (and his SO Jessica Fields), and Jonathan "Jon" Zeolla (and his wife Victoria), and her eight great-children through them: Dakota, Logan, Dominic, Roxanna, Xander, Topanga, Tyrese, and Aaron. My Mom would review all of these names each day so as to remember them and to be able to mention each family member by name in her daily prayers.

Despite her many health problems, she always tried to keep herself in shape. She would go for walks around the neighborhood year-round, regardless of the weather. I can remember her and I going for a walk on a very cold and snowy winter day. My dad thought we were both nuts. In the summer, she would swim at the nearby public pool. Even after her health deteriorated, and she had to use first a cane then a walker, her and my dad would go to a local mall or Walmart, and she would walk there. It was only at the very end that she was not able to keep up with the walking. She also tried to follow a healthy diet most of her life, though I must say, she had some strange ideas of what "healthy" was. But she ate what she felt was best for her.

But much more importantly, my mom had long ago placed her faith in Jesus Christ and His death on the cross for the forgiveness of her sins. She would read her Bible every day, taking notes, and memorizing Bible verses. Her faith pulled her though many hard times, and I know she is in a better place now.

I hadn't seen my mom in several weeks due to first entering a powerlifting contest and then getting sick afterwards, though I had talked with her on the phone, namely to tell her how my contest went. But I made it to the nursing home half an hour before she passed. At that point, she was barely breathing and did not open her eyes. I tried to update her on everything that was happening in my life, letting her know I was doing okay and that I loved her.

I told her I was almost finished writing my latest book (this book) and that I was getting ready to get back into hard training. Otherwise, I prayed for her. I just wished she had opened her eyes just once so I would have known she knew I was there and could hear me.

When her breathing and heartbeat became very shallow, I tried reading Psalm 23 to her, but I was breaking up too much to do so, so I handed my phone to my niece and had her read it. My mom probably passed into Paradise just as my niece finished the Psalm.

You will be missed Mom. But with passing away on my birthday, I will always remember the day you died and will think of you on each birthday and much in-between.

I had my niece read Psalm 23 from the *New King James Version* (NKJV), as that is the version my mom always read, due to my recommendation. The last line is most important—I know my mom will dwell in the house of the LORD forever. Do you, the reader, have this assurance? If not, trust on Jesus Christ today for the forgiveness of your sins. You never know when you will be walking through the valley of the shadow of death.

<A Psalm of David.> [1]The LORD is my shepherd; I shall not want. [2]He makes me to lie down in green pastures; He leads me beside the still waters. [3]He restores my soul; He leads me in the paths of righteousness For His name's sake. [4]Yea, though I walk through the valley of the shadow of death, I will fear no evil; For You are with me; Your rod and Your staff, they comfort me. [5]You prepare a table before me in the presence of my enemies; You anoint my head with oil; My cup runs over. [6]Surely goodness and mercy shall follow me All the days of my life; And I will dwell in the house of the LORD Forever.

Section One
Plant Foods

Creationist Diet

Chapter One
Genesis 1-3
(Fruits, Nuts, Vegetables, Seeds)

The place to begin in developing a Creationist Diet is with the Biblical accounts of Creation and of the Fall. These events are recorded in Genesis 1-3. There are three main passages to be considered in these three chapters. Each of these will be briefly exegeted and then a more detailed discussion of each of the kinds of foods mentioned will follow.

Three Main Passages

The first verse to be considered is Genesis 1:29:

[29]And God said, "Listen! I have given to you* every seed-sowing [fig., bearing] vegetation sowing seed which is upon all of the earth and every tree which has in itself [the] fruit of seed [that is] sown; to you* it will be for food.

Rex Russell, MD, in his book *What the Bible Says about Healthy Living*, comments on the first half of this verse:

> Many plants fit into the categories of Genesis 1:29a: wheat, rice, oats, barley, millet, rye and other grains; legumes of all kinds (e.g., peas, beans); bush and vine-bearing fruits and vegetables (melons, grapes, berries, squash, tomatoes, eggplant, cucumbers, etc.) (p.31).

Thus grains of all kinds, along with certain kinds of fruits and vegetables would be included in this decree. But a point that Russell doesn't mention is that "every seed-sowing [fig., bearing] vegetation sowing seed" would include the seeds themselves when the seeds are edible. Edible seeds include sunflower, pumpkin, sesame, and flax seeds. In reference to the second half of Genesis 1:29, Russell writes:

> This includes every conceivable fruit (apples, pears, apricots, plums, mangoes, avocados, etc.), as well as all nuts,

both large and small (coconuts, almonds, walnuts, cashews, etc.) (p.31).

Thus this part of this verse tells us all kinds of fruits are God-given foods, along with all kinds of nuts.

The second passage is Genesis 2:16. But verses nine and seventeen will also be included for background:

[9]And GOD made to spring up also out of the earth every tree beautiful in appearance and good for food, and the tree of the life in [the] middle of the Paradise, and the tree to know [the] knowing of good and of evil....
[16]And the LORD God commanded Adam, saying, "From every tree in the Paradise you will eat [for] food, [17]but from the tree to be knowing good and evil you* will not eat from it, but in which day you* shall eat from it, you* will die by death [fig., will certainly die]" (Gen 2:9, 2:16,17).

Note that "the Paradise" is traditionally referred to as "the Garden of Eden." Thus God specifically told Adam and Eve they were to eat of "every tree in the Paradise" (or in the Garden of Eden), except for "the tree to know [the] knowing of good and of evil." What grows on trees is fruits and nuts. Thus again, these are definitely God-given foods.

But then Adam and Eve sin against God by eating of the "forbidden fruit" (Gen 3:1-6). This is known theologically as "the Fall." What that fruit was is unknown. By tradition, it is pictured as an apple. But it was probably a special fruit, different from all the others in the Paradise.

In any case, the last pertinent verse in these chapters is given after the Fall, in the second half of Genesis 3:18, "you will eat the vegetation of the field."

Russell comments:

In Genesis 3, note that after Adam and Eve fell into sin God ordered a dietary addition, "You shall eat the herb of the field" (v. 18, NKJV). This was the food previously designated for the animals [see Gen 1:30]. These were herbs without seeds in them, such as lettuce, cabbage, broccoli, cauliflower, spinach, asparagus, etc., and the tubers (yams, potatoes, carrots, beets, etc.) (p.32).

These three passages could be summarized by saying God has given every kind of plant food to us for food: fruits, vegetables, nuts, seeds, grains, and legumes. Therefore, any and all of these would be included in a Creationist Diet.

However, another point relevant to the Creationist Diet principle is when each of these different foods actually began to be consumed by humans and in what form. The Bible does not give specific answers to these questions, but an attempt will be made to glean from the Scriptures the most likely scenario.

Adam and Eve's Diet

The place to begin is in the Garden of Eden. What did Adam and Eve eat before the Fall? Before answering this question, another one needs to be considered: how long were Adam and Eve in the Paradise before the Fall? Unfortunately, the Bible does not give any indication.

Genesis chapter three follows Genesis chapter two without any indication as to how much time has elapsed between the two chapters. It could have been hours, days, weeks, months, years, decades, even centuries between the time Adam and Eve were created and the Fall. Adam and Eve were created to be immortal and did not begin to age until after the Fall, so this question cannot be answered definitely.

However, my opinion is that it is somewhere in the middle of the time ranges. I do not think they were created, told not to eat of the fruit of the tree of the knowledge of good and evil, and then minutes or hours later did so. On the other hand, I doubt seriously they were in the Garden for centuries before giving into temptation.

My guess is they were in the Paradise for a period of months to years. This would give them enough time to explore the Garden, get acquainted with its contents, and for curiosity over the "forbidden tree" to develop. Thus when Satan made his move, they would be susceptible to his trickery. If this timetable is correct, then we can begin to make some educated guesses as to what their diet consisted of.

31

Fruits:

The place to start would be with the verses from Genesis two quoted previously. These include God's description of the Garden and what God told Adam and Eve in regards to food, "⁹And GOD made to spring up also out of the earth every tree beautiful in appearance and good for food.... ¹⁶And the LORD God commanded Adam, saying, 'From every tree in the Paradise you will eat [for] food'" (Gen 2:9, 2:16).

Therefore, Adam and Eve's initial food would have been that which grew on the trees in the Garden. Now, what kind of food grows on trees? The first thing that comes to mind is fruit. It is the most visible tree food and easily eaten raw.

In other words, when Adam and Eve first got hungry and began looking in the Garden for something to eat, the most logical thing for them to notice first would have been very visible and colorful fruit like apples and oranges. To eat an apple merely requires picking it off of the tree and biting into it. Nothing could be simpler.

Now a fruit like an orange would require a little more work—one has to peel it first. But peeling fruit was easily within Adam and Eve's intellectual grasp. As such, it can be assumed that raw fruits were a very important part of Adam and Eve's diet.

Moreover, given the description of the Garden, it can be assumed there was a wide variety of fruit trees in the Garden. As such, raw fruits of all kinds would play an important role in a Creationist Diet, and fruits would not be limited to basic ones like apples and oranges, but more "exotic" fruits like papayas and kiwi.

And fruits do have a prominent place in the Bible, with "fruit" being mentioned 189 times and "fruits" 20 times. Some specific fruits are mentioned as well.

"Apple" is mentioned seven times in the Bible, most often in the affectionate phrase, "the apple of His eye" (see Deut 32:10, Psalm 17:8; Prov 7:2; Zech 2:8). "Apples" is mentioned three times (Prov 25:11; Song 2:5; 7:8). "Apple tree" is also mentioned (Song 2:3; 8:5; Joel 1:12). The last reference also mentions a fig tree. "Fig tree" is mentioned 33 other times in the Bible and "fig trees" six times. Various other fruits are also mentioned, such as grapes (36 times), melons (once; Numbers 11:5), and pomegranate (10 times) or pomegranates (23 times).

Most any nutritionist would agree with the nutritional value of fruits and the benefits of eating them. Fruits are high in natural carbohydrates and sugar, and they are good sources of a wide variety of vitamins, minerals, phytonutrients, and fiber.

Eating fruit provides health benefits — people who eat more fruits and vegetables as part of an overall healthy diet are likely to have a reduced risk of some chronic diseases. **Fruits provide nutrients vital for health and maintenance of your body** (USDA; Why Fruit)

The combination of powerful flavonoids, antioxidants, minerals, vitamins, phytochemicals and the countless micro- and macronutrients make fruits very advantageous for your health. The daily consumption of fresh fruits lowers the risk of strokes, high blood pressure, indigestion, cancer, heart disease, diabetes and other chronic diseases. Fruits keep your skin supple, hydrated and nourish it with essential vitamins, minerals and antioxidants, thereby retaining your radiant skin for a long period of time....

Fruits even ensure healthy hair growth and keep your locks lustrous and soft. Some fruits like bananas contain vital chemicals such as potassium, which helps to prevent strokes, high blood pressure, and anxiety. **Fruit consumption basically eliminates vitamin and mineral deficiencies and their associated symptoms.** Fruits also have high quantities of water and fiber in them, which helps to keep your digestive tract clean and **your weight under control** (Organic Facts; Fruits).

Few things compare to the sweetness of fresh-picked strawberries or the luscious first bite of watermelon that leaves juice dripping down your chin.

Fruits are not only delicious but healthful too. Rich in vitamins A and C, plus folate and other essential nutrients, they **may help prevent heart disease and stroke, control blood pressure and cholesterol, prevent some types of cancer and guard against vision loss.** They're so good for you that Health Canada recommends that most women get seven or eight servings of fruit and vegetables each day (Canadian).

Citrus fruits have long been valued as part of a nutritious and tasty diet. The flavours provided by citrus are among the most preferred in the world, and it is increasingly evident that **citrus not only tastes good, but is also good for people**. It is well established that citrus and citrus products are a rich source of **vitamins, minerals and dietary fibre** (non-starch polysaccharides) that are essential for normal growth and development and overall nutritional well-being. However, it is now beginning to be appreciated that these and other biologically active, non-nutrient compounds found in citrus and other plants (**phytochemicals**) can also help to reduce the risk of many chronic diseases...

The health benefits associated with citrus consumption are clear. Citrus fruits are nutrient-dense foods that can be good sources of carbohydrates, including dietary fibre, and many vitamins and minerals. Citrus fruits are equally valuable among populations who need to overcome and prevent micronutrient deficiencies as well as those concerned with problems of overnutrition, obesity and diet-related chronic diseases. For example, citrus is an ideal component of low-fat, sodium-restricted diets. (FAO).

Many of the studies pool together fruits and vegetables, while some look at fruits directly.

One review of 9 studies found that the risk of heart disease reduced by 7% for each daily portion of fruit.

A study on 9,665 adults in the U.S. found that fruit and vegetable intake was associated with a 46% lower risk of diabetes in women, but there was no difference in men...

There are many other studies showing that fruit and vegetable consumption is associated with a lower risk of heart attacks and stroke, the two most common causes of death in Western countries.

One study looked at how different types of fruit affect the risk of **type II diabetes. Those who consumed the most grapes, apples and blueberries had the lowest risk**, with blueberries having the strongest effect...

That being said, there are also a few randomized controlled trials (real human experiments) showing that **increased fruit intake can lower blood pressure, reduce oxidative stress and improve glycemic control in diabetics**.

Overall, it seems clear from the data that fruits do have significant health benefits.

Bottom Line: **There are many studies showing that fruit intake is associated with a lower risk of serious diseases like heart disease, stroke and type II diabetes** (Authority).

Nuts:

The next thing that grows on trees that would be noticed by Adam and Eve would be various nuts. These are not as noticeable as fruits, as they are not as colorful. They are also harder to prepare. Cracking open a nut requires more work than peeling an orange. But still, the preparation is minimal, and again, nuts can easily be eaten raw. Also again, there would have been a wide variety of nut trees in the Garden.

As such, the second food item that would be a staple in a Creationist Diet would be raw nuts of all kinds: almonds, brazil nuts, cashews, chestnuts filberts, pecans, pistachio nuts, and walnuts. Nuts aren't mentioned too often otherwise in the Bible, but "almond" is mentioned nine times. Six of these are in reference to a "almond blossoms" design being used on utensils for the tabernacle, but three are in reference to an almond tree (Gen 30:37; Eccl 12:5; Jer 1:11). The first also mentions a chestnut tree. "Almonds" are mentioned twice (Gen 43:11 and Numbers 17:8). The first reference also mentions pistachio nuts.

Nuts used to have a "bad rap" because they are high in fat. However, it is now known that the type of fat in nuts is actually beneficial. Nuts contain mainly monounsaturated fat, some polyunsaturated fats, but very little saturated fat.

Monounsaturated fats help to lower blood LDL ("bad") cholesterol levels and to raise HDL ("good") cholesterol levels. It is saturated fats (found mainly in animal products) that raise LDL cholesterol. Polyunsaturated fats also help to lower LDL cholesterol but have no effect on HDL cholesterol (Parsonnet, pp. 22-24).

Thus overall, the best kind of fat to consume is monounsaturated fat, the very kind plentiful in nuts. As a result, "Nuts may help lower total and LDL cholesterol and triglycerides while boosting levels of HDL cholesterol" (Authority Nutrition; Nuts).

In addition, nuts are a good source of protein, vitamins (especially vitamin E), minerals such as magnesium, phosphorus, and iron, along with fiber. As a result, nuts are rightly receiving a resurgence as being a "health food."

In the past, nuts fell into the "bad for you" category. However, **in recent years, studies show that nuts are indeed healthy**.... The bottom line is **all nuts are good for you**... the key is moderation. A healthy handful can lead to good health and longer life. So go nuts! (Fastachi).

Nuts provide key proteins and nutrients, good fats, antioxidants, aid in the reduction of cholesterol and help you live longer.

One way nuts may help your heart health is by lowering the low-density lipoprotein (LDL, or "bad") cholesterol levels. LDL plays a major role in the development of plaque that builds up on the blood vessels. **Eating more nuts has also been linked to lower levels of inflammation linked to heart disease**.

Eating nuts may also reduce your risk of developing blood clots that can cause a fatal heart attack. Nuts also appear to improve the health of the lining of your arteries (Mayo; Nuts).

Two recent studies have touted the benefits of nuts for blood sugar control. One, published in *Diabetes Care*, found that eating pistachio nuts daily may help people at risk of getting diabetes control their blood sugar. A second, published in *PLOS One*, found that tree nuts -- including almonds, Brazil nuts, cashews, and pecans, among others -- may improve blood sugar control in people with type 2 diabetes...

Aside from helping with blood sugar, **nuts have been linked with improving heart health and helping with weight control**. A study from last year even suggested that eating nuts of any type may help you live longer...

Nuts are about 80% fat, but mostly **"good" unsaturated fats**. Other good stuff in nuts includes **magnesium** (which helps maintain the calcium-potassium balance in your body), **folate** (critical for a healthy brain), and **vitamin E** (to maintain a healthy circulatory system). They also have **arginine**, an amino acid that's needed to make nitric oxide, which relaxes the blood vessels (WebMD).

Eating nuts has been associated with plenty of health benefits — from increased cognitive function to protection from Alzheimer's, as well as keeping your heart healthy. Now, scientists have added more benefits to that list: **People who eat a lot of nuts might have a lower risk of mortality and developing chronic diseases**, including respiratory disease, neurodegenerative disease, diabetes, cancer, and heart disease, according to a new study published in the *International Journal of Epidemiology*

In the study, researchers examined data from the Netherlands Cohort Study, which includes information about 120,000 Dutch 55- to 69-year-old men and women from 1986 to the present day. They measured nut intake by asking about portion size and the frequency at which the participants ate tree nuts, peanuts, and peanut butter.

"It was remarkable that substantially lower mortality was already observed at consumption levels of 15 grams of nuts or peanuts on average per day (half a handful)," Professor Piet van den Brandt, the project leader and epidemiologist, said in the press release. **"A higher intake was not associated with further reduction in mortality risk.** This was also supported by a meta-analysis of previously published studies together with the Netherlands Cohort Study, in which cancer and respiratory mortality showed this same dose-response pattern" (Medical Daily).

Nuts (tree nuts and peanuts) are nutrient dense foods with complex matrices rich in unsaturated fatty and other bioactive compounds: high-quality vegetable protein, fiber, minerals, tocopherols, phytosterols, and phenolic compounds.

By virtue of their unique composition, nuts are likely to beneficially impact health outcomes.

Epidemiologic studies have associated nut consumption with a reduced incidence of coronary heart disease and gallstones in both genders and diabetes in women. Limited evidence also suggests beneficial effects on hypertension, cancer, and inflammation. Interventional studies consistently show that nut intake has a cholesterol-lowering effect, even in the context of healthy diets, and there is emerging evidence of beneficial effects on oxidative stress, inflammation, and vascular reactivity.

Blood pressure, visceral adiposity and the metabolic syndrome also appear to be positively influenced by nut consumption. **Thus it is clear that nuts have a beneficial impact on many cardiovascular risk factors.**

Contrary to expectations, epidemiologic studies and clinical trials suggest that **regular nut consumption is unlikely to contribute to obesity and may even help in weight loss.** Safety concerns are limited to the infrequent occurrence of nut allergy in children.

In conclusion, **nuts are nutrient rich foods with wide-ranging cardiovascular and metabolic benefits,** which can be readily incorporated into healthy diets (Ros).

The statement in the next to the last paragraph comes from the fact that nut-eaters do not tend to weigh more than non-nut eaters. This is contrary to popular conception that nuts, due to their high fat content, would be a detriment to controlling bodyweight. The reason for this is nuts have a high satiety value, which is the state of feeling full.

However, it should be obvious that it would be easier to overeat shelled nuts than nuts still in the shell. Having to take the time to crack the nuts open would slow down the rate at which they could be eaten. And salted, roasted nuts seem to be easier to overeat than unsalted, raw nuts. The salt seems to encourage overeating. But there is no reason to overeat nuts, as just a small handful a day will provide their benefits.

Brazil nuts deserve special mention. They are by far the best dietary source of selenium, an essential mineral. "just one Brazil nut provides more than 100% of the RDI [Recommended Dietary Intake] for selenium" (Authority; Nuts). So instead of taking selenium supplements as many are doing today, you could just eat one Brazil nut a day. However, "… toxicity symptoms appear in individuals whose daily intakes are greater than 750 mcg" (Somer, p.115). As such, it would be prudent not to eat more than an average of a couple of Brazil nuts a day.

Olives and Avocados:

A couple of fruits deserve special mention: olives and avocados. These fruits have a high fat content. However, as with nuts, the fat in olives and avocados is also the healthy monounsaturated kind. It is for this reason that olive oil has been found to be heart-protective. It also has many other health benefits.

This is no surprise given that olives have a prominent place in the Bible, with "olive" being mentioned 41 times and "olives" 18 times. However, there are far more than this given that every one of the 202 references to "oil" in the Bible would be to olive oil. I say this as every place in which the NKJV has "oil," my ALT has "olive oil."

> "[13]And He [the LORD] will love you and bless you and multiply you; He will also bless the fruit of your womb and the fruit of your land, your grain and your new wine and your **oil**, the increase of your cattle and the offspring of your flock, in the land of which He swore to your fathers to give you. (Deut. 7:13 NKJV).

> [13]And He will love you, and will bless you, and will multiply you; and He will bless the offspring of your womb, and the fruit of your land, your wheat, and your wine, and your **olive oil**, the herds of your oxen, and the flocks of your sheep, on the land which the LORD swore an oath to your fathers to give to you (Deut 7:13; ALT).

Olives can be eaten whole, but olives are most commonly consumed in the form of oil. Pressing olives into oil is not that difficult of an operation and would be within the intellectual capabilities of the earliest humans, although the first refence to olive oil in the Bible is in Geneses 28:18, "And Jacob rose up in the morning, and took the stone he [had] laid there by his head, and he set it up [as] a pillar, and poured **olive oil** on the top of it."

But an important point is all of the olive oil in Bible times would have been what today is called cold pressed, extra-virgin olive oil. Any further processing would render the resulting oil far different from the olive oil of Biblical times and thus not be God-given. But whole olives and cold pressed, extra-virgin olive oil would fall under the food directives of the first chapters of Genesis as being God-given foods. And not surprisingly, olive oil is very healthy.

True **extra-virgin olive oil** (EVOO) is extracted from olives using only pressure, a process known as **cold pressing**. Extra-virgin olive oil has just 1% acid. It's the oil that comes from the first pressing of the olives, and **is considered the finest, having the freshest, fruitiest flavor** (WebMD. What's).

Olive oil also falls into two distinct categories: refined and unrefined. While unrefined oils are pure and untreated, refined oil is treated to remove flaws from the oil, making it more sellable.

Richard Gawel is an olive oil expert and long-time appointee as Presiding Judge in various major olive oil shows. On the difference of refined and unrefined oils he says, **"Refined oils have little or no olive aroma, flavour, or colour** (what they have gets there via blending in few percent of an extra-virgin oil). They also have no bitterness."

In contrast to unrefined extra-virgin olive oil, **refined oils "lack the important antioxidants and anti-inflammatories that make extra-virgin oil so special"** (Kitchn).

Olive oil is very high in monounsaturated fats and contains a modest amount of vitamins E and K. True extra virgin olive oil is loaded with antioxidants, some of which have powerful health benefits...

Olive oil may be one of the healthiest foods you can eat for heart health. It lowers blood pressure, protects LDL particles from oxidation, reduces inflammation and may help prevent unwanted blood clotting (Authority; Olive Oil).

The health benefits of olive oil are unrivaled, and research reveals more benefits nearly every day. In fact, we are only just beginning to understand the countless ways olive oil can improve our health, and our lives. **Olive oil is the cornerstone of the Mediterranean diet — an essential nutritional mainstay for the world's longest-living cultures** (Olive Oil Times).

Cancer prevention has been one of the most active areas of olive oil research, and the jury is no longer out on the health benefits of olive oil with respect to cancer. Twenty-five studies on olive oil intake and cancer risk—including most of the large-scale human studies conducted up through the year 2010—have recently been analyzed by a team of researchers at the Mario Negri Institute for Pharmacological Research Institute in Milan, Italy. **Firmly established by this research team were the risk-reducing effects of olive oil intake with respect to cancers of the breast, respiratory tract, upper digestive tract and, to a lesser extent, lower digestive tract** (colorectal cancers) (World's).

The FDA says eating 2 tablespoons of olive oil a day may reduce the risk of heart disease, due to its monounsaturated fat content. Extra virgin olive oil also contains polyphenols which act as antioxidants, reducing the oxidative stress throughout your body. A small amount of **Omega-3 and Omega-6 fatty** acids are also present in extra virgin olive oil, which are essential for brain health. **Vitamin E** (also known as tocopherols), which is great for skin health, is also found in extra virgin olive oil. **Many health benefits associated with the consumption of extra virgin olive oil have been discovered** (California).

Avocados are not mentioned in the Bible, which is not surprising since they are native to Mexico, Central and South America. Europeans first became aware of them through the Spanish Conquistadores.

It is evident from miscellaneous reports by Spanish

41

Conquistadores that, at the time of the Spanish conquest, avocados were grown from northern Mexico south through Central America into north-western South America and south in the Andean region as far as Peru (where the avocado had been introduced shortly before the conquest), as well as into the Andean region of Venezuela (What's Cooking).

Avocados are most commonly eaten in the form of guacamole, but they can be used in the place of other fats in recipes and even in the place of mayonnaise on sandwiches.

The health benefits of avocados have not been investigated as much as olive oil, but it is substantial. "**Numerous studies have shown that eating avocado can improve heart disease risk factors** like Total, LDL and HDL cholesterol, as well as blood triglycerides" (Authority Nutrition. Avocado).

Vegetables:

Adam and Eve would definitely have eaten raw fruits and nuts while in Paradise. But what else did they eat? Genesis 1:29 quoted previously included "vine-bearing fruits and vegetables" as God-given foods. And such vegetables would be the next most obvious food for Adam and Eve to find and eat.

Such vegetables would be almost as easy to find as fruits as they grow on vines above ground. Most of these vegetables can also be eaten raw. As such, while still in the Garden, Adam and Eve's diet would have included these kinds of vegetables, at least initially eaten raw.

Then after the Fall, God added "the vegetation of the field" to Adam and Eve's diet. This decree would include all other kinds of vegetables. And again, most of these vegetables could also be eaten raw. Thus raw vegetables would also be considered a staple of the Creationist Diet.

It should be noted that many very healthy foods are included in the previous list of "vegetation of the field." Especially healthy are the cruciferous vegetables. Dr. Kenneth H. Cooper writes about them:

> **Cruciferous vegetables, notably broccoli, brussels sprouts, cauliflower, and cabbage** (the two "Bs" and two "Cs"), have been identified as **strong anticancer weapons**. They are also thought to be **protective against other**

conditions including heart disease, diverticulitis, and constipation" (p. 169).

So maybe God added these foods to the human diet after the Fall as a way for us to ward off the many maladies that would now become common in the fallen earth.

Whatever the case there, most other vegetables are also very healthy foods, and many others have been found to help prevent degenerative disease like cancer.

Women should take note of the following:

"One of the best things you can do to decrease your risk of breast cancer is to eat a large variety of vegetables and fruits," says [Melanine] Polk [R.D. Director of Nutrition Education, American Institute for Cancer Research].

Fruits and vegetables are rich in cancer-fighting substances, including antioxidants such as carotenoids and flavonoids, phytochemicals such as phytoestrogens and indoles, and a variety of vitamins. Antioxidants help to rid the body of waste products believed to increase cancer risk, and phytoestrogens, which are actually weak estrogens, appear to offer protection against breast and prostate cancers, which are affected by hormonal activity (*Women's Health*, p.1).

Some especially healthy vegetables are mentioned in Numbers 11:5: "the leeks and the onions and the garlic." In reference to the last item, Dr. Copper writes:

Various studies have revealed that **garlic may provide health benefits such as these**:

• Lowering of total cholesterol and "bad" LDL cholesterol, and raising of "good" HDL cholesterol....
• Lowering of blood pressure.
• The ability to strengthen the immune system, counter infections, kill fungi, and operate as an anti-septic against oral bacteria.

43

- Functioning as an anticancer agent, especially in animal studies.
- An anticoagulant or anticlotting effect in the blood, which can be protective against thrombosis, the blockage of blood flow by clots, as may happen in stroke (pp., 226-7).

And again, as with fruits, nutritionists say we need to eat more of all kinds of vegetables. They are great sources of vitamins, minerals, phytochemicals, and fiber.

Vegetables, like fruits, are low in calories and fats but contain good amounts of vitamins and minerals. All the Green-Yellow-Orange vegetables are rich sources of calcium, magnesium, potassium, iron, beta-carotene, vitamin B-complex, vitamin-C, vitamin-A, and vitamin K.

As in fruits, vegetables too are home for many antioxidants. These health benefiting phyto-chemical compounds firstly; help protect the human body from oxidant stress, diseases, and cancers, and secondly; help the body develop the capacity to fight against these by boosting immunity.

Additionally, vegetables are packed with soluble as well as insoluble dietary fiber known as non-starch polysaccharides (NSP) such as cellulose, mucilage, hemi-cellulose, gums, pectin...etc. These substances absorb excess water in the colon, retain a good amount of moisture in the fecal matter, and help its smooth passage out of the body. Thus, **sufficient fiber offers protection from conditions like chronic constipation, hemorrhoids, colon cancer, irritable bowel syndrome, and rectal fissures** (Nutrition and You).

Eating vegetables provides health benefits – people who eat more vegetables and fruits as part of an overall healthy diet are likely to have a reduced risk of some chronic diseases. **Vegetables provide nutrients vital for health and maintenance of your body** (USDA; Why Vegetables).

44

The health benefits of vegetables usually show in long run by improving your overall health and keeping the internal systems in perfect condition. The consumption of vegetables takes care of your digestive, excretory, and skeletal system, as well as blood pressure levels. With a diet rich in vegetables, you are being benefited with abundant antioxidants that **keep away diseases like cancer, cardiovascular problems and strokes**. Moreover, vegetables deliver ample amounts of vitamins, including folate, vitamin A, vitamin K and vitamin B6, as well as carotenoids like beta carotene from carrots, lycopene from tomatoes, zeaxanthin from greens, and lutein from spinach and collard greens. **Vegetables also help in keeping your weight under control and promoting healthy skin and hair.** There have been innumerable research studies done all over the world that strongly suggest **having fresh, green vegetables on a regular basis is far better than going for supplementary tablets to get the wholesome nutrition that you need** (Organic Facts; Vegetables).

People who eat fruit and vegetables as part of their daily diet have a reduced risk of many chronic diseases. USDA's MyPlate encourages making half your plate fruits and vegetables.

Vegetables are important part of healthy eating and provide a source of many nutrients, including potassium, fiber, folate (folic acid) and vitamins A, E and C. Options like **broccoli, spinach, tomatoes and garlic provide additional benefits, making them a superfood!**

Potassium may help to maintain healthy blood pressure. **Dietary fiber** from vegetables helps reduce blood cholesterol levels and may lower risk of heart disease.

Folate (folic acid) helps the body form healthy red blood cells. Women of childbearing age who may become pregnant and those in the first trimester of pregnancy need adequate folate to reduce the risk of neural tube defects and spina bifida during fetal development (Dairy Council; Vegetables).

45

Eating 10 portions of fruit and vegetables a day could significantly reduce the risk of heart attack, stroke, cancer and early death, according to new research.

The study, by Imperial College London, says consuming 10 portions per day, or about 800g, could **prevent an estimated 7.8 million premature deaths worldwide**.

The World Health Organization (WHO) currently recommends eating 5 portions, or 400g, of fruit and vegetables every day....

"Our results suggest that although five portions of fruit and vegetables is good, 10 a day is even better," lead author Dr Dagfinn Aune said in a statement released by the college.

The research concluded that eating 10 portions per day was associated with a 24 per cent reduced risk of heart disease, a 33 per cent reduced risk of stroke, a 28 per cent reduced risk of cardiovascular disease, a 13 per cent reduced risk of total cancer, and a **31 per cent reduction in dying prematurely**. It says the risk was calculated in comparison to not eating any fruit and vegetables....

The study found that **apples and pears as well as citrus fruits** and vegetables such as **lettuce, broccoli and cabbage** are particularly effective in preventing strokes, heart disease and early death. Green and yellow vegetables such as **spinach, peppers and carrots** may reduce the risk of cancer (CBS Philly).

Note the amount and variety of fruits and vegetables referred to in the last study. In this regard, a booklet published by *Men's Health* magazine gives some good suggestions:

When you're in the supermarket produce aisle, tear off one of those plastic bags and stuff it will the brightest colored vegetables you see. Vibrant colors usually correspond with more vitamins, says Anne Dubner, R.D. L.D., a nutrition consultant and spokesperson for the American Dietetic Association. This means go easy on the iceberg lettuce, celery, and cucumbers and **load up on carrots, tomatoes, sweet red peppers, and sweet potatoes**. These are higher in vitamins like

A and C. Or go for darker greens. **Romaine lettuce**, for example, has nearly seven times the vitamin C and twice the calcium of its paler iceberg cousin (*Men's Health*, p.20).

Seeds:

Going back to the Garden, as Adam and Eve investigated all the plants around them, they would have discovered they contained seeds. And, as indicated previously, seeds would have been included in the Genesis 1:29 decree.

With some investigation and trial and error, Adam and Eve would have discovered that some of these seeds were edible raw, so raw seeds would also be a Creationist Diet staple. Edible seeds include sunflower seeds, pumpkin seeds, sesame seeds, chia seeds, hemp seeds, and flax seeds. The nutritional contents of seeds would be similar to that of nuts, including having the "good" kind of fat.

One seed of note is flaxseed. Flax itself is mentioned nine times in the Bible. Flaxseed has been getting a good reputation lately as it, " ... contains high amounts of phytoestrogens, as well as omega-3 fatty acids. Both might help prevent heart disease." In addition, "Flaxseed also provides iron, niacin, phosphorous, and vitamin E" (Fargo).

Seeds are packed with dietary fibre, protein, healthy fats and many antioxidants. These are the nutrient-packed seeds you should be eating every day (Best Health; Seeds).

Consider them [seeds] worthy alternatives to the nuts that are commonly enjoyed. (Nuts, in fact, are shelled fruits that contain seeds.) **All contain omega-3 fatty acids, which are associated with everything from a healthy brain and heart to supple skin**. Each also boasts its own distinctive dietary offerings, along with unique flavors that transform everyday eats into food that feels special (Real Simple).

Sunflower seeds provide a rich source of vitamins E and B-1, as well as copper. Adding nuts and seeds to your diet benefits your health. **Individuals who consume these foods on a regular basis enjoy a lower risk of developing**

47

cardiovascular disease or type 2 diabetes, according to the Linus Pauling Institute (Healthy Eating).

Pumpkin seeds have long been valued as a source of the mineral zinc, and the World Health Organization recommends their consumption as a good way of obtaining this nutrient...

While antioxidant nutrients are found in most WHFoods [World's Healthiest Foods], **it's the diversity of antioxidants in pumpkin seeds that makes them unique in their antioxidant support** (World's Pumpkin Seeds).

Sesame seeds—those tiny tasty toppings you may encounter on bagels, breadsticks, and hamburger buns, as well as on sushi rolls and sesame chicken—are called the "queen of oil seeds" for good reason. Though they are not as much in the limelight as flaxseed, chia, and other so-called "super seeds," they **are a notable source of nutrients**, including protein, iron, zinc, copper, vitamin E, thiamin, calcium, magnesium, and manganese, plus unique lignans (sesamin and sesamolin), phytosterols (predominantly B-sitosterol), fiber, and other potentially beneficial compounds (Berkely).

Adding flaxseed to the foods you eat regularly can improve your heart health and digestive system. It also can help control your weight and fight cancer.

For something so small, flaxseed has big benefits. Recent studies have shown that flaxseed, known to the world for thousands of years, may aid in lowering cholesterol, stabilizing blood sugar, reducing bone loss, promoting weight loss, increasing immunity, and fighting cancer, says clinical nutritionist Stella Metsovas of Laguna Beach, Calif (Everyday Health).

Summary:

Raw fruits and certain raw vegetables, along with raw nuts and seeds, would have been staples of the diets of Adam and Eve while they were still in the Garden. Other raw vegetables would have been added after the Fall. However, some vegetables, namely starchy vegetables

48

like white and sweet potatoes, are not easily eaten raw. And this leads to the next question, when did humans begin to cook their food?

Raw vs. Cooked

The Bible does not specially say when food began to be cooked. However, an indication might be found in Genesis 4:22, "And Sella also gave birth to Thobel; he was a hammer-wielding blacksmith of copper and iron; and the sister of Thobel was Noema."

It takes fire and intelligence to forge copper and iron. And if humans learned this early in human history how to use fire to forge copper and iron utensils and tools, they almost certainly also learned very early how to cook foods. However, raw foods would be an "earlier" food than cooked foods. And this point is important.

Whatever the cooking method, there is always some loss of nutrients from cooking. How much nutrients are lost would depend on the type of food, the cooking method, and the length of cooking. But whatever the case, generally speaking, raw foods contain more nutrients than cooked foods. Moreover, while both raw and cooked vegetables are associated with reduced risk of many kinds of cancer, some studies show raw vegetables to have a slightly greater inverse relationship with cancer than cooked vegetables (e.g. Franceschi S, and Levi F).

However, there are exceptions to this general rule. One example is cooked tomatoes. In the form of tomato sauce, cooked tomatoes are more strongly linked to a reduced risk of prostate cancer than raw tomatoes. This is possibly because the antioxidant lycopene found in tomatoes is made more bioavailable by cooking (Cooper, *p.69*).

Since humans ate raw foods earlier than cooked foods, then raw foods should constitute a significant portion of a Creationist Diet. And most of the foods mentioned previously can be eaten raw, namely fruits, vegetables, nuts, and seeds. As such, these foods would be the most basic, God-given foods.

But these same foods can also be eaten cooked. And since humans learned to control fire most probably shortly after the Fall, then cooked versions would have a place in a Creationist Diet, but in lesser amounts than the raw versions.

Moreover, there are vegetables that need to be cooked before eating. As indicated, "starchy vegetables" would fit this category. Thus foods like white and sweet potatoes would have a place in a Creationist Diet, but again, in lesser amounts than raw vegetables.

In addition to starchy vegetables, there are other classes of plant foods that have to be cooked, or at least, are generally eaten cooked rather than raw. Such foods will be looked at in the next chapter.

Bibliography:

Authority Nutrition. 8 Health Benefits of Nuts. https://authoritynutrition.com/8-benefits-of-nuts/

Authority Nutrition. Is Fruit Good or Bad For Your Health? The Sweet Truth. https://authoritynutrition.com/is-fruit-good-or-bad-for-your-health/

Authority Nutrition. 12 Proven Health Benefits of Avocado. https://authoritynutrition.com/12-proven-benefits-of-avocado/ https://www.ncbi.nlm.nih.gov/pubmed/24968103

Berkeley Wellness. Sesame: Little Seeds, Big Benefits/. http://www.bcrkeleywellness.com/healthy-eating/nutrition/article/sesame-little-seeds-big-health-benefits

Best Health; Super Seeds: 7 Types to Eat Daily. http://www.besthealthmag.ca/best-eats/healthy-eating/6-super-seeds-to-eat-every-day/

Canadian Living. The Top 25 Healthy Fruits. http://www.canadianliving.com/health/nutrition/article/the-top-25-healthy-fruits-blueberries-apples-cherries-bananas-and-21-more-healthy-picks

California Olive Ranch. Extra Virgin Olive Oil + Health. https://californiaoliveranch.com/olive-oil-101/extra-virgin-olive-oil-health/

CBS Philly. Eat More Fruit And Veg for A Longer Life, Researchers Say. http://philadelphia.cbslocal.com/2017/02/23/eat-more-fruit-and-veg-for-a-longer-life-researchers-say/

Cooper, Dr. Kenneth H. *Advanced Nutritional Therapies.* Nashville: Thomas Nelson, 1996.

Dairy Council. Health Benefits of Vegetables. http://www.healthyeating.org/Healthy-Eating/All-Star-Foods/Vegetables.aspx

Key TJ, Thorogood M, Appleby PN, Burr ML. *British Medical Journal.* 1996 Sep 28;313(7060):775-9. *Dietary habits and mortality in*

11,000 vegetarians and health conscious people: results of a 17 year follow up.

Fargo, Charlyn. *Valley News Dispatch.* "Flaxseed one of the top 12 trends of 2000," p.B7.

FAO. Nutritional and health benefits of citrus fruits. http://www.fao.org/docrep/x2650T/x2650t03.htm

Fastachi. The Health benefits of Nuts. http://www.fastachi.com/nuts_health_benefits

Franceschi S, Favero A, Parpinel M, Giacosa A, La Vecchia C. *European Journal of Cancer Prevention.* 1998 May;7 Suppl 2:S19-23. *Italian study on colorectal cancer with emphasis on influence of cereals.*

Everyday Health. Tiny Flaxseed Has Big Benefits. http://www.everydayhealth.com/diet-nutrition/tiny-flaxseed-has-big-benefits.aspx

"Health Bulletin" *Men's Health*, April 2000, p.36.

Healthy Eating. What Are the Benefits of Sunflower Seeds? http://healthyeating.sfgate.com/benefits-sunflower-seeds-6529.html

King, Margaret. "Health-food nuts." In *Valley News Dispatch*, January 15, 2000.

Kitchn. What;s the Difference Between Regular Olive Oil and Extra-Virgin Olive Oil? http://www.thekitchn.com/whats-the-difference-between-olive-oil-and-extra-virgin-olive-oil-word-of-mouth-218767

Levi F, Pasche C, La Vecchia C, Lucchini F, Franceschi S. *British Journal of Cancer.* 1999 Mar;79(7-8):1283-7. *Food groups and colorectal cancer risk.*

Mayo Clinic. Nuts and your heart: Eating nuts for heart health. http://www.mayoclinic.org/diseases-conditions/heart-disease/in-depth/nuts/art-20046635

Medical Daily. Benefits Of Nuts: Eating 10 Grams Of Nuts And Peanuts A Day Lowers Death Risk Of Major Causes. http://www.medicaldaily.com/benefits-nuts-eating-10-grams-nuts-and-peanuts-day-lowers-death-risk-major-causes-337576

Men's Health: 101 Nutrition Secrets. By the editors of *Men's Health*, Emmaus, PA; Rodale, 1999.

Nutrition and You. Vegetable nutrition facts. http://www.nutrition-and-you.com/vegetable-nutrition.html

Nutrition Action HealthLetter, Vol. 27, No. 3, April, 2000, "Multiple Choice: How to Pick a Multivitamin, pp. 1,5-13.

Olive Oil Times. Olive Oil Health Benefits. https://www.oliveoiltimes.com/olive-oil-health-benefits

Organic Facts. Benefits Of Fruits. https://www.organicfacts.net/health-benefits/fruit/fruits.html

Organic Facts. Benefits Of Vegetables. https://www.organicfacts.net/health-benefits/vegetable/vegetables.html

Parsonnet, Mia, M.D. *What's in Our Food?* New York: Madison Books, 1996.

Real Simple. The Health Benefits of Popular Seeds. http://www.realsimple.com/health/nutrition-diet/healthy-eating/chia-seeds-benefits/chia-seeds-benefits-3

Ros, Emilio. *Nutrients.* 2010 Jul; 2(7): 652–682. PMCID: PMC3257681

Health Benefits of Nut Consumption. https://www.ncbi.nlm.nih.gov/pmc/articles/PMC3257681/

Russell, Rex MD. *What the Bible Says about Healthy Living.* Grand Rapids, MI: Baker Book House, 1999.

Sabate, J. *American Journal of Clinical Nutrition.* 1999 Sep;70(3 Suppl):500S-503S. *Nut consumption, vegetarian diets, ischemic heart disease risk, and all-cause mortality: evidence from epidemiologic studies.*

USDA. Why is it important to eat fruit? https://www.choosemyplate.gov/fruits-nutrients-health

USDA. Why is it important to eat vegetables? https://www.choosemyplate.gov/vegetables-nutrients-health

WebMD. What's in Your Olive Oil? http://www.webmd.com/food-recipes/features/olive-oil-health-benefits#1

What's Cooking America? Avocados – Learn All About Avocados. https://whatscookingamerica.net/avocado.htm

World's Healthiest Foods. Olive oil, extra virgin. http://www.whfoods.com/genpage.php?tname=foodspice&dbid=132

World's Healthiest Foods. Pumpkin Seeds. http://www.whfoods.com/genpage.php?tname=foodspice&dbid=82

Women's Health Reporter. "Diet, Exercise, and Breast, Cancer." Vol. 1, No. 3, March 2000, pp.1,3.

Chapter Two:
Grains and Legumes

This chapter will look at the two major remaining classes of plant foods: grains and legumes.

Grains

Grains are the next class of plant foods to be considered. As indicated in Chapter One, grains would have been included among the "every seed-sowing [fig., bearing] vegetation sowing seed" decree of Genesis 1:29. Thus grains are God-given foods. But did Adam and Eve, or at least their earliest descendants, eat grain foods? The answer to this question is a bit difficult.

The first possible reference to a grain food is in Genesis 3:19, as part of the curse God pronounced upon Adam for his disobedience. In part, God told Adam, "In sweat of your face will you eat your **bread** until you return to the earth out of which you were taken; for earth you are and to earth you will depart [or, return]."

Note the word "bread" in the first part of the verse. If this is a reference to bread as we know it, then it would mean that Adam and Eve had already figured out how to grind grain and bake bread before leaving the Garden. As such, it would make cooked grain foods another staple of the Creationist Diet.

The word translated "bread" here in the ALT is from the Greek word in the LXX, which is most often rendered as bread. It is so rendered in every occurrence in the ALT. The same goes for the Hebrew word, which is rendered as "bread" in most every occurrence in the NKJV (e.g., Gen 14:18; 18:5; 21:14). But both words can more generally mean "food," and it is sometimes so rendered in many occurrences in the NASB, NIV, and ESV (Gen 24:33; 43:31; 47:15). As such, it is unsure if a grain food is being referred to in Genesis 3:19.

If not, then the question of whether Adam and Eve ate grain foods is more difficult to answer. Making bread is a rather complex operation. It requires many steps in its production. However, grains do not have to be made into bread to be eaten. Some grains, like rice require fewer steps, just boiling water. But even boiling water requires the knowledge of making fire and the ability to make some kind in vessel to boil the water in.

As previously indicated, there is some indication that humans learned how to control fire and forge metal shortly after the Fall. But there is no indication that Adam and Eve did so while still in the Garden, so it is unlikely they were making bread or cooking rice in the Garden.

However, it is possible to eat some kinds of grains raw, at least in limited amounts. An example of this is seen in Luke 6:1:

[1]Now it happened on the second-first Sabbath [fig., the first Sabbath of the second month], He [was] passing through the grain fields, and His disciples were picking the heads of grain and were eating, rubbing [the husk from the grain] with their hands."

Therefore, it is possible that Adam and Eve ate grains in the Garden in the same fashion as the apostles did many millennia later. Today, the most popular way grains are eaten raw is in the form of sprouts.

But whatever the case in the Garden, it is likely that sometime after the Fall humans did figure out ways to make cooked grain foods. There is little doubt that the correct rendering is "bread" in Genesis 14:18, "And Melchizedek king of Salem brought out bread and wine, and he was the priest of the Most High God."

Moreover, bread has an important place in the Bible, being mentioned 346 times. An indication of its importance can be seen in Jesus calling bread a "good gift" (Matt 7:9-11) and Himself "the bread of life" (John 6:35, 48).

Wheat is the most popular Biblical grain, being mentioned 49 times. But other grains are also mentioned. Barley is the next most popular grain, being mentioned 36 times.

Spelt is mentioned three times (Exodus 9:32, Isaiah 28:25, Ezekiel 4:9). I found these references interesting as when I was working on the First Edition of this book, I had only recently learned what "spelt" was:

Spelt is an ancient grain widely recognized for its many health benefits. *Triticum spelta*, the scientific name for spelt, is a hardier and more nutritious cousin to modern wheat

(*Triticum aestivum*). Some taxonomists classify spelt as a parent of wheat (Nature's Legacy).

I guess I just passed over the Biblical references without much thought. But then I bought some cereals from a "health food store," and one of these was *Spelt Flakes*. I found the taste to be even better than cereal flakes made from other kinds of grains. Spelt flakes have a light, crispy texture.

Otherwise, some of today's more popular grains are not specifically mentioned in the Bible, such as oats, rice, rye, and corn. But these too would have been included in the decree of Genesis 1:29. And it should be noted; there are many kinds of grains besides the ones generally eaten in western society.

Besides spelt, grains such as buckwheat, amaranth, kamut, quinoa, and others have been utilized in various ways, in various cultures. All of these different grains have varying nutritional qualities, but in their whole grain forms, they are all good sources of a variety of nutrients including carbohydrates, protein, vitamins, minerals, and fiber.

Moreover, an important point about there being such a wide range of grains available is certain people cannot tolerate some kinds of grains for various reasons. However, these reasons are being overblown of late.

The first reason is celiac disease. "Celiac disease, also known as gluten intolerance, is a genetic disorder that affects at least 1 in 133 Americans" (Celiac.com). The 1 in 133 number is less than 1% of the US population.

However, some try to make a distinction between celiac disease and gluten intolerance (or sensitivity), claiming the latter is more prevalent. But "the data suggest that almost two-thirds of people who think they are gluten-intolerant really aren't" (Medical Examiner).

And in a double-blind study, people who thought they were gluten intolerant were given pills to take with a controlled diet and told the pills contained gluten. They reported feeling sick as a result, but the pills were placeboes. "Gluten wasn't the culprit; the cause was likely psychological. Participants expected the diets to make them sick, and so they did" (Real Clear Science).

Related to this would be a wheat allergy. But, "... it's estimated that approximately 0.4 percent of children and 0.5 percent of adults are allergic to wheat" (Allergist). So a true wheat allergy is even rarer than true celiac disease or gluten intolerance.

> **Gluten is a protein in wheat (all kinds, including spelt, Kamut® khorasan, einkorn and farro/emmer), barley, rye and triticale (a rye/wheat hybrid) that is hard for some people to digest.**
> This group includes the estimated **1-2% of the population with celiac disease** – an autoimmune form of gluten intolerance – who must eat a gluten-free diet for life. Other people may not have celiac disease, but may be **allergic to wheat (about 0.2-0.4% of people)** or may have what's termed **non-celiac gluten sensitivity** (a group some experts estimate at from **1% to 6% of the population) -- though new research shows NCGS may not actually be the issue it was once thought to be**.
> **There's no reason for the rest of us to go gluten-free**, no matter what fear-mongering books like *Wheat Belly* and *Grain Brain* may say (Oldways; Gluten Free).

Adding together the most liberal numbers, at most 8.5% of the US population suffers from conditions that would require them to avoid wheat. Or looking at it the other way, for at least 91.5% of Americans there would be no benefit from eliminating wheat from their diets.

> A gluten-free diet is essential for people suffering from celiac disease or gluten intolerance, but **for the average person, going gluten-free doesn't make a lot of sense**. Gluten-laden whole grains such as wheat, barley, and rye are linked to a reduced risk for heart disease, cancer, and diabetes; and gluten may also boost immune system functioning (Fox News).

> People with celiac disease, gluten sensitivity or a wheat allergy should avoid gluten. But **there's no evidence that avoiding gluten will help people without these conditions lose weight or have any benefit on heart health** (Live).

That said; if you have been diagnosed by a medical doctor via clinical tests with celiac disease, gluten intolerance, or a wheat allergy, then you must eliminate wheat and other gluten containing grains from your diet. But the following grains and flours can be consumed by those with Celiac Disease: amaranth, brown rice flour, buckwheat flour and groats (kasha), corn meal (and polenta), millet (pilaf and flour), poha (poha is beaten rice that has the texture of oatmeal when used in recipes), potato starch, potato flour, quinoa flour, rice cereal, soy (Gluten Free and Casein Free).

As for oats, they do contain gluten, however studies show that it should not be a problem for those with celiac disease. There are several articles on Celiac.com in this regard. One states, "Recent evidence from a number of studies has supported the idea that oats are safe for people with celiac disease" (Another). But cross-contamination with gluten containing grains can be an issue and must be considered.

Spelt is another grain about which there is controversy if it can be consumed by those with celiac disease or who are allergic to wheat:

The word 'allergy' covers a broad spectrum of reactions to certain foods, such as wheat. A true allergy can be life threatening, leading to anaphylactic shock. If you have a known wheat allergy or sensitivity, consult your doctor before introducing spelt into your diet. Many people who consider themselves allergic to certain foods, experience non-life threatening symptoms such as headaches, rashes, and stomach aches. According to the World's Healthiest Foods website: **"Spelt does not seem to cause sensitivities in many people who are intolerant of wheat**." Many of our customers who are sensitive to wheat have verified this. And remember, not all spelt is processed in dedicated, wheat-free processing plants. If you are allergic to wheat, be sure to look for 100% pure spelt.

… **the gluten in spelt has a different molecular make-up than the gluten in modern wheat**. It is more fragile and more water soluble, which makes it **easier to digest**. Spelt is also higher in fiber than wheat, and the extra fiber aids in the digestion of the gluten. **Modern wheat has been bred to contain a high gluten content** for the production of high-volume commercial baked goods. **The content and character**

of the gluten in spelt has not been modified from its natural state (Nature's Legacy).

Sprouted grains are also said by some to be easier to digest than regular grains. As such, some believe sprouted grains can be eaten by celiacs (Living). But both of these claims are controversial as spelt and sprouted grains contain gluten, so others say they must be avoided by those with celiac disease (Very Well). Given these controversies, talk with your doctor if you are in any way sensitive to gluten or wheat before trying these alternatives.

However, on another important point there is no controversy—all of the grains consumed in the antediluvian age, and for that matter throughout most of history since then, up until the beginning of the last century, would have been whole grains. It has only been in the last century or so that refined grains have become popular.

There is a significant distinction between whole and refined grains. Whole grains, which contain the outer bran and inner germ of the wheat kernel, are a storehouse of fiber, vitamins, and minerals. The refining process eliminates the most nutritious parts of the grains and thus most of the nutrients.

The invention of industrialized roller mills in the late 19th century changed the way we process grains. **Milling strips away the bran and germ, making the grain easier to chew and digest, but such highly processed grains are much lower in nutritional quality**. Refining wheat creates fluffy flour that makes light, airy breads and pastries, but **the process strips away more than half of wheat's B vitamins, 90 percent of the vitamin E, and virtually all of the fiber** (Harvard).

And "enriched" grains are anything but. In the "enriching" process only a few of the many nutrients in whole grains that are lost in processing are restored. How much of a difference is there between whole grains and "enriched" grains? The book *The Essential Guide to Vitamins and Minerals* by Elizabeth Somer has the following chart.

White bread contains:
22% of the magnesium in whole wheat bread

38% of the zinc
28% of the chromium
42% of the copper
12% of the manganese
 4% of the vitamin E
18% of the vitamin B6
63% of the folic acid
56% of the pantothenic acid (p.263).

So what happens to the nutritious elements of grains that are refined out? A short article in a cookbook I received with a Vitamix blender I purchased a while back answers this question. The article is titled "The Poverty of Enrichment" and states:

> The practice of refining whole wheat gave birth to several other businesses—all motivated by answers to this question: "What to do with the discarded (and most nutritious) parts of the wheat—the bran, wheat germ oil, and endosperm?" Simple. **Extol the wholesome virtues of these by-products and package them for sale**. The resulting "new" products today represent millions of dollars in annual sales—**wheat germ oil, bran flakes, vitamin E tablets, vitamin supplements, cosmetics, laxatives, and wheat germ**.
> Isn't it interesting how big business has taken whole grain—a food you can buy for 20 to 30 cents a pound, broken it down into its individual parts, and sells it for $2 a pound ($1 an ounce for wheat germ oil)? (Vitamix, p.12).

In addition to being devoid of the nutrition of whole grains, refined grains are not associated with decreased risks of various disease, while whole grains are associated with reduced risks.

The difference between refined grains and whole grains is actually quite extreme, with refined grains being significantly modified from their whole grain starting points. Primarily, this modification involves the mechanical removal of the bran and the germ, either through grinding or selective sifting. In addition, **the refining process can include mixing,**

59

bleaching, and even adding potassium bromate, a known carcinogen...

Why then is grain refined and adulterated?

The bran (the fiber of the grain) is removed primarily for aesthetic reasons -- to make the grain flour look whiter, prettier, and cook with a lighter texture. **The germ, on the other hand is removed to extend shelf life.** The germ is the "heart" of the cereal kernel (the embryo of the seed) and is a concentrated source of essential nutrients including a number of vitamins and minerals. But most importantly, **it contains key oils such as Vitamin E and the essential fatty acids, which explains why it is removed -- to prevent the refined grain from turning rancid and spoiling** (Baseline).

Eating more whole grains is an easy way to add a layer of "health insurance" to your life. **Whole grains are packed with nutrients**, including protein, fiber, B vitamins, antioxidants, and trace minerals (iron, zinc, copper, and magnesium). A diet rich in whole grains has been shown to **reduce the risk of heart disease, type 2 diabetes, obesity, and some forms of cancer. Whole-grain diets also improve bowel health** by helping to maintain regular bowel movements and promote growth of healthy bacteria in the colon.

Yet only 10% of Americans consume the recommended minimum of three servings a day (WebMD; Guide)

Studies show that eating whole grains instead of refined grains lowers the risk of many chronic diseases. While benefits are greatest with at least 3 servings daily, some studies show reduced risks from as little as one serving daily. The message: **every whole grain in your diet helps!**...

The benefits of whole grains most documented by repeated studies include:

1. stroke risk reduced 30-36%
2. type 2 diabetes risk reduced 21-30%
3. heart disease risk reduced 25-28%
4. better weight maintenance (Oldways; Benefits)

A growing body of research shows that choosing whole grains and other less-processed, higher-quality sources of carbohydrates, and cutting back on refined grains, **improves health in many ways**....

As researchers have begun to look more closely at carbohydrates and health, they are learning that **the quality of the carbohydrates you eat is at least as important as the quantity**. Most studies, including some from several different Harvard teams, show a connection between whole grains and better health (Harvard).

Whole grains are rich sources of vitamins, minerals, dietary fiber, lignans, beta-glucan, several phytochemicals, phytosterols, phytin, and sphingolipids, **all of which may have individual, synergistic, or additive actions that positively affect health. In addition, whole grains' phytochemicals complement the phytochemicals in fruits and vegetables when they're consumed together.**

Most of the beneficial phytochemicals in whole grains are found in the bran and germ, the components that often are milled out during refinement, resulting in grains composed mainly of the nutrient-poor endosperm. **Refined wheat flour loses** 83% of total phenolic acids, 79% of total flavonoids, 93% of ferulic acid, 78% of total zeaxanthin, 51% of total lutein, and 42% of total beta-crytoxanthin compared with whole wheat flour.

Overall, studies show that consuming **two to three servings of whole grain foods per day will provide health benefits**, possibly reducing the risk of cardiovascular disease, hypertension, type 2 diabetes, colon cancer, and obesity. In prospective studies, **the protection from these diseases that results from consuming whole grains far exceeds the protection expected from the individual nutrients and phytochemicals found in whole grains** (Today's Dietician).

There is thus a syncretistic effect from all of the beneficial elements to be found in whole grains, and these work together in a synchronistic

61

fashion with beneficial elements in other whole foods. That is why taking a supplement in way makes up for a diet deficient in whole, natural foods.

Lastly on whole grains, a 2017 study found whole grains can help people to lose weight as compared to refined grains:

> For the study, researchers recorded the weight, metabolic rate, blood glucose, fecal calories, hunger and fullness for 81 participants over an eight week period. After an initial period of two weeks where all participants were given the same foods, **the researchers fed some of the participants a diet with whole grains and some a diet with refined grains**. The study was conducted at the Energy Metabolism Laboratory at the Jean Mayer USDA Human Nutrition Research Center on Aging (HNRCA)at Tufts University.
>
> According to a statement released by Tufts University announcing the study, the scientists found that **those who ate whole grain foods burned an extra 100 calories per day** because of their increased resting metabolic rate and greater fecal losses when compared to the group that ate mostly refined grains. The extra calories lost by the whole grain eaters equaled the calories burned in a brisk walk or a small cookie, according to the study's author (ABC).

Putting all of this information together, whole grains, but not refined grains, would be included in a Creationist Diet. But since they entered the human diet later than fruits, vegetables, nuts, and seeds, they would have less of an importance than those more original foods.

Legumes

The last main class of plant foods would be legumes, also called beans or pulses. These are unique plant foods in that generally speaking they cannot be eaten raw. As such, it is unlikely Adam and Eve ate legumes in the Garden.

However, as with grains, humans in the antediluvian age probably rather quickly figured out how to prepare legumes for food, with the first reference to a legume being in Genesis 25:34a, "Now Jacob gave bread to Esau, and **a stew of lentil[s]**; and he ate and drank, and he arose and departed."

Lentils are also mentioned in 2Samuel 23:11, while beans in general are mentioned twice in the Bible (2Sam 17:28 and Ezek 4:9). Both of these verses also mention lentils. As such, legumes would have a place in a Creationist Diet, but after whole grains.

The following should be noted:

> Previously known by their maiden names—kidney bean, navy bean, pinto bean, garbanzo bean, dried French green bean (flageolets), black-eyed and split pea, lentil, and peanut— **pulses are legumes** harvested only for the dry seed, unlike green peas or soybeans, which are vegetable crops (Men's Fitness).

But by whatever name, beans are an incredibly nutritious food with many health benefits:

> **Beans can be the least expensive source of protein,** especially when compared to fresh meat. Aside from protein, complex carbs and fiber, **beans contain a powerhouse of nutrients** including antioxidants, and vitamins and minerals, such as copper, folate, iron, magnesium, manganese, phosphorous, potassium and zinc (Huffington Post).

> Beans may get a bad rap for making people gassy, but that's no reason to cut them out of your diet. **Experts recommend you consume up to 3 cups of the legumes a week—because they are so good for your health**. And the more you eat, the less likely you are to have tummy trouble. **"People who eat beans on a consistent basis experience less gas and bloating than people who consume them less often,"** says Cynthia Sass, MPH, RD (Health).

> Eating beans as part of a heart healthy diet and lifestyle may help improve your blood cholesterol, a leading cause of heart

disease. **Adding beans to your diet may help keep you feeling full longer.**

Drain canned beans in a colander and rinse with water to remove some of the excess salt; or buy canned beans with no salt added if they have them at your store. Or, you can make your own salt-free beans from scratch (AHA).

According to an analysis of 21 clinical trials, 940 subjects ate just a 3/4-cup serving of pulses daily—but didn't change anything else diet-or activity-wise—yet in six weeks, they **still lost about three-fourths of a pound**, the *American Journal of Clinical Nutrition* reports.

Bonus: **Pulses also help you:**

1. Feel fuller
2. Supply fiber
3. Provide non-animal protein
4. Cut cholesterol (Men's Fitness).

Beans are nutritional powerhouses packed with protein, fiber, B vitamins, iron, potassium, and are low in fat; but this mighty food can also pose potential health risks.

Health Benefit: Beans can prevent heart disease.
Health Benefit: Beans can fight cancer.
Health Benefit: Beans can lower cholesterol.
Health Benefit: Beans can help you lose weight.
Health Benefit: Beans can help manage diabetes.

Health Risk: Beans can cause migraines.
Health Risk: Beans can raise blood pressure.
Health Risk: Beans can interfere with vitamin absorption.
Health Risk: Beans can trigger gout.
Health Risk: Beans can make you gassy (Reader's Digest).

On the last risk, if you're using canned beans, simply rinsing them off before use removes the gas producing compounds. I've found this works very well. If you're using dried beans, then change the water a couple of times in the soaking process.

As for the blood pressure risk, that is only for those who are taking "monoamine oxidase (MAO) inhibitor to treat depression." If you are, talk to your doctor. But if not, then it is not a concern.

On interfering with vitamin absorption, this is only for soybeans. That legume will require special attention later. But first, another legume also deserves special mention.

Peanuts:

Although generally called "nuts," peanuts are technically legumes. But nutritionally, they have more in common with nuts than legumes. They are high in monounsaturated fats, and have vitamin, mineral, fiber, and protein contents similar to most nuts.

However, the preparation time of peanuts would be similar to that of other legumes. But even if best eaten roasted than raw, again, antediluvian humans knew how to make fire and roast things, so peanuts would be included in a Creationist Diet and would have the same benefits as nuts.

In fact, a study conducted at this writer's alma mater, Penn State, found that consumption of peanuts and peanut butter was associated with a reduced risk of heart disease, just as nuts are. The study reported, "Besides monounsaturated fats, peanuts and peanut butter contain many other heart-healthy nutrients such as vitamin E, folic acid, soluble fiber, arginine, plant sterols, copper, zinc, selenium and magnesium" (PRNewswire). There are other benefits to peanuts as well.

In addition to their monounsaturated fat content, **peanuts feature an array of other nutrients that, in numerous studies, have been shown to promote heart health**. Peanuts are good sources of vitamin E, niacin, folate, protein and manganese. In addition, **peanuts provide resveratrol, the phenolic antioxidant also found in red grapes and red wine** that is thought to be responsible for the French paradox: the fact that in France, people consume a diet that is not low in fat, but have a lower risk of cardiovascular disease compared to the U.S.

With all of the important nutrients provided by nuts like peanuts, it is no wonder that numerous research studies, including the Nurses' Health Study that involved over 86,000 women, have found that **frequent nut consumption is related to reduced risk of cardiovascular disease** (World's).

Peanuts are a type of nuts, **originating in South America**. Scientifically known as Arachis hypogea, **peanuts go by a variety of names, such as groundnuts, earth nuts, and goobers.** However, peanuts are technically not nuts. They actually belong to the legume family and are therefore related to beans, lentils, and soy.

In the US, peanuts are rarely eaten raw. Instead, they are most often consumed as roasted and salted whole peanuts or peanut butter. Other products made from peanuts include peanut oil, peanut flour, and peanut protein. Peanut products are used in a variety of foods; desserts, cakes, confectionery, snacks, and sauces.

Not only do peanuts taste good, they are also rich in protein, fat, and various healthy nutrients (Authority; Peanuts).

Studies show that peanuts may be useful for weight loss, and are linked to reduced risk of cardiovascular disease.

But **in those who ate peanuts, their mortality risk was lowered**. It's been known for some time that nuts — which are rich in essential nutrients like fiber, protein, minerals, monounsaturated and polyunsaturated fatty acids, and antioxidants — have plenty of health benefits….

It turns out that eating pure peanuts instead of peanut butter is better: **The researchers found no improvement among people who ate peanut butter, which typically contains non-healthy additives like salt and vegetable oils.** But in those who ate peanuts, their mortality risk was lowered (Medical Daily; Nuts).

The last paragraph requires comment. Grinding peanuts into butter was not done in Biblical times. It was first done in the 1800s. But such would not be beyond the technical expertise of people in Biblical times, and there is no loss of nutrients when doing so. But as mentioned, a problem can occur due to what is often added: salt, sugar, refined vegetable oils, and artificial ingredients.

But it is possible to purchase all-natural peanut butter that is pure peanuts. In that case, the oil tends to separate to the top and needs to be stirred back into the rest of the product. It is because of that "difficulty" that manufacturers add the above ingredients. But it really is simple to do, but it needs to be done before the peanut butter is refrigerated. And yes, all-natural peanut butter should be refrigerated.

It should also be noted that butter made from tree nuts is also available, such as almond or cashew butter. Such is more expensive than peanut butter, but they are a tasty alternative.

Soybeans:

A second legume deserving special mention is soybeans. Like peanuts, soybeans are best eaten cooked. In fact, "Soybeans **must** be cooked, as they are poisonous when raw" (Authority; Soy, bolding in original). But there is much controversy in regards to soybeans. Some studies show potential benefits, such as a reduction in the risk of heart disease, but the evidence is not clear cut. And there are also potential drawbacks to soy consumption.

One reason for the potential problems with soy is soybeans contain isoflavones (aka, phytoestrogens), which are estrogen-like substances. On the one hand, for some pre-menopausal women, isoflavones can disrupt their menstrual cycles. On the other hand, for some women isoflavones can lessen the severity of the symptoms of menopause. There is also debate if these isoflavones lower testosterone levels in men and if they increase or decrease the risk of breast cancer in women.

Second, a relatively high number of people are allergic to soybeans. And third, soybeans tend to be hard to digest. How soybeans are prepared might have a bearing on this latter point. Roasted soybeans tend to be harder to digest than tofu.

But one definite good point is soybeans contain complete protein, while most all other plant foods contain incomplete protein. This is why soybeans are found in many vegetarian foods as they are a good source of high quality protein.

Soybeans are high in quality protein; 175 ml (¾ cup) of cooked soybeans contains as much protein as 75 g (125 ml (½ cup) of cooked meat, chicken or fish. Like meat, **soybeans contain all the essential building blocks, or amino acids, in amounts we need for health.**

Soy is higher in fat than other legumes, which are generally almost fat-free; **however, it's mainly good fat** (monounsaturated and polyunsaturated fats, including omega-3 fatty acids). All legumes, including soy, have no cholesterol.

Soy is an excellent source of the minerals calcium and iron…

There has been a lot of research done on the potential health benefits and safety of soy. **The two areas where soy has been found to have beneficial roles are heart health and breast cancer** (Dieticians).

Here are **7 health benefits of soybeans**:
1. Soybeans can help individuals control weight.
2. Soybeans can contribute to improving an individual's sleep.
3. Soybeans may help prevent and manage diabetes.
4. Soybeans can help improve circulation and oxygenation.
5. Soybeans may help improve an individual's digestive health.
6. Soybeans can help prevent birth defects.
7. Soybeans have a significant vitamin and mineral density (Dove Med).

Soy appears to help midlife women deal with hot flashes and night sweats, according to a new report.

However, **the evidence for other potential benefits of soy** -- such as effects on heart and bone health -- **is not clear**, a panel of experts has concluded (WebMD; Soy).

Soy is definitely one of the most controversial foods in the world. Depending on who you ask, **it is either a wonderful superfood or a hormone disrupting poison.** As with most things in nutrition, there are good arguments on both sides…

Over 90% of soy produced in the U.S. is genetically modified and the crops are sprayed with the herbicide Roundup, which may be associated with adverse effects on health...

The isoflavones found in soy can activate and/or inhibit estrogen receptors in the body, which can disrupt the body's normal function....

Animal studies show that soy isoflavones can cause breast cancer. There are also human studies showing that soy isoflavones can stimulate the proliferation and activity of cells in the breasts.... These changes may indicate an increased risk of breast cancer, which is the most common cancer in women. However, many observational studies show that women who consume soy actually have a reduced risk of breast cancer...

Many believe that soy can reduce testosterone levels, but the effect appears to be weak and inconsistent Some studies show a small reduction, while others find no effect (Authority; Soy).

Soybeans are a common allergen. Raw or sprouted soya beans contain substances called goitrogens, which can interfere with thyroid gland activity. Soya also contains oxalate. Individuals with a history of oxalate containing kidney stones should avoid overconsumption. Women who have or have had oestrogen-sensitive breast tumours should restrict their soya intake to no more than four servings per week.

Although studies don't give us any clear guidance on eating soya-rich foods, women with oestrogen receptor positive breast tumours should restrict their soya intake to no more than four servings per week and should avoid soya isoflavone supplements. Before changing your diet, it is advisable that you speak to your GP [general practitioner] or alternative health professional (Good Food).

The bottom line, if you have never eaten soybeans before, it would be best not to begin to do so. There are simply too many questions and not enough support for benefits. Soybeans are not mentioned in the

Bible, nor were they consumed in Biblical times. But since they are a legume, they can be included in the Creationist Diet. But if you choose to consume them, introduce them slowly and watch closely for any reactions.

But other legumes, including peanuts, would have a place in a Creationist Diet. But since they are a later food than all of the previously mentioned foods, the proportion of them in the diet would be less than fruits, vegetables, nuts, seeds, and even whole grains.

Bibliography:

ABC. New Study Suggests Eating Whole Grains Can Aid Weight Loss. http://abcnews.go.com/Health/study-suggests-eating-grains-aid-weight-loss/story?id=45361969

AHA (American Heart Association). The Benefits of Beans and Legumes. https://recipes.heart.org/Articles/1026/The-Benefits-of-Beans-and-Legumes

Allergist. Wheat Allergy. http://acaai.org/allergies/types/food-allergies/types-food-allergy/wheat-gluten-allergy

Authority Nutrition. Peanuts 101: Nutrition Facts and Health Benefits. https://authoritynutrition.com/foods/peanuts/

Authority Nutrition. Is Soy Bad For You, or Good? The Shocking Truth. https://authoritynutrition.com/is-soy-bad-for-you-or-good/

Brown-Driver-Briggs-Gesenius Hebrew and English Lexicon. As contained in *BibleWorks™ for Windows™.* Copyright © 1992-1999 BibleWorks, L.C.C. Big Fork, MT: Hermeneutika. Programmed by Michael S. Bushell and Michael D. Tan.

Celicac.com. Home page and "Another Study Okays Oats for Celiac Patients" - https://www.celiac.com/articles/21550/1/Another-Study-Okays-Oats-for-Celiac-Patients/Page1.html

Dove Med. 7 Health Benefits of Soybeans. http://www.dovemed.com/7-health-benefits-of-soybean/

Gluten Free and Casein Free Web site: Part Three. http://www.gfcfdiet.com/section_three.htm

Dieticians of Canada. What are the health benefits of soy?
http://www.dietitians.ca/Your-Health/Nutrition-A-Z/Soy/Health-Benefits-of-Soy.aspx

Fox News Health. 5 pieces of basically useless nutrition advice.
http://www.foxnews.com/health/2017/01/05/5-pieces-basically-useless-nutrition-advice.html

Good Food. The health benefits of... soya.
http://www.bbcgoodfood.com/howto/guide/ingredient-focus-soya

Harvard. Whole Grains.
https://www.hsph.harvard.edu/nutritionsource/whole-grains/

Health. 9 Reasons You Should Eat More Beans.

Huffington Post. 11 Health Benefits Of Beans.
http://www.huffingtonpost.com/2012/08/16/beans-health-benefits_n_1792504.html

Journal of the American Medical Association," 281, pp.1998,1999; reported in *Nutrition Action Healthletter* October, 1999, p.10.

"Know your beans," in the *Valley News Dispatch,* January 29, 2000.

Levi F, Pasche C, La Vecchia C, Lucchini F, Franceschi S. *British Journal of Cancer.* 1999 Mar;79(7-8):1283-7. *Food groups and colorectal cancer risk.*

Live Science. Are Any Fad Diets Actually Healthy? What the Research Shows.
http://www.livescience.com/58036-fad-diets-heart-disease.html

Living Beyond Organic. TV show on TBN.

Malkmus, Rev. George H., with Michael Dye. *God's Way to Ultimate Health.* Shelby, NC: Hallelujah Acres Publishing, 1995, 1998.

Medical Daily. Benefits Of Nuts: Eating 10 Grams Of Nuts And Peanuts A Day Lowers Death Risk Of Major Causes.
http://www.medicaldaily.com/benefits-nuts-eating-10-grams-nuts-and-peanuts-day-lowers-death-risk-major-causes-337576

Medical Examiner. Why Do So Many People Think They Need Gluten-Free Foods?
http://www.slate.com/articles/health_and_science/medical_examiner/2013/02/gluten_free_diet_distinguishing_celiac_disease_wheat_allergy_and_gluten.html

Men's Fitness. 5 Health Benefits of Beans.
http://www.mensfitness.com/nutrition/what-to-eat/5-health-benefits-beans

Nature's Legacy. What is spelt?
https://natureslegacyforlife.com/faqs/what-is-spelt/
Nutrition Action HealthLetter, Vol. 26, No. 7. November 1999, p. 10.

"Oats." Celiac.com (http://www.celiac.com/oats.html). Citing, *New England Journal of Medicine*. October 19, 1995, Vol. 333, No. 16, "A Comparison of Diets with and without Oats in Adults with Celiac Disease"
(http://www.nejm.org/content/1995/0333/0016/1033.asp). Also Scott Adams' "June 27, 1999 Post Regarding Oats. Gluten-Free Grains and Cross-Contamination."

PRNewswire. *"Good" Fat Peanut Diet Beats Low-Fat Diet for Heart Health*. Arlington, Va., Nov. 22, 1999.

Oldways Whole Grains Council. Gluten Free Whole Grains.
http://wholegrainscouncil.org/whole-grains-101/whats-whole-grain-refined-grain/gluten-free-whole-grains

Real Clear Science. Non-Celiac Gluten Sensitivity May Not Exist.
http://www.realclearscience.com/blog/2014/05/gluten_sensitivity_may_not_exist.html

Reader's Digest. 5 Health Benefits of Beans—and 5 Surprising Risks.
http://www.rd.com/health/conditions/health-benefits-of-beans/

Somer, Elizabeth, M.A., R.D. *The Essential Guide to Vitamins and Minerals*. New York: Harper Paperback, 1992.

Today's Dietician. The Impact of Whole Grains on Health.
http://www.todaysdietitian.com/newarchives/050113p44.shtml

Very Well. Are Sprouted Grains Gluten-Free?
https://www.verywell.com/are-sprouted-grains-gluten-free-562843

Vita-Mix Corporation. *Whole Grains Cookbook*, 1999.

WebMD. Benefits of Soy: A Mixed Bag.
http://www.webmd.com/food-recipes/news/20110630/benefits-of-soy-a-mixed-bag#1

WebMD; Guide to a Healthy Kitchen.
http://www.webmd.com/diet/healthy-kitchen-11/reaping-benefits-whole-grains

World's Healthiest Foods. Peanuts.
http://www.whfoods.com/genpage.php?tname=foodspice&dbid=101

Chapter Three:
Problems with Restrictive Diets

The most likely interpretation of the evidence is that Adam and Eve, while in the Garden, ate a 100% raw foods diet, consisting of raw fruits and vegetables, raw nuts and seeds, and possibly raw grains.

Would such a diet be healthy today? It sustained Adam and Eve for however long they were in the Garden. Moreover, such a diet would consist solely of God-given foods in the raw form in which God most originally gave them to be eaten. Therefore, it would seem it would be. But is it? Many people today seem to think so.

Raw Foods Movement

There is a vibrant "raw vegan foods" movement on the Internet. Websites like "Living and Raw Foods" discuss many of the claimed benefits of such a diet, while presenting testimonies of people who have thrived on it. An article on this site even makes the following claims:

> **When food is cooked** above 118 degrees F for three minutes or longer, **its protein has become coagulated, its sugar has become caramelized, its natural fibers have been broken down**, which means it will take longer to move through the intestinal tract, **30% to 50% of its vitamins and minerals have been destroyed and 100% of its enzymes have been destroyed. Cooked food depletes our body's enzyme potential** and drains the energy we need to maintain and repair our tissues and organ systems and **shortens our lifespan**....
>
> When we treat foods with thermal fire, **we lose up to 97% of the water soluble vitamins** (Vitamins B and C) and **up to 40% of the lipid soluble vitamins** (Vitamins A, D, E and K). **We need only one-half the amount of protein in the diet if raw protein foods are eaten** rather than protein foods which are cooked. **Heating also changes the lipids**. These changed fats are incorporated into the cell wall and interfere with the

respiration of the cell, **causing an increase in cancer and heart disease**....

If you consult the ancient scriptures and sacred writings, you will read that in Eden, people did not eat cooked food with "burning fire." In fact, **Chinese, Egyptian, Indian and Hebrew accounts, indicate that people were expelled from Paradise for using fire to cook food**. **Methuselah**, it is contended, because he **ate only raw foods**, lived to an old age (Living. Why).

To comment first on the last paragraph first, we already saw that the sin of Adam and Eve in the Garden was eating of the "forbidden fruit." There is no mention or even hint in the Hebrew Scriptures, i.e., the Book of Genesis, that their sin was cooking food. We also already saw that soon after the fall, human beings learned to control fire and thus were probably cooking food. Therefore, the long lives of Methuselah and the other antediluvians were not due to eating a raw foods diet.

As for the other claims, it should first be noted that this article cites no references to support its claims. The same goes for every other article I checked on this website. They simply make outrageous assertions with no support whatsoever for them.

Nutrients in Raw vs. Cooked Foods

It has already been admitted that there is a loss of nutrients when food is cooked. But how much is lost depends on many factors: the length of cooking, the form of cooking, the exact food, and the nutrients under consideration. However, it has also already been asserted that the bioavailability of some nutrients is increased by cooking. These points are elaborated on in the following studies and quotes:

> **Vitamin C is highly water-soluble and sensitive to heat**. These properties make it susceptible to processing technologies as well as cooking in the home....
>
> Depending on the cooking method used, **losses of ascorbic acid [vitamin C] during home cooking range from 15 to 55%**....

Howard et al. compared uncooked and microwave-cooked fresh refrigerated, frozen and canned carrots. Interestingly, the **cooked versions did not always contain lower amounts of ascorbic acid. Microwave cooking may increase the content of ascorbic acid in a food**, although no overall pattern was observed. Since results were expressed on a wet weight basis, **the apparent increase may be attributed to loss of soluble solids**: the authors suggest that the rate of diffusion of ascorbic acid out of the cell may be slower than that of other solids such as sugars. This poses an avenue for future research. Of the products compared, **cooked canned carrots contained the lowest amounts of vitamin C, although the results may be nutritionally insignificant, since carrots are not good sources of the vitamin**...

Next to vitamin C, thiamin is the least stable of the vitamins to thermal processing, so its losses are the most studied of the B vitamins...

Cooking vegetables can result in thiamin losses ranging from 11 to 66% WW, depending on the commodity and cooking process. **Retention of other B vitamins is generally high**, although losses due to leaching can be significant, depending on cooking conditions (Rickman).

Raw food diets are predominantly plant-based diets that are practiced with the intention of preventing chronic diseases by virtue of their high content of beneficial nutritive substances such as carotenoids. However, **the benefit of a long-term adherence to these diets is controversial since little is known about their adequacy**. Therefore, we investigated vitamin A and carotenoid status and related food sources in raw food diet adherents in Germany. Dietary vitamin A, carotenoid intake, plasma retinol and plasma carotenoids were determined in 198 (ninety-two male and 106 female) strict raw food diet adherents in a cross-sectional study...

Long-term raw food diet adherents showed normal vitamin A status and achieve favourable plasma beta-carotene concentrations as recommended for chronic disease prevention, but showed low plasma lycopene levels.

Plasma carotenoids in raw food adherents are predicted mainly by fat intake (Garcia).

The objective of the present study was **to evaluate the effect of three common cooking practices (i.e., boiling, steaming, and frying) on phytochemical contents** (i.e., polyphenols, carotenoids, glucosinolates, and ascorbic acid), **total antioxidant capacities (TAC)**, as measured by three different analytical assays **[Trolox equivalent antioxidant capacity (TEAC), total radical-trapping antioxidant parameter (TRAP), ferric reducing antioxidant power (FRAP)]** and physicochemical parameters of three vegetables (carrots, courgettes, and broccoli). Water-cooking treatments better preserved the antioxidant compounds, particularly carotenoids, in all vegetables analyzed and ascorbic acid in carrots and courgettes. Steamed vegetables maintained a better texture quality than boiled ones, whereas boiled vegetables showed limited discoloration. Fried vegetables showed the lowest degree of softening, even though antioxidant compounds were less retained. **An overall increase of TEAC, FRAP, and TRAP values was observed in all cooked vegetables**, probably because of matrix softening and increased extractability of compounds, which could be partially converted into more antioxidant chemical species. **Our findings defy the notion that processed vegetables offer lower nutritional quality** and also suggest that for each vegetable a cooking method would be preferred to preserve the nutritional and physicochemical qualities (Miglio).

It's true that cooking methods alter the nutritional composition of fruits and vegetables, but that's not always a bad thing. **Several studies have shown that while cooking can degrade some nutrients, it can enhance the availability of others.** As a result, **no single cooking or preparation method is best, and that includes eating vegetables raw**...

A March 2007 study looked at the effects of boiling, steaming, microwaving and pressure cooking on the nutrients in broccoli. Steaming and boiling caused a 22 percent to 34 percent loss of vitamin C. **Microwaved and pressure-cooked vegetables retained 90 percent of their vitamin C...**

The bottom line is that no one cooking or preparation method is superior for preserving 100 percent of the nutrients in a vegetable. And since **the best vegetables are the ones you will actually eat**, taste should also be factored in when deciding on a cooking method. **The best way to get the most out of your vegetables is to enjoy them in a variety of ways -- raw, steamed, boiled, baked and grilled**. If you eat a variety of fruits and vegetables on a regular basis, you don't have to worry about the cooking method (NYT; Does).

Egg proteins contribute substantially to the daily nitrogen allowances in Western countries and are generally considered to be highly digestible. However, information is lacking on the true ileal digestibility of either raw or cooked egg protein. The recent availability of stable isotope-labeled egg protein allowed determination of the true ileal digestibility of egg protein by means of noninvasive tracer techniques....

In summary, using the 15N-dilution technique we demonstrated that **the assimilation of cooked egg protein is efficient**, albeit incomplete, and that **the true ileal digestibility of egg protein is significantly enhanced by heat-pretreatment** (Evenepoel).

We review evidence showing that **cooking facilitates mastication, increases digestibility, and otherwise improves the net energy value of plant and animal foods** regularly consumed by humans (Carmody).

This study investigated the **total antioxidant capacity (TAC)** of meats (beef, chicken, pork and fish) and its changes on thermal treatment.... **Upon heating at 180°C, TAC of meats increased** to an apparent maximum at 5 min followed by sudden decreases until 15 min, while the final stage of heating was characterized by slight increases (Serpen).

The effects of five domestic cooking methods, including steaming, microwaving, boiling, stir-frying, and stir-frying followed by boiling (stir-frying/boiling), on the nutrients and health-promoting compounds of broccoli were investigated….

Steaming had minimal effects on chlorophyll, soluble proteins and sugars, and vitamin C as well as glucosinolates. On the other hand, stir-frying and stir-frying/boiling, two popular Chinese cooking methods, caused great losses of these compounds. To best retain nutritional values at maximum level, Chinese consumers may process the broccoli by steam cooking, a 'friendly' and 'better' process, instead of traditional stir-fry or stir-fry/boil cooking (Gao-feng Yuan).

It can be seen, there is some loss of select nutrients with certain cooking methods, but nowhere near the 97% the raw foodists claim. Moreover, some cooking methods increase the bioavailability of certain nutrients. This is especially the case with protein; the exact opposite of what the raw foodists claim.

These studies did not look at nuts and seeds, but the same would probably be true. There would be some loss of nutrients when nuts and seeds are roasted, but other nutrients would be made more bioavailable.

As one quote indicates, the best approach is to eat a variety of foods prepared in a variety of different ways, and most of all, in the form that you most enjoy them. And that is exactly what the Creationist Diet advocates. God gave us a wide variety of foods for our nourishment and enjoyment and the intelligence to prepare them in different ways. So yes, eat raw fruits, vegetables, nuts, seeds, and even grains. But also eat these foods cooked in various ways, along with legumes.

Enzymes in Raw Foods

The quote that opened this chapter claimed:

When food is cooked … 100% of its enzymes have been destroyed. **Cooked food depletes our body's enzyme potential and drains the energy we need to maintain and repair our tissues and organ systems and shortens our lifespan** (Living. Why).

The idea here is the enzymes in a raw food help to digest that food and absorb its nutrients, but these enzymes are destroyed by cooking. Therefore, if we eat all cooked foods, our bodies will run out of enzymes, and we will not get full nourishment from the food.

Although the enzyme-producing organs continue to function over the entire course of a healthy life, they eventually wear down, especially with the "standard American diet" (which, in the naturopathic community, we call SAD.) Dr. Francis M. Pottenger's nutritional studies have shown that **a regular diet of cooked or canned foods causes the development of chronic degenerative diseases and premature mortality.** Professor Jackson of the Dept. of Anatomy, University of Minnesota, has shown that rats fed for 135 days on an 80 percent cooked food diet resulted in an increase pancreatic weight of 20 to 30 percent.

What this means is that the pancreas is forced to work harder with a cooked food diet. "Although the body can manufacture enzymes, **the more you use your enzyme potential, the faster it is going to run out**..." wrote Dr. Edward Howell, who pioneered research in the benefits of food enzymes. A youth of 18 may produce amylase levels 30 times greater than those of an 85 year old person (Living. Enzymes).

I first heard such claims from an alternative doctor I went to at one time. He would use this claim to get people to buy his digestive enzyme supplements. But here, the claim is we need to eat an all or at least mostly raw foods diet for food to be properly digested, nutrients absorbed, and for our bodies not to run out of enzymes. But are these claims true?

First, **the enzymes in plants are for the plants**. They help with germination, photosynthesis, respiration, decomposition, and so on. **They cannot help with any human body functions, including digestion.** Our bodies produce their own digestive enzymes for that, about 22 of them. Second, **the hydrochloric acid your stomach produces to break down food** is so concentrated that one drop will eat a hole in a piece of wood.

79

Very few of the enzymes in raw foods make it through that acid bath into the intestines, where nutrients are absorbed. Don't believe me? Want to see my sources? **Pick up any high-school biology textbook** (Jane Says).

In the 1920's, Edward Howell, M.D., asserted his idea that the enzymes in raw foods help us to break down these same foods and reduce the need to produced enzymes internally. Further, he claimed that the normal, continuous, internal manufacture of enzymes by the body taxes its limited energy stores.

But healthy people have no difficulty synthesizing enzymes, provided the body gets enough protein and other essential nutrients. And healthy people normally experience no shortage of digestive enzymes, or any difficulty digesting frozen or cooked foods....

Nor is there any evidence for Dr. Howell's claim that diets high in cooked foods tax the body's digestion or overall metabolism, promote disease, or accelerate aging.

In brief, we can find little or no persuasive evidence for Dr. Howell's core claims, which were largely based on limited, unpersuasive research conducted in the 1920's and 1930's.
here are several major problems with Dr. Howell's hypothesis.

First, the enzymes present in food are not equipped to act as digestive enzymes. Second, almost all of the enzymes present in raw foods are broken down into their components (amino acids) by our own digestive processes. Last, the healthy human body has no shortage of the amino acids and proteins needed to construct enzymes internally (Vital Choice.).

What about the claim by some raw-foodistas that our bodies have a limited lifetime supply of enzymes—and that by eating more foods with their enzymes intact, we'll be able to spare our bodies from using up their supply? **"The reality is that you don't really have a finite number of enzymes; you'll continue to make enzymes as long as you live,"** says Davis.

Enzymes are so vital to life, she adds, **"the human body is actually quite efficient at producing them"** (Eating Well).

The pancreas makes pancreatic juices. These juices contain enzymes that help break down and digest food. The juices flow through a system of ducts leading to the main pancreatic duct. The pancreatic juices flow through the main duct to the duodenum, **the first part of the small intestine.** (Pancreatic.org).

The bottom line of these quotes is that enzymes in foods get broken down by the stomach's hydrochloric acid (HCL) long before they reach the small intestines where digestive enzymes are needed and nutrients are absorbed. As such, it is simply impossible that the enzymes in food could contribute to the digestion of the foods they are contained in or aid in the absorption of the nutrients in those foods. The same goes for digestive enzyme supplements. They are broken down and rendered useless by the stomach's HCL before they reach the small intestines, so such supplements are a waste of money. Furthermore, the human body will continue to produce enzymes as long as the person is alive and consumes sufficient protein.

To claim otherwise is to show a complete lack of knowledge of human biology. That should have been a tip off to me that the doctor who made such claims was a quack, as is anyone else who does so. But it is possible that the diets of raw foodist are low in protein, and that might be the source of these myths. But before getting to that, a quick look at how raw foods diets are promoted would be helpful.

Testimonials

The preceding information does not prevent books like Rev. George H. Malkmus' *God's Way to Ultimate Health* from presenting the testimonies of many who report overcoming numerous diseases, from arthritis to cancer, by following his "Hallelujah Diet." This diet consists of eating solely or at least mostly raw vegan foods. His website "Hallelujah Acres" (www.hacres.com) also has such testimonies. The testimonial section of the website states:

People have found results by using the principles of the Hallelujah Diet to rebuild their self-healing bodies. **If you're battling high cholesterol, heart disease, weight issues or even cancer**, the testimonies below will inspire, motivate and encourage. These are normal people who have regained their health, restored their lives and reclaimed their vitality. This could be you too!

But what you do not see are any actual scientific studies showing that his diet works better other diet plans that are not so restrictive. This is par for the course for raw foodists and others who advocate restrictive diets—they rely on testimonies but not on actual scientific evidence.

This is important as the placebo effect cannot be discounted, and neither can self-deception. Some people simply convince themselves a diet plan will work and thus claim that it does, even when it is obvious to others that it is not.

For instance, I remember hearing a man call into a talk show a while back who was concerned for his wife. She had been following the Hallelujah Diet for some time, even to the point of becoming one of its advocates, promoting the diet in churches. But she was in fact not healthy at all. She was frail, skinny to the point of looking anorexic, had little energy, and was constantly sick. But her husband could not persuade her that there was a problem, as she had been convinced she was following "God's ideal diet." But he was in great anguish over her failing health.

Potential Problems

There are many potential problems with a raw foods diet, as one longtime raw foodist admits:

If you are a newcomer to the Gen 1:29 Diet [a form of a raw foods diet], this article may not make much sense right now. Newcomers to the diet often feel like a frisky colt in the early going. Some even overcome serious disease on the diet.

But if you've been on the diet for several years like we were, this article may be a godsend. **After only three years on the diet, we sadly admitted to ourselves that we were losing**

82

ground; going backwards in our health, not forward. If you've experienced new and troubling symptoms in your health on the Gen 1:29 Diet, take heart. **You haven't failed the diet. The diet has probably failed you**.

The Gen 1:29 Biblical Health movement is built on one single verse in the Bible, and sets itself at odds with the entire spectrum of Biblical teaching on diet. Although there is no moral harm in personal experimentation with the vegan diet, **there is everything wrong with teaching the vegan diet as "God's Ideal Diet" that leads to "ultimate health."**

In this paper, we will closely examine a research paper by Michael Donaldson, PhD and **highlight the nutritional deficiencies he found in 141 Hallelujah vegetarian dieters**. As we shall see, the diet is not "ideal" because it has several deficiencies. It is:

- Too high in carbohydrates
- **Too low in protein**
- **Low in energy (calories)**
- Completely missing two essential micronutrients and low in seven others
- **Requires eating voluminous amounts of vegetables** (over a gallon per day) if properly done (Chet Day's).

Such potential problems are common with those who strictly follow a raw foods diet. This is especially so for those who take the idea of raw foods to the extreme of fruitarianism (i.e. eating only raw fruits), or even diets like the Hallelujah Diet.

Rev. Malkmus advocates eating mostly raw vegetables and fruits, with very little nuts and seeds or cooked foods. Specifically, Malkmus advocates eating at least 85% raw foods, and less than 15% cooked. Although, he says the "ideal" would be "an all-raw diet" (p.244). And his wife Rhonda writes in reference to nuts and seeds:

If you must eat them, use sparingly. Almonds are the least harmful. Peanuts should be avoided. They are a legume, not a nut, and do not easily digest. In seeds and nuts about 80-90% of the calories come from fat (Malkmus, pp. 257,8).

These statements run counter to the benefits of nuts presented previously, and they show an ignorance of the beneficial type of fat found in nuts, seeds, and peanuts.

Some of these potential problems are even outlined in articles on the Living and Raw Foods website. One such article is titled *Troubleshooting: Avoiding or Overcoming Problems in Raw and Living Foods Diets* by Thomas E. Billing. This article lists the following potential problems, among others:

1. I'm always hungry, even though I overeat! (gluttony)
2. I have cravings for "undesirable" foods. How can I resist?
3. I'm underweight and emaciated.
4. I'm always cold!
5. I'm frequently very weak/fatigued.

Many of these problems are related to the issue of inability to consume sufficient calories. Raw fruits and vegetables are great! They are highly nutritious. However, they are not very high in calories, so eating only fruit as in fruitarianism, or only raw fruits and vegetables, as in Malkmus' Hallelujah Diet or in other forms of raw foods diets, can make it very difficult to consume sufficient calories.

Now for those who are trying to lose weight, this might sound great. And in fact, many of the health improvements reported on raw foods diets can be attributed to the loss of excess bodyfat. However, such restrictive diets are not the best way to lose weight, as they can be deficient in many nutrients and can be quite monotonous.

Moreover, not everyone is trying to lose weight. And for those who are not, trying to survive on just fruits and vegetables would be tough. The consumption of nuts and seeds would help to alleviate this problem somewhat. But even with the nuts and seeds, a diet of just raw fruits, vegetables, nuts, seeds, and maybe grain sprouts can get monotonous. And this could be part of the reason for the food cravings many report on raw foods diets.

Along with monotony and inability to consume sufficient calories, other problems can also be associated with diets that are too restrictive. For instance, another potential problem with raw foods diets Billing mentions is "sugar addiction." This is especially the case with fruitarians.

Fruits are great! But to eat nothing but fruits is simply put, too much of a good thing. Fruits are high in natural sugar (fructose). In moderate amounts and consumed with other foods, this is not a problem. But when fruits constitute the bulk of a diet, it can lead to addiction to sugar and insulin problems and even cravings for others kinds of sugary foods.

Another problem with being too restrictive in one's diet is nutrient deficiencies. No one food or class of foods provides all the nutrients humans needs. In the case of vegan raw foods diets, protein is just one of many possible nutrients that will be deficient. But a varied diet not only can prevent monotony, but also prevent nutrient deficiencies.

Billings next compares eating patterns often seen in those following raw foods diets with behaviors found in those with eating disorders:

> Behaviors Found In Eating Disorders (Anorexia, Bulimia) and Raw Foods: - **lying about eating** (common in fruitarianism) - **obsession with food** (fueled by constant hunger/sugar addiction) - backsliding (**"cheating"**), **eating in secret, binges - feeling guilty about eating** - perfectionist attitude and resultant poor self-image - **eating is a stressful act** (anorectic: will it make me fat? raw fooder: will it produce mucus? will it constipate me? did I combine foods correctly?) - acceptance of severe underweight because of delusions/dogma (anorectic: **I'm FAT!** raw fooder: the lost weight is mucus/toxins; glad it's gone!)

All of these behaviors are serious. And they relate to the points already mentioned: styling one's diet to be too restrictive. What this does is to make the list of "forbidden" foods so all-encompassing that it is virtually impossible to avoid them. And with hunger and nutrient deficiencies driving you to eat such self-imposed, forbidden foods, it is very easy for you to "cheat" and eat a forbidden food. This can lead to unnecessary guilt, a feeling of being out of control, and consequentially "giving up" and binge eating. Then more guilt follows; then you get more determined to follow the restrictive diet, until the next time you "cheat" and the cycle continues.

On the Beyond Vegetarianism website (www.beyondveg.com) there are many testimonies of former raw foodists. These are listed on the page "Dietary Problems in the Real World." People describe the health problems they encountered while following a raw foods diet, and how their health improved when they abandoned such a restrictive diet.

Personal Experience

I tried something similar to a raw foods diet for ten days. This was part of a "detox" that another alternative doctor put me on. And my experiences here might prove instructive.

I was supposed to eat nothing but raw fruits and vegetables for ten days. I did so for a week, and it did really "clean me out" as I had large bowel movements, but that could have been due to the laxatives he also put me on. But after a week, I just couldn't stand the hunger anymore. Simply put, I was getting famished. I had lost five pounds. I know this sounds appealing for many, but I really didn't need to lose any weight. I was eating over 20 servings of fruits and vegetables a day, but this required literally stuffing myself at each meal. But even that couldn't provide sufficient calories.

Moreover, I began to be obsessed with eating and to get some strong junk food cravings. To try to counteract this hunger, I added in raw nuts and seeds. But even with that addition, the having to stuff myself, hunger, food obsession, and junk food cravings continued. Therefore, after the ten days, I was delighted to go back to my normal diet. But it took me several weeks to regain the weight I had lost.

This experience should explain why I am so hard on restrictive diets. If just one week on such a diet caused such difficulties, I can see how someone could easily develop an eating disorder from trying to stick long-term with such a diet.

I am very sensitive to this as I once suffered with an eating disorder, but with the help of the LORD, I had overcome it a few years prior to this time, and it had not been a problem since then. But the stuffing of myself, the obsession with food, and the junk food cravings were all reminiscent of the years I had struggled with the eating disorder. But such things were no longer a problem, until this detox diet. And if I had continued with a raw foods diet much longer, I can see how I could have easily relapsed into the eating disorder.

Less Restrictive Creationist Diet

All of this is very physically and psychologically damaging and is totally unnecessary. By recognizing that cooked food is not "poison" as many in the raw foods movement call it, and by recognizing that God has not been so restrictive in His food decrees, but has given to us all kinds of plant foods for food, such cravings can be avoided.

This is why the Creationist Diet is not that restrictive. It does not stop reading the Bible at Genesis 1:29 or even Genesis chapter three, but it continues on into the rest of the antediluvian age, and beyond.

And, as has been indicated, shortly after the Fall, humans most likely began cooking their foods. As such, the Creationist Diet includes not just raw fruits, vegetables, nuts, seeds, and grains, but also cooked versions of these foods, particularly whole grains. And legumes would also be included. And eating a wider variety of foods helps to avoid both the problem of insufficient calories and of tediousness.

But would a diet that includes all possible plant foods in both raw and cooked forms be a healthy diet? We turn to that question in the next chapter.

Bibliography:

Billing, Thomas E. *Troubleshooting: Avoiding or Overcoming Problems in Raw and Living Foods Diets.*
http://www.living-foods.com/articles/troubleshooting.html

Carmody RN1, Wrangham RW. Cold Spring Harb Symposium. *Quant Biol*. 2009;74:427-34. doi: 10.1101/sqb.2009.74.019. Epub 2009 Oct 20.

Chet Day's Tips. Hallelujah Acres Research Cast Doubt On "Ideal Diet. By Greg Westbrook.
http://www.chetday.com/hallelujah-diet-dangers.htm

Cooking and the human commitment to a high-quality diet.
https://www.ncbi.nlm.nih.gov/pubmed/19843593

Eating Well. The 13 Biggest Nutrition and Food Myths Busted.
http://www.eatingwell.com/nutrition_health/nutrition_news_informati on/the_13_biggest_nutrition_and_food_myths_busted?page=5

Creationist Diet

Evenepoel, P1, et. al., *Journal of Nutrition*. 1998 Oct;128(10):1716-22. Digestibility of cooked and raw egg protein in humans as assessed by stable isotope techniques.
https://www.ncbi.nlm.nih.gov/pubmed/9772141

Garcia AL, et. al. *British Journal of Nutrition*. 2008 Jun;99(6):1293-300. Epub 2007 Nov 21. Long-term strict raw food diet is associated with favourable plasma beta-carotene and low plasma lycopene concentrations in Germans.
https://www.ncbi.nlm.nih.gov/pubmed/18028575

Gao-feng Yuan, et. al., *J Zhejiang Univ Sci B*. 2009 Aug; 10(8): 580–588. Effects of different cooking methods on health-promoting compounds of broccoli.
https://www.ncbi.nlm.nih.gov/pmc/articles/PMC2722699/

Living and Raw Foods. Enzymes: The Difference Between Raw and Cooked Foods.
http://www.living-foods.com/articles/rawvscooked.html

Living and Raw Foods. Why All Should Eat Only Raw Foods Always.
http://www.living-foods.com/articles/eatonlyraw.html

Jane Says: Raw Foodism Is a Raw Deal.
http://www.takepart.com/article/2013/05/08/jane-says-raw-foodism-raw-deal/

Malkmus, Rev. George H., with Michael Dye. *God's Way to Ultimate Health*. Shelby, NC: Hallelujah Acres Publishing, 1995, 1998.

Miglio, Cristiana, et. al., Effects of Different Cooking Methods on Nutritional and Physicochemical Characteristics of Selected Vegetables. *Journal of Agricultural Food Chemistry.*, 2008, 56 (1), pp 139–147.
http://pubs.acs.org/doi/full/10.1021/jf072304b

New York Times. Ask Well: Does Boiling or Baking Vegetables Destroy Their Vitamins?
http://well.blogs.nytimes.com/2013/10/18/ask-well-does-boiling-or-baking-vegetables-destroy-their-vitamins/

Pancreatic.org. The Pancreas.
http://pancreatic.org/pancreatic-cancer/about-the-pancreas/the-pancreas/

Rickman, Joy C and Diane M Barrett and Christine M Bruhn. *Journal of the Science of Food and Agriculture*. 87:930–944 (2007)/

Nutritional comparison of fresh, frozen and canned fruits and vegetables. Part 1. Vitamins C and B and phenolic compounds. Department of Food Science and Technology, University of California – Davis, Davis, CA 95616, US
http://ucce.ucdavis.edu/files/datastore/234-779.pdf

Serpen Al, Gökmen V, Fogliano V. *Meat Science.* 2012 Jan;90(1):60-5. doi: 10.1016/j.meatsci.2011.05.027. Epub 2011 Jun 7. Total antioxidant capacities of raw and cooked meats.
https://www.ncbi.nlm.nih.gov/pubmed/21684086

Vital Choice. Enzymes in Raw Food: Do They Matter?
https://www.vitalchoice.com/article/enzymes-in-raw-food-do-they-matter

Creationist Diet

Chapter Four:
Potential Benefits and
Drawbacks of a Vegan Diet

As might be surmised, what has been described so far in this book is a vegetarian diet, or more correctly, a vegan diet. A vegan diet is one that includes no animal foods of any sort, but it includes all kinds of plant foods, both raw and cooked.

How is "Vegan" Pronounced"

Before continuing, it might be good to answer what should be a simple question—how is "vegan" pronounced? This question was addressed in the FAQ page for the now defunct "rec.food.veg" newsgroup:

> The word was invented by the UK [United Kingdom, i.e., Great Britain] Vegan society in the 1940's. They pronounced it "vee-gn." This is the most common pronunciation in the UK today. No one can say this pronunciation is "wrong," so this is also the politically correct pronunciation.
>
> In the US, common pronunciations are "vee-jan" and "vay-gn" in addition to "vee-gn," though the American Vegan Society says the correct pronunciation is as per the UK.
>
> The UK and US and other places have other pronunciations. This is sometimes a touchy subject, so be prepared to change your pronunciation (Answer to question 2:15).

Interestingly, at one time this writer had two "talking" dictionaries on my computer. One was an *American Heritage Dictionary*, and the other a *Webster's Dictionary*. The former pronounced it as "vay-gn," and the latter as "vee-gn." Currently, YourDictionary.com pronounces it as "vee-gn," while Dictionary.com gives both pronunciations.

Healthy?

In any case, a similar diet would be an ovo-lacto vegetarian diet. This diet includes eggs and dairy and usually honey, along with all plant foods. In most cases, such a diet is simply called a vegetarian diet and will be so in this book. Thus a vegan diet excludes all animal foods, while a vegetarian diet includes dairy, eggs, and honey. But are vegan and vegetarian diets healthy?

Well, a vegan diet is what all people throughout the entire antediluvian age ate. And that covers a period of about 1,500 years. Further, the recorded age of people at that time was over 900 years! It would thus seem like a vegan diet supported the antediluvians very well. Moreover, consider the following statement by the American Dietetic Association (ADA):

It is the position of the American Dietetic Association that **appropriately planned vegetarian diets, including total vegetarian or vegan diets, are healthful, nutritionally adequate, and may provide health benefits in the prevention and treatment of certain diseases**. Well-planned vegetarian diets are appropriate for individuals during all stages of the life cycle, including pregnancy, lactation, infancy, childhood, and adolescence, and for athletes. A vegetarian diet is defined as one that does not include meat (including fowl) or seafood, or products containing those foods.

This article reviews the current data related to key nutrients for vegetarians including protein, n-3 fatty acids, iron, zinc, iodine, calcium, and vitamins D and B-12. **A vegetarian diet can meet current recommendations for all of these nutrients.** In some cases, **supplements or fortified foods can provide useful amounts of important nutrients**. An evidence-based review showed that vegetarian diets can be nutritionally adequate in pregnancy and result in positive maternal and infant health outcomes. **The results of an evidence-based review showed that a vegetarian diet is associated with a lower risk of death from ischemic heart disease.** Vegetarians also appear to have lower low-density lipoprotein cholesterol levels, lower blood pressure, and lower rates of hypertension and type 2 diabetes than nonvegetarians. Furthermore, **vegetarians tend to have a lower body mass index and lower overall cancer rates.** Features of a vegetarian diet that may reduce risk of chronic disease include **lower intakes of saturated fat and cholesterol and higher intakes of fruits, vegetables, whole grains, nuts, soy products, fiber, and phytochemicals.**

Thus "appropriately planned vegetarian diets" can be healthy, even beneficial. They can provide adequate levels of all necessary nutrients.

Nutrients

The key phrase here is "appropriately planned." A not-so-well-planned vegetarian diet could be detrimental, especially in the long-term. This point is confirmed in the following abstracts:

The quality of vegetarian diets to meet nutritional needs and support peak performance among athletes continues to be questioned. **Appropriately planned vegetarian diets can provide sufficient energy and an appropriate range of carbohydrate, fat and protein intakes to support performance and health.** The acceptable macronutrient distribution ranges for carbohydrate, fat and protein of 45-65%, 20-35% and 10-35%, respectively, are appropriate for vegetarian and non-vegetarian athletes alike, especially those who perform endurance events.

Vegetarian athletes can meet their protein needs from predominantly or exclusively plant-based sources when **a variety of these foods are consumed daily and energy intake is adequate. Muscle creatine stores are lower in vegetarians than non-vegetarians.** Creatine supplementation provides ergogenic responses in both vegetarian and non-vegetarian athletes, with limited data supporting greater ergogenic effects on lean body mass accretion and work performance for vegetarians.

The potential adverse effect of a vegetarian diet on iron status is based on the bioavailability of iron from plant

foods rather than the amount of total iron present in the diet. Vegetarian and non-vegetarian athletes alike must consume sufficient iron to prevent deficiency, which will adversely affect performance. **Other nutrients of concern for vegetarian athletes include zinc, vitamin B12 (cyanocobalamin), vitamin D (cholecalciferol) and calcium.** The main sources of these nutrients are animal products; however, they can be found in many food sources suitable for vegetarians, including **fortified soy milk and whole grain cereals.**

Vegetarians have higher antioxidant status for vitamin C (ascorbic acid), vitamin E (tocopherol), and beta-carotene than omnivores, which might help reduce exercise-induced oxidative stress. Research is needed comparing antioxidant defences in vegetarian and non-vegetarian athletes (Venderley).

Recently, vegetarian diets have experienced an increase in popularity. A vegetarian diet is associated with many health benefits because of its **higher content of fiber, folic acid, vitamins C and E, potassium, magnesium, and many phytochemicals and a fat content that is more unsaturated.** Compared with other vegetarian diets, vegan diets tend to contain less saturated fat and cholesterol and more dietary fiber. **Vegans tend to be thinner, have lower serum cholesterol, and lower blood pressure, reducing their risk of heart disease.** However, eliminating all animal products from the diet increases the risk of certain nutritional deficiencies. **Micronutrients of special concern for the vegan include vitamins B-12 and D, calcium, and long-chain n-3 (omega-3) fatty acids.** Unless vegans regularly consume foods that are fortified with these nutrients, **appropriate supplements should be consumed.** In some cases, **iron and zinc status of vegans may also be of concern** because of the limited bioavailability of these minerals (Craig. American).

Every day, vegetarians consume many carbohydrate-rich plant foods such as fruits and vegetables, cereals, pulses, and nuts. As a consequence, their diet contains more antioxidant vitamins (vitamin C, vitamin E, and beta-carotene) and copper than that of omnivores. Intake of zinc is generally comparable to that by omnivores. However, **the bioavailability of zinc in vegetarian diets is generally lower than that of omnivores**. Dietary intake of selenium is variable in both groups and depends on the selenium content of the soil. Measurements of antioxidant body levels in vegetarians show that a **vegetarian diet maintains higher antioxidant vitamin status (vitamin C, vitamin E, beta-carotene) but variable antioxidant trace element status as compared with an omnivorous diet.** To evaluate the antioxidative potential of a vegetarian diet versus an omnivorous diet, more studies are needed in which the total antioxidant capacity is determined rather than the status of a single antioxidant nutrient (Rauma).

Vegetarians exhibit a wide diversity of dietary practices, often described by what is omitted from their diet. When a vegetarian diet **is appropriately planned and includes fortified foods**, it can be nutritionally adequate for adults and children and can promote health and lower the risk of major chronic diseases.

The nutrients of concern in the diet of vegetarians include vitamin B(12), vitamin D, omega-3 fatty acids, calcium, iron, and zinc. Although a vegetarian diet can meet current recommendations for all of these nutrients, **the use of supplements and fortified foods provides a useful shield against deficiency.**

A vegetarian diet usually provides a low intake of saturated fat and cholesterol and a high intake of dietary fiber and many health-promoting phytochemicals. This is achieved by an **increased consumption of fruits, vegetables, whole-grains, legumes, nuts, and various soy products.**

As a result of these factors, vegetarians typically have lower body mass index, serum total and low-density lipoprotein cholesterol levels, and blood pressure; reduced rates of death from ischemic heart disease; and decreased incidence of hypertension, stroke, type 2 diabetes, and certain cancers than do nonvegetarians (Craig. Nutrition).

95

Note again the words "appropriately planned" in the first and last abstracts. That is one purpose of this book, to help not just those following vegan or vegetarian diets but any kind of diet to appropriately plan their diets. But note the nutrients of concern in vegan or vegetarian diets: iron, zinc, vitamin B12, vitamin D, calcium, omega 3 fatty acids, and trace elements. As indicated, "The main sources of these nutrients are animal products." This will be seen as we proceed. But here, much care must be taken by vegans and vegetarians to consume sufficient amounts of these nutrients.

Going back to the statement by the ADA, it notes that "a vegetarian diet is associated with a lower risk of death from ischemic heart disease" and "vegetarians tend to have a lower body mass index and lower overall cancer rates." Most studies bear out these observations, as indicated in the last abstract. However, there are a couple of caveats.

First, such studies usually compare those following vegan or vegetarian diets with those following the Standard American Diet, which has the appropriate acronym of SAD. As will be seen later in this book, the diets of most Americans are "sad" as they contain far too few fruits, vegetables, and other beneficial plant foods and far too much saturated fats and refined carbohydrates (carbs). Whereas, as noted in the statement, vegans and vegetarians tend to consume "lower intakes of saturated fat and cholesterol and higher intakes of fruits, vegetables, whole grains, nuts, soy products, fiber, and phytochemicals." The latter is the reason they tend to have "higher antioxidant vitamin status."

However, you do not have to follow a vegan or vegetarian diet to limit consumption of saturated fat or to consume copious amounts of these beneficial plant foods. An omnivore diet can be low in saturated fat and high in these plant foods, as will be detailed later.

Second, the type of animal foods that are commonly consumed by Americans is an important issue that will also be detailed later.

Third, those who are so health conscious as to be undertaking the difficult proposition of eliminating animal foods from their diets tend to be more health conscious in other areas of their lives, such as in regards to exercise, stress control, sleep habits, and smoking. But again, you do not need to be a vegan or vegetarian to stop smoking, to start exercising, and the like.

Finally, it should be noted that most of these abstracts recommend the use of supplements or fortified foods by vegetarians to guard against potential nutrient deficiencies. But if you must use such to make your diet work, then it could be a sign the diet is not that ideal after all. And there is one vitamin for which vegans must take a supplement.

Vitamin B12

As stated previously, if a vegetarian diet is "varied and well-planned" it can meet the nutrient needs of even athletes. However, there is one nutrient that can be of particular concern to those following a vegan diet: vitamin B12.

The problem is, vitamin B12 only occurs in animal foods. Now an interesting question is, where did the antediluvians get their vitamin B12 from? It is possible there were physiological changes to the human body at the time of the Flood. In fact:

> Bacteria in the human intestinal tract do make vitamin B12. However, the majority of these bacteria are found in the large intestine. Vitamin B12 does not appear to be absorbed from the large intestine (Wasserman and Mangels).

> Vitamin B12 is a product of bacterial metabolism. Although bacteria in the colon also produce vitamin B12, it cannot be absorbed at that site (Encyclopedia Britannica; Human Digestion).

But before the Flood, maybe humans could create their own B12 in a manner that was absorbable, but something happened as a result of the Flood that caused humans to lose this ability. It is possible that the mere fact that humans began eating animal foods caused them to lose the ability to create absorbable vitamin B12. Since the vitamin is found in abundance in animal foods, the body would not need to create it; so maybe after generations of not needing to make the vitamin, humans simply lost the ability to create absorbable vitamin B12.

Another theory, and this does sound a little gross, is that antediluvians got their B12 from dirt, yes, dirt. If plant foods are not cleaned thoroughly there will be some dirt residue on them. And vegans sometimes claim dirt contains B12, and a little bit of residue would be enough to provide the B12.

> B12 is synthesized by bacteria and is therefore found in areas of bacterial growth, namely dirt and soil. **Humans have been getting their B12 from the dirt** for hundreds of thousands of years by eating plants that still had bits of soil on them (Peaceful Dumpling).

I repeated this idea in the First Edition of this book, but researching this Second Edition, I discovered this is not true. The only way dirt contains vitamin B12 is if it contains fecal matter.

> **Human faeces contain appreciable quantities of vitamin B12** or vitamin B12-like material presumably produced by bacteria in the colon, **but this is unavailable to the non-coprophagic individual** (Albert).

Note that the word coprophagia means "the eating of feces or dung" (Oxford). Some animals attain their vitamin B12 from eating their own feces, such as rabbits. I learned this from watching the holiday movie *Christmas Bunny*. It is a heartwarming movie I would highly recommend. The little girl who stars in the movie calls what the rabbits eat "poopsicles."

How do animals get B12?
- They absorb B12 made by their gut bacteria, in the case of ruminants like cows and sheep.
- **They eat poop (coprophagia)**, like some rodents do. (Please don't get any bright ideas from this fact!)
- They have bacterial contamination of their food.
- They eat animal-sourced foods like other animal flesh, milk, or eggs (CNS).

However, human beings do not and would not eat feces, human or otherwise. Now from an evolutionary viewpoint with its conception of ancient humans being dumb, grunting cavemen, then I can see how some might think they would have eaten food contaminated with feces.

98

But from a creationist viewpoint, human beings have always been intelligent, and intelligent people would not eat poop.

But whatever the case in the far past, the only reliable source of vitamin B12 today is animal foods. And this fact argues against a vegan diet being the most "natural" diet for human beings today. This is not an issue that vegans can brush off, as a deficiency of vitamin B12 is very serious:

Vitamin B12 is synthesized by microorganisms that occur in the rumen (the first stomach chamber) of cows and sheep. From the rumen it is transferred to the muscle and other tissues, which other animals and humans eat. Good dietary sources of vitamin B12 are eggs, meat, and dairy products.
In humans, a lack of the vitamin results in defective formation of the papillae (small projections) of the tongue, giving an appearance of abnormal smoothness. A deficiency of vitamin B12 often causes defective function of the intestine, resulting in indigestion and sometimes constipation or diarrhea. **A very serious effect is degeneration of certain motor and sensory tracts of the spinal cord**; if the degeneration **continues for some time, treatment with vitamin B12 may not correct it. Initial numbness and tingling of fingers or toes may, without treatment, progress to instability of gait or paralysis**.
Because vitamin B12 is found in animal but not vegetable foods, **strict vegetarians (vegans) who do not eat dairy products, meats, fish, eggs, or vitamin B12-fortified foods may develop a deficiency if they do not receive supplements of the vitamin** (Encyclopedia Britannica; Vitamin B12).

A **deficiency of vitamin B12 can lead to anemia**. A mild deficiency may cause no symptoms. But **if untreated, it may progress and cause symptoms such as:**

- Weakness, tiredness, or lightheadedness
- Heart palpitations and shortness of breath
- Pale skin

- A smooth tongue
- Constipation, diarrhea, a loss of appetite, or gas
- **Nerve problems** like numbness or tingling, muscle weakness, and problems walking
- **Vision loss**
- **Mental problems** like depression, memory loss, or behavioral changes (WebMD. Vitamin B12 Deficiency).

However, some vegans claim seaweed contains vitamin B12, and that is how ancient humans attained their vitamin B12. Again, that is an idea I repeated in the First Edition of this book, but it is in no way a reliable source of vitamin B12:

What foods might naturally contain B12?
- **Animal foods, including meat, milk, and eggs, contain B12 and are essentially the exclusive source of the vitamin in the American food supply** (not counting supplements or fortification).
- Two varieties of edible algae (Dried green (Enteromorpha sp.) and purple (Porphyra sp.) seaweed (nori)) have been found to have active B12, but **other algae have inactive B12-analog compounds** that have no apparent benefit in animal metabolism.
- Some varieties of mushrooms and some foods made with certain fermentation processes have very small amounts of active B12.
- **Plants found in our food supply do not contain B12**, though plants grown in experimental settings with B12-enriched soils or water (with hydroponic processes, for example) do actually take up B12....

I don't eat my own poop, or anyone else's poop. How do I get B12?
- I'm pleased with your basic hygiene choices. But if you don't eat animal-sourced foods, you aren't getting B12 except through **foods that have been artificially fortified**

with B12 (nondairy milks, cereals, etc.), which is potentially insufficient.

- **I mentioned a few rare plants or fermented foods before that may have B12, but I absolutely do not think these are a reliable way to get B12 for the average person**.
- This is why I recommend a daily supplement for those people with a reduced intake of animal foods (CNS).

Therefore, taking a supplement is the only reliable way for vegans to attain vitamin B12. But I must reiterate—if you need to take a supplement to make your diet work, that is evidence your diet really is not that natural.

But I should mention, there are medical conditions that can lead to a vitamin B12 deficiency. Therefore, even if you are not a vegan, if you have any of the preceding symptoms, you might want to talk to your doctor about having your vitamin B12 blood levels tested. And if you are a vegan, you most definitely should get tested.

Neither Beneficial Nor Detrimental

A couple of additional abstracts are worth pursuing:

> **The aim of this study was to assess and compare dietary intake and nutritional status of vegetarian and omnivorous preschool children and their parents**. Fifty-six omnivores (28 children and 28 parents) and 42 vegetarians (21 preschool children with 18 lacto-ovo-vegetarians and 3 ovo-vegetarians; 21 parents with 16 lacto-ovo-vegetarians, 2 ovo-vegetarians, 1 lacto-vegetarian, and 2 vegans) were recruited....
>
> Both omnivorous parents and their children had significantly higher fat and lower fiber intakes than vegetarian parents and children. Omnivorous children had significantly higher protein and lower vitamin C intakes than vegetarian children, whereas omnivorous parents had significantly lower vitamin A and iron intakes than vegetarian parents. Vegetarians and omnivores in both parent and child groups had mean calcium consumption less than 75% of the Taiwan dietary intakes. **All mean hematologic and biochemical nutrient**

status indices were within the reference range in any groups. However, both vegetarian parents and children had significantly lower mean total cholesterol and serum ferritin concentrations than those of omnivorous parents and children. **Our vegetarian and omnivorous preschool children had normal growth and adequate nutritional status. However, both parents and children had inadequate calcium intakes,** which may potentially affect bone health, especially for preschool children in the growing stage (Yen CE).

Seven randomized controlled trials and one cross-sectional study met the inclusion criteria. No distinguished differences between vegetarian-based diets and omnivorous mixed diets were identified when physical performance was compared. **Consuming a predominately vegetarian-based diet did not improve nor hinder performance in athletes.** However, with only 8 studies identified, with substantial variability among the studies' experimental designs, aims and outcomes, further research is warranted (Craddock).

The first study shows that both vegetarian and non-vegetarian children and their parents had adequate nutrient levels, and both types of children had normal growth rates. The second study shows there is no difference in performance between vegetarians and non-vegetarian athletes. Therefore, in these instances, vegetarian diets were shown to be neither beneficial nor detrimental as compared to omnivore diets.

Protein Intake

But there is an area where vegan and vegetarian diets are often criticized for—that of protein intake. The FAQ page for the former "rec.food.veg" newsgroup explains, "Should I be worried about getting enough protein on a vegetarian diet? The short answer is: 'No, sufficient protein can be obtained by eating a variety of foods.'"

As for the issue of complete vs. incomplete proteins, the FAQ page explains:

Protein that contains all essential amino acids is called "complete" protein. Protein that contains some, but not all essential amino acids is called "incomplete" protein. It used to be believed that all amino acids must be eaten at the same time to form complete proteins. We now know that **incomplete proteins can be stored in the body for many days to be combined with other incomplete proteins.** As long as all essential amino acids are in the diet, it does not matter if the proteins are complete or incomplete.

What is said here is true. Most plant proteins are incomplete, meaning they lack one or more of the eight essential amino acids. But if different plant foods with different amino acid profiles are included in the diet, then they complement each other. That means the amino acid that is lacking in one food is found in over-abundance in the other, and vice-a-versa. Thus together, the foods provide a complete protein. Moreover, these two complementary foods do not need to be eaten at the same time. But what this page claims next is more questionable.

The reality is that the average American takes in twice the amount of protein he or she needs. **Excess protein has been linked with osteoporosis, kidney disease, calcium stones in the urinary tract, and some cancers.** Despite all this, many people still worry about getting enough protein.

Such claims of harm from excessive protein intake is common among vegetarians and can be found on many vegetarian websites, and I repeated this claim in the First Edition of this book. But recent research proves such claims are not true.

The aim of this review was to assess the impact of a vegetarian diet on indices of skeletal integrity to address specifically whether vegetarians have a normal bone mass. Analysis of existing literature, through a combination of observational, clinical and intervention studies were assessed in relation to bone health for the following: lacto-ovo-vegetarian and vegan diets versus omnivorous, predominantly meat diets, consumption of animal versus vegetable protein, and fruit and vegetable consumption. Mechanisms of action for a dietary "component" effect were examined and other potential dietary differences between vegetarians and non-vegetarians were also explored.

Key findings included: (i) **no differences in bone health indices between lacto-ovo-vegetarians and omnivores**; (ii) **conflicting data for protein effects on bone with high protein consumption** (particularly without supporting calcium/alkali intakes) **and low protein intake (particularly with respect to vegan diets) being detrimental to the skeleton**; (iii) growing support for a **beneficial effect of fruit and vegetable intake on bone**, with mechanisms of action currently remaining unclarified (New).

What this study is saying is it is unclear if a high protein intake is detrimental to bone health, but it is just as possible the exact opposite is true—that a low protein intake as found in vegan diets is detrimental. Thus things are not as clear cut as the vegan sites make it out to be. It is in fact their diets that could be detrimental. However, it is clear that eating fruits and vegetables is good for the bones.

The reason or this discrepancy might be explained by the following study:

Vegetarian and vegan diets contain low amounts of protein and calcium. For this reason, they are supposed to cause low bone mineral density (BMD) and osteoporosis. But this is not the case, except for vegans with a particularly low calcium intake. **The absence of osteoporosis or low BMD can be explained by the low acid load of these diets.**

Nutritional acid load is negatively correlated with bone mineral density (BMD) and positively with fracture risk. Low acid load is correlated with lower bone resorption and higher BMD. **It is linked to high intake of potassium-rich nutrients, such as fruits and vegetables, as found in vegetarian diets.**

The total nutritional acid load, which not only depends on the potassium content of the nutrition, was recently assessed in several studies on vegetarian and vegan diets and was found to be very low or absent, while the diet of Western-style omnivores produces daily 50 to 70 mEq of acid. This might be an important factor for the protection of vegetarians from osteoporosis (Burckhardt).

Note that the low protein intake of vegetarian and vegan diets was expected to result in low bone mineral density (BMD), but it did not due to the low acid load of these diets, mainly due to a high intake of fruits and vegetables. But I must reiterate, you do not need to be a vegetarian or vegan to eat copious amounts of fruits and vegetables. That vegans and vegetarians do so is simply an indication of their propensity to be more health conscious. But omnivores can be health conscious and consume lots of fruits and veggies as well.

The next study is even clearer on the issue of BMD:

OBJECTIVES:

To compare the bone mineral density [BMD] and dietary intake of elderly Chinese vegetarian women with omnivores, to compare the bone mineral density of Chinese 'vegans' and 'lactovegetarians', and to study the relationship between nutrient intake and BMD in vegetarians....

RESULTS:

The dietary calorie, protein and fat intake were much lower, but the sodium/creatinine ratio was much higher in vegetarians than omnivores. **The BMD at the spine was similar between vegetarians and omnivores. However, the BMD at the hip was significantly lower in vegetarians at some sites** ($P < 0.05$). There was no significant difference in BMD between 'vegans' and 'lactovegetarians.' **BMD in vegetarians appeared to be positively correlated with energy, protein and calcium intake**; and negatively associated with urinary sodium/creatinine levels (Lau).

Thus this study found that vegetarians and vegans had a lower BMD at the hip than omnivores. Furthermore, the more energy (calories), protein, and calcium that they consumed, the better their BMD was. This means greater not less protein is better for bone health.

As for kidney disease, there is no evidence whatsoever that a high protein intake causes kidney disease. A search of PubMed turned up no evidence in this regard. The closest I could find is the following:

> Traditional strategies for management of patients with **chronic kidney disease (CKD)** have not resulted in any change in the growing prevalence of CKD worldwide. A historic belief that eating healthily might ameliorate kidney disease still holds credibility in the 21(st) century. **Dietary sodium restriction to <2.3 g daily, a diet rich in fruits and vegetables and increased water consumption** corresponding to a urine output of 3-4 l daily might slow the progression of early CKD, polycystic kidney disease or recurrent kidney stones. Current evidence suggests that a **reduction in dietary net acid load could be beneficial in patients with CKD**, but the supremacy of any particular diet has yet to be established (Jain).

Notice the recommendations to reduce acid load for those who already have chronic kidney disease. But acid in foods can come from many sources other than just meat. And again, that is only for people who already have kidney disease, and even that recommendation is qualified. There is better evidence for reducing salt and drinking lots of water and eating lots of fruits and vegetables.

As for the claim of "calcium stones in the urinary tract," there is again no evidence that a high protein diet *causes* kidney stones, although there is some evidence that a low protein might help those with recurring kidney stones. But even then, it is as not clear cut as the vegetarians would make it.

> Diet interventions may reduce the risk of urinary stone formation and its recurrence, but **there is no conclusive consensus in the literature regarding the effectiveness of dietary interventions and recommendations about specific diets for patients with urinary calculi**....

> CONCLUSIONS:
> ... Dietary calcium restriction is not recommended for stone formers with nephrolithiasis. Diets with a calcium content ≥ 1

g/day (and **low protein-low sodium) could be protective against the risk of stone formation in hypercalciuric stone forming adults**.... A diet low in oxalate and/or a calcium intake normal to high (800-1200 mg/day for adults) reduce the urinary excretion of oxalate, conversely a diet rich in oxalates and/or a diet low in calcium increase urinary oxalate. **A restriction in protein intake may reduce the urinary excretion of oxalate although a vegetarian diet may lead to an increase in urinary oxalate.** ...

CHILDREN:...

Despite the low level of scientific evidence, a low-protein (< 20 g/day) low-salt (< 2 g/day) diet with high hydration (> 3 liters/day) is strongly advised in children with cystinuria....

ELDERLY:...

A lower content of animal protein in association to an higher intake of plant products decrease the acid load and the excretion of uric acid has **no particular contraindications in the elderly patients, although overall nutritional status has to be preserved**. (Prezioso).

Even with looking at the best available evidence, note the phrases: no conclusive consensus, could, may, low level of scientific evidence. Note also that a vegetarian diet is not recommended as it "may lead to an increase in urinary oxalate." What this means is that even for those who already have had kidney stones, there really is no clear evidence that a low protein intake let alone a vegetarian diet is best to prevent reoccurrence. In fact, a vegetarian diet might make things worse.

As for cancer, it would be difficult to tease out the difference between plant protein intake and animal food intake, and a diet high in animal foods would invariably be high in protein. The issue of meat and cancer will be addressed later.

What all of this means, there really is no evidence that for those without preexisting problems that a vegan diet with its low protein intake would be preferable to an omnivore diet with its higher protein intake for bone or kidney health and may even be detrimental. But claims of such benefits are still made on vegan and vegetarian websites.

Other Claimed Benefits

There are also many other claimed benefits to a vegan diet. For instance, a blog on Nursingdegree.net states, "Following a healthy, balanced vegan diet ensures a host of health benefits as well as prevention of some of the major diseases striking people in North America." It then lists "57 Health Benefits of Going Vegan."

However, among these claimed "health benefits" are consumption of less protein being healthier and even preventing osteoporosis, which we just saw is not true. Other claimed benefits have already or will be addressed. It also does not list potential problems with a vegan diet.

Similarly, Medical News Today website states, "Eating animal fats and proteins has been shown in studies to raise a person's risk of developing cancer, diabetes, rheumatoid arthritis, hypertension, heart disease, and a number of other illnesses and conditions."

But again, such studies compared those following a vegan diet to those following a SAD diet, not to those following a healthy omnivore diet. They also do not take into account the types of animal foods consumed. And we just say that a high protein intake is not problematic.

But to look at one of the claimed benefits, that of diabetes, a vegan diet can actually be detrimental in this regard:

> Diabetes is considered an oxidative stress and a chronic inflammatory disease. The purpose of this study was to investigate the correlations between **vitamin B-12 status and oxidative stress and inflammation in diabetic vegetarians and omnivores**....
>
> **Diabetic vegetarians with higher levels of vitamin B-12 (>250 pmol/L) had significantly lower levels of fasting glucose, HbA1c and higher antioxidant enzyme activity (catalase) than those with lower levels of vitamin B-12 (≤ 250 pmol/L)**. A significant association was found between vitamin B-12 status and fasting glucose ($r = -0.17$, $p = 0.03$), HbA1c ($r = -0.33$, $p = 0.02$), oxidative stress (oxidized low density lipoprotein-cholesterol, $r = -0.19$, $p = 0.03$), and antioxidant enzyme activity (catalase, $r = 0.28$, $p = 0.01$) in the diabetic vegetarians; **vitamin B-12 status was significantly correlated**

with inflammatory markers (interleukin-6, $r = -0.33$, $p <$ 0.01) in diabetic omnivores.

As a result, we suggest that **it is necessary to monitor the levels of vitamin B-12 in patients with diabetes, particularly those adhering to a vegetarian diet** (Lee).

To be clear, this study is saying that vegetarians with low vitamin B12 status had higher fasting blood glucose and inflammation and lower antioxidant activity. These are all bad things. But these were reversed in vegetarians with higher vitamin B12 status and in omnivores. The potential for vegetarian and especially vegan diets being low in vitamin B12 was mention in previous abstracts, and here we see additional problems low vitamin B12 levels can cause.

And so it goes, for each of the claimed benefits of a vegan diet there are confounding factors that the claimants do not take into account, but which have been or will be discussed in this book.

Saturated Fat

Before beginning discussions on saturated fat and cholesterol, the following information should be noted:

There are two main types of cholesterol [found in the blood]:

•Low-density lipoprotein (LDL): LDL, or "bad," cholesterol can build up in the walls of your arteries, making them hard and narrow.

•High-density lipoprotein (HDL): HDL, or "good," cholesterol picks up excess cholesterol and takes it back to your liver (Mayo: Trans fat).

Blood triglycerides also need to be considered:

Triglycerides provide unique information as a marker associated with the risk for heart disease and stroke (AHA: Triglycerides)

Creationist Diet

With that in mind, there is an area in which claims of benefits about vegan diets might be real, but it is also an area that many people think is no longer an issue. It is the lower intake of saturated fat and cholesterol found in a vegan diet versus an omnivore diet and especially the SAD.

This is an often claimed benefit of a vegan diet, and there is no doubt vegans consume less saturated fat and cholesterol than omnivores. This is due to many animal foods containing saturated fats, while most plant foods contain little or no saturated fat, and it is due to only animal foods containing cholesterol.

This leads to vegetarians and vegan having lower blood cholesterol levels. However, both LDL and HDL cholesterol are lower.

Eleven trials were included in the meta-analysis. **Vegetarian diets significantly lowered blood concentrations of total cholesterol, low-density lipoprotein cholesterol, high-density lipoprotein cholesterol, and non-high-density lipoprotein cholesterol**, and the pooled estimated changes were -0.36 mmol/L (95% CI -0.55 to -0.17; P<0.001), -0.34 mmol/L (95% CI -0.57 to -0.11; P<0.001), -0.10 mmol/L (95% CI -0.14 to -0.06; P<0.001), and -0.30 mmol/L (95% CI -0.50 to -0.10; P=0.04), respectively. **Vegetarian diets did not significantly affect blood triglyceride concentrations**, with a pooled estimated mean difference of 0.04 mmol/L (95% CI -0.05 to 0.13; P=0.40) (Wang; Effects).

The reason for these results is that saturated fat raises both LDL and HDL cholesterol. Thus some of the positive effects of the lowered LDL in vegetarians is offset by the negative effect of lowered HDL. But still, vegetarians tend to have a better lipid profile than omnivores due to consuming less saturated fat and cholesterol.

However, due to some well-publicized studies, many people now think saturated fats do not elevated LDL cholesterol and subsequent heart disease risk. But this simply is not true, as those studies were misrepresented in the media, and newer studies have verified that saturated fats are problematic. The doubts about saturated fat were based on a well-publicized meta-analysis from 2010 that concluded:

110

There is no significant evidence for concluding that dietary saturated fat is associated with an increased risk of CHD [coronary heart disease] or CVD [cardiovascular disease]" (Siri-Tarino; Meta-analysis).

"More recently, Chowdhury and colleagues published a separate meta-analysis in the Annals of Internal Medicine, and reached similar conclusions to that of Siri-Tarino and colleagues regarding the association between saturated fat and coronary heart disease" (McDougall).

But as a video on the American Heart Association's website points out, those meta-analyses were of observational (epidemiological) studies, not clinical trials. The latter are more reliable and have consistently showed saturated fat increases LDL levels and heart disease risk (AHA; Saturated Fats).

One such clinical trial showed, "an important mechanism by which reductions in dietary saturated fatty acids decrease LDL-cholesterol in humans is through an increase in LDL-receptor number" (Mustad, e.t al.). Thus the exact mechanism by which saturated fats increase LDL is known.

For those who are still skeptical about saturated fat increasing heart disease risk, consider the following:

Cutting back on saturated fat will likely have no benefit, however, if people replace saturated fat with refined carbohydrates—white bread, white rice, mashed potatoes, sugary drinks, and the like. Eating refined carbs in place of saturated fat does lower "bad" LDL cholesterol—but it also lowers the "good" HDL cholesterol and increases triglycerides. The net effect is as bad for the heart as eating too much saturated fat—and perhaps even worse for people who have insulin resistance because they are overweight or inactive (Harvard; Fats).

Substituting polyunsaturated fat for saturated fat reduces LDL cholesterol and the total cholesterol to high-density lipoprotein cholesterol ratio. **However, replacement of**

111

saturated fat by carbohydrates, particularly refined carbohydrates and added sugars, increases levels of triglyceride and small LDL particles and reduces high-density lipoprotein cholesterol, effects that are of particular concern in the context of the increased prevalence of obesity and insulin resistance (Siri-Tarino; Saturated fatty acids).

There is evidence suggesting that the substitution of MUFA [monounsaturated fatty acids] instead of carbohydrate for SFA [saturated fatty acids] calories may favorably affect CVD [cardio-vascular disease] risk.... Compared with SFA, MUFAs lower total and LDL cholesterol levels, and relative to carbohydrate, they increase HDL cholesterol levels and decrease plasma triglyceride levels (Kris-Etherton).

It's true that researchers found little differences in heart disease rates when comparing those who ate the most vs. the least saturated fat. But the results are not so clear cut. The study did not look at what else people were eating. So if eating less saturated fat means eating more refined starch and sugar, then no wonder there's little or no improvements. However, if saturated fat is replaced with polyunsaturated fat or monounsaturated fat in the form of olive oil, nuts and other plant oils, there's a lot of evidence that heart disease risk will be reduced (US News; 5 Shades).

The best way to prevent heart disease may be to eat more whole, unprocessed foods. So eat fish, beans, fruits, vegetables, brown rice, nuts, seeds, vegetable oils and olive oils, and even some animal products like yogurt and high-quality meat and cheese (WebMD; Is Butter Back?).

What probably happened in the two meta-analyses is they were comparing high saturated fat diets with high processed carb diets; that is why there was no difference in the CVD rate. This happened as the SAD is high in processed carbs, and more so for people who follow low-fat diets by consuming processed low-fat foods, which generally replace fat with sugar and other processed carbs (which is why I've always considered such foods silly). But if you compare a high saturated fat diet with a diet high in unsaturated fats and unprocessed carbs using foods like the ones mentioned in the last quote, then the latter diet will have a lower heart disease risk. And those types of foods constitute the bulk of the Creationist Diet.

Note also that the same researchers who conducted the 2010 meta-analysis (Siri-Tarino, et, al.) later that same year found this beneficial effect of replacing saturated fats with unsaturated fats. As such, it is disingenuous to cite their research to support a high saturated fat diet. In fact, in that later study, they write about their former analysis:

> … the lack of association between saturated fat and risk of CHD [coronary heart disease] observed in epidemiologic studies can be interpreted as **the lack of benefit of substitution of carbohydrates for saturated fat**" (Siri-Tarino, et. al. Saturated fatty acids).

Moreover, a more recent evaluation of the same studies included in both meta-analyses found, "The findings reviewed here support the hypothesis that **saturated fat increases the risk of coronary heart disease mortality**" (McDougall).

Cholesterol

As indicted, cholesterol is only found in animal foods. However, a vegetarian diet could be as high in cholesterol as an omnivore diet if eggs and whole fat dairy products are consumed, but vegans consume little or no cholesterol. But does this translate into lower blood cholesterol levels? The answer is not as clear cut as might be thought.

> The recommended daily allowance [of less than 300 mg of cholesterol] has sometimes come into question. The reason for this is because **dietary cholesterol is only responsible for about 15 percent of total blood cholesterol. The rest is manufactured by the body.** Other factors that contribute to blood cholesterol levels include smoking, obesity, physical activity **and the consumption of saturated fat** (Livestrong).

113

Cholesterol levels in the human body tend to be affected less by cholesterol in our diets than they are by the saturated fats and trans fats we eat, according to Tara Linitz, a registered dietitian at Massachusetts General Hospital who also has a master's degree in exercise science (Boston Globe).

The 2015 Dietary Guidelines Advisory Committee (DGAC) has already garnered headlines because its members are advocating revisions to a decades-old warning about cholesterol consumption. An overview of the committee's Dec. 15, 2014 meeting says, "**Cholesterol is not considered a nutrient of concern for overconsumption.**" …

As for cholesterol, the changes being considered there are backed by many studies that have questioned the relationship between dietary cholesterol and heart disease. Experts now believe that **saturated fats in foods like red meat and cheese have a bigger impact on blood cholesterol levels than the cholesterol in foods like eggs** (Fiscal Times).

Moreover, I remember back at Penn State a professor teaching that the body will decrease its production of cholesterol when dietary cholesterol is increased. At that time, the professor was not sure how much the body could down-regulate its production. But "Your liver can produce about 1,000 mg of cholesterol a day. A little more is added by the small intestines" (How Stuff Works). There is thus a limit to how much the body can reduce its production, but it is much more than the generally recommended limit of 300 mg.

This makes sense as some recent studies show that eating up to three eggs (about 600 mg of cholesterol) a day does not significantly increase cholesterol levels (Authority; Eggs).

What all of this means is, a lower cholesterol intake is not necessarily an advantage of a vegan diet. Moreover, it could actually be a detriment, as can the lower saturated fat intake. But before explaining how, some details on the primary male hormone will be helpful.

Effects of Testosterone

Testosterone is the primary male hormone. It is found in females, but it has its greatest affect in males, so what follows will primarily be for men. In fact, it is primarily the presence of testosterone that causes men to have greater musculature than women. Testosterone is also responsible for a man's sex drive, and can affect bodyweight, both the levels of body fat and of muscle.

Testosterone is the primary male sex hormone and an anabolic steroid. In men, testosterone plays a key role in the development of male reproductive tissues such as the testis and prostate, as well as promoting secondary sexual characteristics such as increased muscle and bone mass, and the growth of body hair. In addition, **testosterone is essential for health and well-being, and for the prevention of osteoporosis. Insufficient levels of testosterone in men may lead to abnormalities including frailty and bone loss** (Wikipedia).

Testosterone's effects can be classified as either anabolic (related to protein synthesis and growth) or virilizing (related to the biological development of male sex characteristics). However, the two categories are closely related:

Anabolic effects involve **growth of muscle mass, increased bone density**, and stimulation of linear growth and bone maturation.

Virilizing effects (also known as androgenic effects) include maturation of the sex organs, particularly the growth of the penis and the formation of the scrotum in the male fetus. During puberty, testosterone also coordinates development of masculine characteristics such as deepening of the voice and growth of facial hair.

Greatly differing amounts of testosterone prenatally, at puberty, and throughout life account for a share of biological differences between males and females. On average, the adult male human produces about 20 to 30 times the amount of testosterone synthesized by an adult female (Larsen, et al. 2002). Nonetheless, like men, **women rely on testosterone**

115

(albeit in significantly smaller quantities) to maintain libido, bone density, and muscle mass throughout their lives (New World).

After age 30, most men begin to experience a gradual decline in testosterone. A decrease in sex drive sometimes accompanies the drop in testosterone, leading many men to mistakenly believe that their loss of interest in sex is simply due to getting older…
Low testosterone scores often lead to drops in bone density, meaning that bones become more fragile and increasingly prone to breaks (WebMD; Low).

At some point in their 40s, men's testosterone production begins to slow. By some estimates, levels of this hormone drop by about 1% a year. As men get into their 50s, 60s, and beyond, they may start to have signs and symptoms of low testosterone. These include reduced sex drive and sense of vitality, erectile dysfunction, decreased energy, lower muscle mass and bone density, and anemia. When severe, these signs and symptoms characterize a condition called hypogonadism (Harvard; Testosterone).

Testosterone is the hormone most responsible for sex drives and high libidos in men. A decrease in testosterone can mean a decrease in libido, fewer spontaneous erections, and a slightly lower sperm count.…
Decreases in testosterone can lead to physical changes including the following:

- increased body fat
- decreased strength/mass of muscles
- fragile bones
- decreased body hair
- swelling/tenderness in the breast tissue
- hot flashes
- increased fatigue

- effects on cholesterol metabolism

Despite that fact that it can cause lower energy levels, **low testosterone can also cause insomnia** and other changes in your sleep patterns (Healthline).

Thus decreasing testosterone levels men experience as we age can be very detrimental in many aspects of our lives. Therefore, it would seem logical that steps should be taken to prevent this loss. It is for this reason that male hormone replacement therapy (HRT) is becoming popular. But there is a more natural way to improve testosterone levels.

But before continuing, a caveat is needed. Some authorities believe high testosterone levels increase the risk of prostate cancer and thus conversely, a lower level would decrease the risk. But there is little agreement in this regard, and the best evidence to date is that it does not. But still, if you are at high risk of prostate cancer or currently have prostate cancer, talk to your doctor before making any dietary changes.

One of the most heated debates centers on whether testosterone fuels prostate cancer. If that's true, say some experts, then **why do men develop prostate cancer when they are older, at the same time their testosterone levels are dropping?** (Harvard; Testosterone).

Testosterone, whether occurring naturally or taken as replacement therapy, does not cause prostate cancer or spur increases in prostate-specific antigen (PSA) levels in men, according to a new meta-analysis.

The results are "encouraging," but longer-term data from randomized trials are needed to strengthen the finding, said lead author Peter Boyle, PhD, DSc, who is president of the International Prevention Research Institute in Lyon, France (Medscape).

Testosterone and Dietary Fat

The reason for the preceding discussion about testosterone is dietary fat and cholesterol increase testosterone levels, while low-fat and vegan diets lower it, as seen in the following studies. Note that "androgen" is a general term for male sex hormones, which includes testosterone.

The results from several investigations strongly suggest that **dietary fat has a significant impact on T [testosterone] concentrations**; however, the influence of different types of lipids on T is not as clear. In the present investigation, **dietary fat, SFA [saturated fatty acids], and MUFA [monounsaturated fatty acids] were the best predictors of resting T concentrations** (Volek).

It is known that diet interacts with androgen levels (known to be related to **reduced androgen concentrations in vegetarians and reduced androgen levels in cohorts with lower fat intakes**), which is thought to be related to dietary fat since putting men on **a low-fat (high fiber) diet reduces circulating androgens** whereas the opposite exists as well (**higher fat diet at 41% of calories, with a higher intake of saturated fat, increasing testosterone**). The magnitude of these changes is **a low fat diet reducing testosterone in older men by 12% and an increase in dietary fat in young men increasing testosterone by 13%** (Examine).

Vegetarian group showed a higher levels of sex hormone-binding globulin (SHBG) while the free androgen index (FAI; calculated by the ratio testosterone/SHBG) was lower in this group. Although the concentrations of androsterone glucuronide were higher in vegetarian group, the **vegetarians had a 25-50% lower level** of androstane-3 alpha, 17 beta-diol glucuronide and androstane-3 beta,17 beta-diol glucuronide. Our data further indicate that both, androstane-3 alpha,17 beta-diol glucuronide and androstane-3 beta,17 beta-diol glucuronide concentrations are significantly correlated with SHBG levels and with the FAI values. The increases in androstane-3 alpha,17 beta-diol glucuronide and androstane-3 beta,17 beta-diol glucuronide levels in the omnivorous group are probably a consequence of the elevation of the FAI. **Our**

data suggest that in a vegetarian group, less testosterone is available for androgenic action (Belanger).

Urinary steroid hormone content was determined in Black and White North American men and in rural Black South African **men between 40 and 55 years of age** and in Black South African **men over 60 years of age** when maintained on their customary diets or when transferred to a vegetarian or Western diet, respectively.

When eating their customary diets, Black South African men had lower levels of urinary estrogens and androgens than did Black and White North American men. The **total androgen content decreased significantly in Black North American men on the vegetarian diet and increased in Black South African men fed a Western diet** (Hill).

To validate our hypothesis that reduction in dietary fat may result in changes in androgen metabolism, 39 middle-aged, white, healthy men **(50-60 yr of age)** were **studied while they were consuming their usual high-fat, low-fiber diet and after 8 wk modulation to an isocaloric low-fat, high-fiber diet**. Mean body weight decreased by 1 kg, whereas total caloric intake, energy expenditure, and activity index were not changed.

After diet modulation, mean serum testosterone (T) concentration fell (P < 0.0001), accompanied by small but significant decreases in serum free T (P = 0.0045), 5 alpha-dihydrotestosterone (P = 0.0053), and adrenal androgens (androstendione, P = 0.0135; dehydroepiandrosterone sulfate, P = 0.0011). Serum estradiol and SHBG showed smaller decreases. Parallel decreases in urinary excretion of some testicular and adrenal androgens were demonstrated. Metabolic clearance rates of T were not changed, and production rates for T showed a downward trend while on low-fat diet modulation. **We conclude that reduction in dietary fat intake (and increase in fiber) results in 12% consistent lowering of circulating androgen levels without changing the clearance** (Wang; Low Fat).

We conducted a controlled feeding study to evaluate the effects of fat and fiber consumption on plasma and urine sex hormones in men. The study had a crossover design and included **43 healthy men aged 19-56 y**. Men were initially randomly assigned to **either a low-fat, high-fiber or high-fat, low-fiber diet** for 10 wk and after a 2-wk washout period crossed over to the other diet. The energy content of diets was varied to maintain constant body weight but averaged approximately 13.3 MJ (3170 kcal)/d on both diets.

The low-fat diet provided 18.8% of energy from fat with a ratio of polyunsaturated to saturated fat (P:S) of 1.3, whereas **the high-fat diet provided 41.0% of energy from fat** with a P:S of 0.6. Total dietary fiber consumption from the low- and high-fat diets averaged 4.6 and 2.0 g.MJ-1.d-1, respectively.

Mean plasma concentrations of total and sex-hormone-binding-globulin (SHBG)-bound testosterone were 13% and 15% higher, respectively, on the high-fat, low-fiber diet and the difference from the low-fat, high-fiber diet was significant for the SHBG-bound fraction ($P = 0.04$). **Men's daily urinary excretion of testosterone also was 13% higher with the high-fat, low-fiber diet than with the low-fat, high-fiber diet ($P = 0.01$).** Conversely, their urinary excretion of estradiol and estrone and their 2-hydroxy metabolites were 12-28% lower with the high-fat, low-fiber diet ($P <$ or $= 0.01$). **Results of this study suggest that diet may alter endogenous sex hormone metabolism in men** (Dorgan).

Monounsaturated fats are the good guys that you want more of in your body. Not only do monounsaturated fats raise testosterone, but they may also reduce the risk of heart disease. Essentially, you are reaping the benefits of saturated fats without having to endure the flip side of the coin....

In one study, 12 male subjects were subjected to 20 minutes of high-intensity exercise consisting of bench presses and jumping squats. After a five minute rest, their testosterone serum levels were tested. All subjects submitted a detailed report of the foods they consumed for 17 days straight prior to the exercise session.

The results showed that those who consumed a higher fat content, especially monounsaturated fats, exhibited the highest levels of free testosterone at rest. Surprisingly, **those that consumed the highest levels of protein had the lowest T count.** This runs in contradiction with the mainstream belief that high protein is essential for building lean muscle and maintaining peak athletic performance (Test Shock).

Diets containing greater amounts of fats were correlated with higher resting testosterone levels. Specifically, the **consumption of saturated fats was strongly correlated with higher resting levels of testosterone. Monounsaturated fats were the next highest predictor of resting serum testosterone levels.**

The absolute levels of **polyunsaturated fats had no effect on serum testosterone levels.** Protein intake = lower testosterone, but it's thought that **meat is better at maintaining testosterone than other proteins** (PaleoHacks).

To summarize, total dietary fat, saturated fat, and monounsaturated fat increase testosterone levels, while low-fat and vegan diets lower it. The relationship of protein and testosterone levels will be explored in more detail later. But here, note the last sentence of the last quote.

Another point to note is, "cholesterol is the building block of testosterone" (Testosterone Week).

There are two possible pathways to testosterone [T] production:
Cholesterol » pregnenolone » progesterone » androstenedione » T
Cholesterol » pregnenolone » DHEA » androstenediol » T
(Bodybuilding.com).

The body can produce only a limited amount of cholesterol, so dietary cholesterol is needed for optimal testosterone production, but a vegan diet provides zero cholesterol. This is another reason vegetarians tend to have lower testosterone levels than omnivores (Volek, et.al).

121

However, there is little evidence that a high cholesterol intake correlates with high testosterone levels. This makes sense as if the intake is excessively high, the body will decrease its production of cholesterol.

Putting all of this information together, the best evidence is that total fat, saturated fat, and monounsaturated fat intake increase testosterone levels, while a low-fat, low cholesterol, vegan diet lowers it.

However, there is a tradeoff. Given the role of saturated fat and cholesterol in heart disease, too high of an intake of either could be detrimental, but too low is also detrimental.

However, monounsaturated fats also elevate testosterone levels, and those are found in abundance in vegan foods like nuts and olive oil. Thus a copious intake of them might help to offset the low saturated fat and cholesterol intake of vegans. But still, some cholesterol intake would be helpful. And the general recommendation is to keep saturated fat levels to less than 10% of calories. And that level would allow for the consumption of some animal fat. But before discussing animal foods, we will conclude this first section of this book on plant foods.

"Failure to Thrive"

A problem that is sometimes seen in long-time vegetarians and vegans is a condition known as "failure to thrive."

"Failure to thrive" is usually mild and unrecognized as such at first. However, there is another side to the vegetarian story that rarely gets talked about, which is the phenomenon known as **"failure to thrive" (FTT)**. Normally this term is used to describe infants who fail to do well or to meet minimum standards for growth and development, due to some shortfall in the standard of care received. However, the term can also be applied to anyone not doing well health-wise when they might otherwise be expected to.

Where vegetarianism is concerned, it means that despite following prudent recommendations for the diet, some people simply do not experience the best health, or, put differently perhaps, "well-being." This can range anywhere from mild symptoms such as:

- Lassitude or "being hungry all day" and "not feeling satisfied," as described above; to
- Poor sex drive or poor-quality sleep; to
  Behavioral effects such as not being able to get one's mind off food (not uncommon if one is not feeling physically satiated or otherwise satisfied on the diet), or
- The yo-yo syndrome of not being able to stay on the diet consistently due to cravings; to
- Emotional effects such as a vague, nonspecific loss of zest for life (which is usually more apparent to other people than to the person themselves); to
- Actual deficiencies in some cases (Beyond Veg. Why).

Even a book published by *Natural Health* magazine (which generally advocates a plant-based diet) admits to this problem:

> There is little question that adopting a varied plant-based diet will improve your chances of avoiding such chronic ailments as cancer and heart disease. Animal foods can, however, still play a minor part in your diet, if you so choose. **Even some longtime vegetarians have found that eating meat occasionally provides some health benefits**. Anne Louise Gitterman M.S., a nutritional counselor specializing in woman's health, says strict vegetarianism has its limits. ... Gitterman says **some of her longtime vegetarian clients experience fatigue, protein deficiencies, and loss of hair** (Mayell, pp.7,8).

Many testimonials can be found on the internet of long-time vegans who simply began not feeling good, but the re-inclusion of animal foods into their diets improved their health. In fact, a study of "seventy-seven former vegetarians" found "thirty-five percent of our participants indicated that declining health was the main reason they reverted back to eating flesh" (Psychology Today; Why). And consider the following:

> What about organizations that promote a 100 percent vegan diet strictly for health reasons? I think that these organizations

123

can thrive because many people who first make the conversion from a highly processed and animal-based diet to a strict vegan diet typically experience incredible improvement with their health. **For a few months or even a year or two, many people can thrive on a strict vegan diet**, making it easy for them to believe that they have discovered a diet that will best support their health for the rest of their lives. **But then, as most of them predictably become deficient in nutrients that are difficult to obtain from plant foods alone, they usually become confused about why their health is suffering** (Chet Day's; Vegan Diet).

In spite of all the rhetoric from vegan diet teachers, **there has never been a civilization in the entire world that has been able to survive on the vegan diet. Every culture depends on some type of animal products to a degree,** be it eggs, milk, cheese, or meat (even insects in third world countries). This includes the Hunza people who are often falsely represented as vegan even though they eat dairy and some meat (Chet Day's; Hallelujah).

Dr. Klaper discusses this condition in an article formerly posted on the Earth Save website. In summary form, his theory is that humans can create certain nutrients that are found in meat, "like carnitine (required for energy production) and some long-chain fatty acids (EPA, DHA, etc., needed for hormone function, membrane synthesis, etc.)."

When people are raised on a meat-based diet, they get these substances from their food, so their bodies stop producing them. Then when they go "cold turkey" (no pun intended) onto a meatless diet, their body is unable to start producing these substances again. And over time, the lack of these nutrients causes the poor health.

Evidence for this theory is that Robbins reports about the "failures to thrive" syndrome, "In my experience, these problems are not encountered in people raised on vegetarian diets from infancy." For the person who was raised on a meat-based diet, a way to avoid this problem might to be slowly decrease one's intake of animal foods rather than eliminating them all at once. This would give the body time to adapt to the lack of meat and start to produce the needed substances (Klaper).

I could not find any evidence as to whether Dr. Klaper's claims are true or not. But as a general principle, it is good advice to make slow changes in one's diet, as slow changes will give a person a chance to gradually "discover" a new way of eating, rather than having to replace all former foods at once.

Moreover, the opposite is probably true, as well. People who have been vegans for a long period of time could experiences difficulties in resuming meat eating.

I, personally, have **been vegetarian since around 5 yrs old**. During High School/College I had several friends try it out only lasting a few months or years. Personally, **meat makes me feel sick**. Not entirely sure why, but I was thinking that maybe it is because **I have not eaten meat in so long that my gut has adjusted to the diet that I have been eating. Probably, if I did eat meat, my body would eventually adjust** (not sure though). Once I ate some meat in High School at friend's house because I didn't want to be "different," but I became so sick a few hours later in the night that I threw up and had to go home. That was when I told my friends that I had actually not eaten meat for ten years (Anonymous comment on Psychology Today).

Cheating on a Vegan Diet

Eating small amounts of animal foods would solve both the vitamin B12 and possibly the failure to thrive problems. And in fact, this is probably what is happening in people who claim to have been following a vegan diet for many years and are thriving on it.

I believe that people can survive for many years on a strict vegan diet, but almost always with one or more significant health problems. And I believe that **some people who are truly thriving without any health problems, and claim to have been strict vegans for many years usually eat some animal foods, even if it is a small amount**. The fact is, you and I can never know with certainty what another person eats on a moment-to-moment basis. **The only dietary regimen that you**

125

can know with absolute accuracy is your own. Even your dog or cat probably eat things that you don't know about (Chet Day's; Vegan).

In other words, many longtime vegans cheat on occasion. Not often enough that they no longer consider themselves to be vegans, but often enough so as consume needed nutrients that are missing in their otherwise plant-based diet.

On any given day, **how much meat does the average vegetarian eat**? Since vegetarians, by definition, don't eat meat, this question should be boring because of course the answer is zero. This question isn't boring at all, though, because it has a very specific, very not-zero answer—**83.2 grams, about one standard serving**....

This first figure—seriously, **the average vegetarian in the U.S. eats one serving of meat per day!**—comes from a 2003 analysis of data collected by the U.S. Department of Agriculture in the late 90's. The researchers examined responses from a representative sample of nearly 10,000 Americans who had detailed everything they ate over two separate and nonconsecutive 24-hour periods. And **vegetarians, it turns out, eat meat**. About 40 percent of what the typical American reported—220 grams or so—but meat all the same....

Another survey from the USDA, also conducted by phone, put **the number of vegetarians who've eaten meat in the last day at about two-thirds**. Based on a 1995 survey of wealthy, well-educated Americans from the East Coast, **only 1.5 percent said they never eat poultry or fish, but 7 percent called themselves vegetarians**. Surveys by Canada's National Institute of Nutrition put the number of **Canadian vegetarians who eat chicken at about 60 percent and red meat at about 32 percent** (Daily Beast).

Vegetarians are going to have a cow over this. Oh, wait, they already are.

A new survey [of 1,789 British vegetarians] says more than **a third of vegetarians eat meat when they've had too much**

to drink. What's more, they're sneaky about it, with 69 percent saying they don't fess up...

According to a study by the Humane Research Council, many American vegetarians are bad to the bone as well: **around 84 percent stray from a strict vegetarian diet** (Huffington Post).

But sometimes, cheating vegans do fess up, and they do so publicly:

When people hear the word "cheater," they might think of gross celebrities who've cheated in relationships, or kids who'll never actually know how to spell since they've cheated on every test ever. Those kinds of cheaters are pretty bad.

I'm a cheater, too–just of a different kind. I am a vegan, but that is just 95 percent of the real story. **The other five percent is kind of a lie**. I've been vegan for years, which means I don't eat or use any animal products at all no meat (obviously!), no poultry or fish, no milk products, no eggs, honey, leather, fur–you get the idea. Some of my good friends are vegan, too, which makes it easy. We cook together, we sip soy milk together, it's like a big happy scene.

Thing is, without my vegan posse, things get a little more complicated and I . . . cheat....

I didn't want to be the no-fun militant vegan at my friend's party! And if you think I only cheated that once, you're wrong. Like most cheaters, my cheating wasn't a one-time deal (Gurl, ellipses in original).

As **more and more people, including athletes and celebrities, openly admitting they cheat on their vegetarian or vegan diet**, one has to question the claim the vegetarian move is on the rise. **Olympian Venus Williams admits she has cheated on her vegan diet. She is not alone**. Actor and singer Jared Leto admits in a *Rolling Stone* interview he is also a "cheating vegan." In fact, confessing you cheated is now a brand new trend. Yep, **cheagan is the newest name tag to adorn** (National).

Confessions of a Cheating Vegan. I myself am a vegan of sorts and I'm here to tell you that it's not an easy life – that's why **it's OK to cheat**...

You're OK when you can cook your own food (really), but going out is hard. Most restaurants offer very limited, unappetizing fare for people who don't eat meat or dairy. Grocery stores, while better than they used to be, still aren't great.

And you have to get used to that sickening silence on the other end of the line when you tell the person who's inviting you to dinner that you don't eat meat, cheese, fish, soup made from beef stock, or anything else he or she was planning to cook.

The way I handle that is...I cheat. I'll order fish in a restaurant and eat what I'm served in someone else's home. And when I go to a ballgame, I declare hotdogs a vegetable for the day. **Mostly, though, I'm a vegan** (Alternet).

Not only is it okay to cheat, but vegans are probably be better off if they do so. A small amount of animal foods on occasion would go a long way towards preventing the potential drawbacks of a vegan diet.

Frankly, **most of the pure vegans that I know personally do not appear to be particularly healthy**. My pure vegan friends all have kind of dull skin and hair, most have dark circles around their eyes, and they all seem to get colds and flus more often than I do. They seem rather tired and listless much of the time, too; almost depressed. **My vegetarian friends who also consume milk, cheese, eggs, and sometimes fish seem much, MUCH healthier to me**, and have more energy (anonymous comment on Psychology Today).

What all of this means is, though the potential drawbacks of vegan and vegetarian diets can be overcome, it is not easy to follow them, and there are no clear-cut benefits when all factors are taken into account. This is probably why "84% of Vegetarians and Vegans Return to Meat." Moreover:

The proportion of true vegetarians and vegans in the United States is surprisingly small. Only about 2% of respondents did not consume any meat – **1.5% were vegetarians and 0.5% were vegans**. These finding are generally consistent with other studies.

… **the fact that five out of six vegetarians go back to eating meat suggests that an all-veggie diet is very hard for most people to maintain over the long haul** (Psychology Today).

Therefore, it must be asked if the difficulties of following a vegan or vegetarian diet is worthwhile. Only the reader can answer that question for yourself.

Summary of Edenic and Antediluvian Diets

The Creationist Diet at this point presents two options. First, one could follow the diet of Adam and Eve while they were in the Garden of Eden and eat nothing but raw fruits and vegetables and raw nuts and seeds. Since this was the diet they ate in the Garden of Eden, a good name for this type of diet would be the "Edenic Diet."

Such a diet could be beneficial for someone trying to overcome specific health problems, such as heart problems or cancer. But it should be looked at as more of a short-term diet, as it was for Adam and Eve, not as a long-term diet.

The second option would be to follow the diet of the antediluvians (who lived between the time of the Fall and the Flood) and eat the above foods, along with cooked versions thereof, especially whole grains, plus legumes. This second version would avoid some of the possible long-term problems of the former, and thus can be looked upon as a life-long dietary strategy. Since this was the diet eaten in the antediluvian era, then it could be called the "Antediluvian Diet."

That covers the major plant foods. But when did animal foods enter the picture? Do they have a place in a Creationist Diet? These questions will be looked at in Section Two. But first, a couple of important issues in regards to plant foods need to be addressed.

Bibliography:

AHA (American Heart Association); Saturated Fats. http://www.heart.org/HEARTORG/HealthyLiving/HealthyEating/Nutrition/Saturated-Fats_UCM_301110_Article.jsp#.WHC8ui_QeUk

AHA: Triglycerides: Frequently Asked Questions. https://my.americanheart.org/idc/groups/ahamah-public/@wcm/@sop/@smd/documents/downloadable/ucm_425988.pdf

Albert, MJ, et. al. *Nature*. 1980 Feb 21;283(5749):781-2. Vitamin B12 synthesis by human small intestinal bacteria. https://www.ncbi.nlm.nih.gov/pubmed/7354869

Alternet. Confessions of a Cheating Vegan. http://www.alternet.org/story/155380/confessions_of_a_cheating_vegan

American Heritage® Dictionary of the English Language, Third Edition copyright © 1992 by Houghton Mifflin Company. Electronic version licensed from InfoSoft International, Inc. All rights reserved.

Art of Manliness. Testosterone Week: A Short Primer on How T Is Made. http://www.artofmanliness.com/2013/01/15/how-testosterone-is-made/

Authority Nutrition; Eggs and Cholesterol - How Many Eggs Can You Safely Eat? https://authoritynutrition.com/how-many-eggs-should-you-eat/

Bélanger A, et.al. *Journal of Steroid Biochemistry*. 1989 Jun;32(6):829-33. Influence of diet on plasma steroids and sex hormone-binding globulin levels in adult men. https://www.ncbi.nlm.nih.gov/pubmed/2526906

Beyond Veg. Why "failure to thrive" on vegetarian diets is rarely talked about. http://www.beyondveg.com/nicholson-w/veg-prob/veg-prob-scen1b.shtml

Bodybuilding.com. All About Testosterone. http://www.bodybuilding.com/fun/vm12.htm?clickid=wvGysiwQQ0Zn2WfUT-zls0m0UkkSDSSVRRJ8xA0&irpid=97201

Boston Globe. Six myths about nutrition and health. http://www.bostonglobe.com/lifestyle/2015/01/23/six-myths-about-nutrition-and-health/BRiFwWBn6l8rFZQbdaYD1O/story.html

Encyclopedia Britannica. Vitamin B$_{12}$.

https://www.britannica.com/science/vitamin-B12

Burckhardt, P. *Swiss Medical Weekly*. 2016 Feb 22. The role of low acid load in vegetarian diet on bone health: a narrative review. https://www.ncbi.nlm.nih.gov/pubmed/26900949

Chet Day's Tips. Hallelujah Acres Research Cast Doubt On "Ideal Diet. By Greg Westbrook. http://www.chetday.com/hallelujah-diet-dangers.htm

Chet Day's Tips. Vegan Diet: Recipe for Disaster? Dr. Ben Kim. http://www.chetday.com/strictvegandiet.htm

Craddock JC1, Probst YC, Peoples GE. *International Journal of Sports Nutrition and Exercise Metabolism* 2016 Jun;26(3):212-20. Vegetarian and Omnivorous Nutrition - Comparing Physical Performance. https://www.ncbi.nlm.nih.gov/pubmed/26568522

Craig WJ. *American Journal of Clinical Nutrition*. 2009 May;89(5):1627S-1633S. doi: 10.3945/ajcn.2009.26736N. Epub 2009 Mar 11. Health effects of vegan diets. https://www.ncbi.nlm.nih.gov/pubmed/19279075

Craig WJ. *Nutrition in Clinical Practice*. 2010 Dec;25(6):613-20. doi: 10.1177/0884533610385707. Nutrition concerns and health effects of vegetarian diets. https://www.ncbi.nlm.nih.gov/pubmed/21139125

CNS. Center for Nutritional Studies. 12 Questions Answered Regarding Vitamin B12. http://nutritionstudies.org/12-questions-answered-regarding-vitamin-b12/

Daily Beast. Why Drunk Vegetarians Eat Meat. http://www.thedailybeast.com/articles/2015/10/11/why-drunk-vegetarians-eat-meat.html

Dorfman, Lisa. *The Vegetarian Sports Nutrition Guide*. Quoted in *Natural Health* magazine, March 2000, "Can Vegetarians be Champions? p.37.

Dorgan JF. *American Journal of Clinical Nutrition*. 1996 Dec;64(6):850-5. Effects of dietary fat and fiber on plasma and urine androgens and estrogens in men: a controlled feeding study. https://www.ncbi.nlm.nih.gov/pubmed/8942407

Examine. Is saturated fat bad for me? https://examine.com/nutrition/is-saturated-fat-bad-for-me/

Farley, Dixie. *Vegetarian Diets: The Plusses and the Pitfalls*. US Food and Drug Administration:
http://www.fda.gov/bbs/topics/CONSUMER/CON00138.html

Fiscal Times; Why the Government's New Dietary Guidelines Could Set Off a Food Fight.
http://www.thefiscaltimes.com/2015/02/18/More-Eggs-Less-Meat-Why-Government-s-New-Nutrition-Guidelines-Could-Set-Food-Fight

Giem P, Beeson WL, Fraser GE. *Neuroepidemiology*. 1993;12(1):28-36. *The incidence of dementia and intake of animal products: preliminary findings from the Adventist Health Study*.

Gurl. Confession: I Say I'm Vegan, But I Totally Cheat.
http://www.gurl.com/2012/01/27/i-am-not-always-vegan/

Healthline. Low Testosterone in Men.
http://www.healthline.com/health/side-effects-of-low-testosterone#Overview1

Hill P, et.al., *Cancer Resources*. 1979 Dec;39(12):5101-5. Diet and urinary steroids in black and white North American men and black South African men.
https://www.ncbi.nlm.nih.gov/pubmed/498137

How Stuff Works: Health. What's the difference between LDL and HDL cholesterol?
http://health.howstuffworks.com/diseases-conditions/cardiovascular/cholesterol/difference-between-ldl-and-hdl-cholesterol1.htm

Huffington Post. Surprising Number Of Drunk Vegetarians Secretly Eat Meat.
http://www.huffingtonpost.com/entry/vegetarians-eat-meat-drunk-survey_us_56167f34e4b0e66ad4c69f50

Kjeldsen-Kragh J. *American Journal of Clinical Nutrition*. 1999 Sep;70(3 Suppl):594S-600S. *Rheumatoid arthritis treated with vegetarian diets*.

Kris-Etherton. AHA Science Advisory. Monounsaturated Fatty Acids and Risk of Cardiovascular Disease. Originally published September 14, 1999.
http://circ.ahajournals.org/content/100/11/1253.full

Harvard School of Public Health. Fats and Cholesterol.
https://www.hsph.harvard.edu/nutritionsource/what-should-you-eat/fats-and-cholesterol/

Harvard. Testosterone supplementation after prostate cancer?
http://www.harvardprostateknowledge.org/testosterone-supplementation-after-prostate-cancer

Lau EM1, Kwok T, Woo J, Ho SC. *European Journal of Clinical Nutrition.* 1998 Jan;52(1):60-4. Bone mineral density in Chinese elderly female vegetarians, vegans, lacto-vegetarians and omnivores.
https://www.ncbi.nlm.nih.gov/pubmed/9481534

Lee YJ, et.al. *Nutrients.* 2016 Feb 26;8(3):118. Associations between Vitamin B-12 Status and Oxidative Stress and Inflammation in Diabetic Vegetarians and Omnivores.
https://www.ncbi.nlm.nih.gov/pubmed/26927168

Livestrong. How Many Milligrams of Cholesterol Should I Have a Day?
http://www.livestrong.com/article/254182-how-many-milligrams-of-cholesterol-should-i-have-a-day/

Mayo Clinic: Trans fat is double trouble for your heart health.
http://www.mayoclinic.org/diseases-conditions/high blood cholesterol/in-depth/trans-fat/art-20046114

Medical News Today. Vegan Diet: Health Benefits Of Being Vegan.
http://www.medicalnewstoday.com/articles/149636.php

Medscape. Meta-analysis: Testosterone Is Not a Risk for Prostate Cancer, But...
http://www.medscape.com/viewarticle/844907

McDougall, Dr. Clearing Up The Confusion Surrounding Saturated Fat.
https://www.drmcdougall.com/misc/2014nl/apr/saturatedfat.htm

Mustad, V A, et. al. *Journal of Lipid Research.* Reducing saturated fat intake is associated with increased levels of LDL receptors on mononuclear cells in healthy men and women.
http://www.jlr.org/content/38/3/459.abstract

National Hog Farmer. Stylish ways vegans justify eating meat.
http://www.nationalhogfarmer.com/blog/stylish-ways-vegans-justify-eating-meat

New SA. *Osteoporosis International.* 2004 Sep;15(9):679-88. Epub 2004 Jul 16. Do vegetarians have a normal bone mass?
https://www.ncbi.nlm.nih.gov/pubmed/15258721

New World Encyclopedia. Testosterone.

http://www.newworldencyclopedia.org/entry/Testosterone

Nicholson AS, Sklar M, Barnard ND, Gore S, Sullivan R, Browning S. *Preventative Medicine.* 1999 Aug;29(2):87-91. *Toward improved management of NIDDM: A randomized, controlled, pilot intervention using a lowfat, vegetarian diet.* Copyright 1999 American Health Foundation and Academic Press.

Nieman, DC. *American Journal of Clinical Nutrition.* 1999 Sep;70(3 Suppl):570S-575S. *Physical fitness and vegetarian diets: is there a relation?*

rec.food.veg Newsgroup. *Frequently Asked Questions* page – http://www.veg.org/veg/FAQ/rec.food.veg.html

Nursingdegree.net. 57 Health Benefits of Going Vegan. http://www.nursingdegree.net/blog/19/57-health-benefits-of-going-vegan/

Oxford Dictionary. As found on Microsoft *Word 365.*

PaleoHacks. Saturated fat or Monounsaturated to boost testosterone? https://www.paleohacks.com/fats/saturated-fat-or-monounsaturated-to-boost-testosterone-21080

Peaceful Dumpling. Eat Your Dirt: Vitamin B12. http://www.peacefuldumpling.com/vitamin-b12-eat-your-dirt

Psychology Today. 84% of Vegetarians and Vegans Return to Meat. https://www.psychologytoday.com/blog/animals-and-us/201412/84-vegetarians-and-vegans-return-meat-why

Prezioso D, *Archives of Italian Urology Androl.* 2015 Jul 7;87(2):105-20. doi: 10.4081/aiua.2015.2.105. Dietary treatment of urinary risk factors for renal stone formation. A review of CLU Working Group. https://www.ncbi.nlm.nih.gov/pubmed/26150027

Rauma AL, Mykkänen H. *Nutrition.* 2000 Feb;16(2):111-9. Antioxidant status in vegetarians versus omnivores. https://www.ncbi.nlm.nih.gov/pubmed/10696634

Robbins, John. *Save Your Health: One Bite at a Time* – http://www.earthsave.org/news/19980915.htm

Siri-Tarino, Patty W, et. al., *American Journal of Clinical Nutrition.* 2010 Mar; 91(3): 535–546. Published online 2010 Jan 13. Meta-analysis

of prospective cohort studies evaluating the association of saturated fat with cardiovascular disease.
https://www.ncbi.nlm.nih.gov/pmc/articles/PMC2824152/

Siri-Tarino, Patty W. et. al., *Current Atherosclerosis Rep.* 2010 Nov; 12(6): 384–390. Saturated Fatty Acids and Risk of Coronary Heart Disease: Modulation by Replacement Nutrients.
https://www.ncbi.nlm.nih.gov/pmc/articles/PMC2943062/

Suzuki H. *Journal of Nutrition Science, Vitaminol (Tokyo).* 1995 Dec;41(6):587-94. *Serum vitamin B12 levels in young vegans who eat brown rice.*

Testosterone Week: A Short Primer on How T Is Made.
http://www.artofmanliness.com/2013/01/15/how-testosterone-is-made/

Test Shock. Skyrocket Your Testosterone Levels With a Diet Rich in Monounsaturated Fats.
http://www.testshock.com/skyrocket-your-testosterone-levels-with-a-diet-rich-in-monounsaturated-fats/

US News; 5 Shades of Grey in Nutrition.
http://health.usnews.com/health-news/blogs/eat-run/2015/04/16/5-shades-of-grey-in-nutrition

Vegan Society of the UK.*Why Vegan?* -
http://www.vegansociety.com/why/whyhealth.html

Vegetarian Pages Web site. *How to win an argument with a meat eater.*
http://www.veg.org/veg/FAQ/extinction.html

Venderley AM1, Campbell WW. *Sports Medicine.* 2006;36(4):293-305. Vegetarian diets : nutritional considerations for athletes.
https://www.ncbi.nlm.nih.gov/pubmed/16573356

Volek, Jeff S. *Journal of Applied Physiology.* Testosterone and cortisol in relationship to dietary nutrients and resistance exercise.
http://jap.physiology.org/content/82/1/49

Wang, F, et.al. *Journal of the American Heart Association.* 2015 Oct 27;4(10):e002408. Effects of Vegetarian Diets on Blood Lipids: A Systematic Review and Meta-Analysis of Randomized Controlled Trials.
https://www.ncbi.nlm.nih.gov/pubmed/26508743

Wang C, et.al. *Journal of Clinical Endocrinology Metabolism.* 2005 Jun;90(6):3550-9. Epub 2005 Mar 1. Low-fat high-fiber diet decreased serum and urine androgens in men.

Creationist Diet

https://www.ncbi.nlm.nih.gov/pubmed/15741266

Wasserman, Debra and Nutrition Section by Reed Mangels, Ph.D., R.D. *Simply Vegan: Quick Vegetarian Meals.* Vegetarian Resource Group, P.O. Box 1463, Baltimore, MD 21203, 1990/1991, as quoted on the "rec.good.veg" Newsgroup FAQ page.

WebMD; Is Butter Back? The Truth About Saturated Fats.
http://www.webmd.com/cholesterol-management/features/truth-about-saturated-fats

WebMD. Low Testosterone: How Do You Know When Levels Are Too Low?
http://www.webmd.com/men/features/low-testosterone-explained-how-do-you-know-when-levels-are-too-low#3

WebMD. Vitamin B12 Deficiency.
http://www.webmd.com/food-recipes/guide/vitamin-b12-deficiency-symptoms-causes#1

Webster's Talking Dictionary/ Thesaurus. Licensed property of Parson's Technology, Inc. v. 1.0b. Software Copyright 1996 by Exceller Software Corp. Based on Random House *Webster's College Dictionary.* Copyright 1995 by Random House, Inc.

Wikipedia. Testosterone.
https://en.wikipedia.org/wiki/Testosterone

WPXI TV News cast. *Healthcast* segment. 1/21/2000.

Yen CE, et. al., Nutrition Res. 2008 Jul;28(7):430-6. doi: 10.1016/j.nutres.2008.03.012. Dietary intake and nutritional status of vegetarian and omnivorous preschool children and their parents in Taiwan.
https://www.ncbi.nlm.nih.gov/pubmed/1908344

Chapter Five
Organic and Non-GMO Foods

Before leaving this section on plant foods, a couple of general points of importance about plant foods need to be addressed.

Organic Versus Commercial Produce

It goes without saying, Adam and Eve did not spray chemical fertilizers, pesticides, and herbicides on the trees and plants in the Garden of Eden. For that matter, nobody throughout human history did, until about a century ago. Plants were fertilized naturally using manure.

If the idea of using manure as fertilizer seems strange to the reader, it shouldn't as that is how plants were fertilized throughout most of human history. This can be seen in the Bible, in a parable that Jesus told:

[6]Then He spoke this parable: "A certain [man] had a fig tree having been planted in his vineyard, and he came looking for fruit on it and did not find [any]. [7]Then he said to the vineyard keeper, 'Look! Three years I [have] come looking for fruit in this fig tree and do not find [any]. Cut it down! Why does it even use up the ground?' [8]But answering, he says to him, 'Lord, let it alone this year also, until which [time] I dig around it and **put piles of manure** [fig., fertilizer] [on it]. [9]And if then it produces fruit [fine], but if not, in the coming [year] you will cut it down'" (Luke 13:6-9).

As with most Scripture quotes in this book, this verse is quoted from this writer's *Analytical Literal Translation* (ALT). As the name indicates, it is a very literal translation of the original Greek text. That is why it has "put piles of manure." But as the bracketed note indicates, the meaning here is "fertilizer." I include this note as many today do not seem to know that manure is used to fertilize plants. That is why most modern-day Bible translation have just "fertilize" here.

The point is, using manure rather than chemical fertilizers is the natural and Biblical method of fertilizing plants. And that is how all organic famers today fertilize their soil. It would thus be more natural and Biblical to consume organic rather than commercial produce.

Pesticides and herbicides are of course used to reduce infestation by pests and bacterial and fungal growth. But there are natural methods to do so. Granted these are not as effective, which is why organic produce costs more than commercial produce. The farmers have to charge more to make up for their losses.

But are organic foods worth the extra cost? There is some evidence that organic produce is more nutrient packed than commercial produce, though there are disagreements.

An article by Walter J. Crinnion in *Alternative Medicine Review* is titled, "Organic Foods Contain Higher Levels of Certain Nutrients, Lower Levels of Pesticides, and May Provide Health Benefits for the Consumer." The abstract states:

The multi-billion dollar organic food industry is fueled by consumer perception that organic food is healthier (greater nutritional value and fewer toxic chemicals). **Studies of the nutrient content in organic foods vary in results** due to differences in the ground cover and maturity of the organic farming operation. Nutrient content also varies from farmer to farmer and year to year.

However, **reviews of multiple studies show that organic varieties do provide significantly greater levels of vitamin C, iron, magnesium, and phosphorus than non-organic varieties of the same foods**. While being higher in these nutrients, they are also **significantly lower in nitrates and pesticide residues**. In addition, with the exception of wheat, oats, and wine, **organic foods typically provide greater levels of a number of important antioxidant phytochemicals** (anthocyanins, flavonoids, and carotenoids).

Although *in vitro* [in a test tube] studies of organic fruits and vegetables consistently demonstrate that organic foods have greater antioxidant activity, are more potent suppressors of the mutagenic action of toxic compounds, and inhibit the proliferation of certain cancer cell lines, *in vivo* **[within a living organism] studies of antioxidant activity in humans have failed to demonstrate additional benefit**. Clear health benefits from consuming organic dairy products have been demonstrated in regard to allergic dermatitis.

Other researchers have come to similar conclusions:

Demand for organic foods is partially driven by consumers' perceptions that they are more nutritious. However, **scientific opinion is divided on whether there are significant nutritional differences between organic and non-organic foods**, and two recent reviews have concluded that there are no differences. In the present study, we carried out meta-analyses based on **343 peer-reviewed publications that indicate statistically significant and meaningful differences in composition between organic and non-organic crops/crop-based foods**. Most importantly, the **concentrations of a range of antioxidants such as polyphenolics were found to be substantially higher in organic crops/crop based foods**....

Many of these compounds have previously been linked to a reduced risk of chronic diseases, including CVD [cardiovascular disease] and neurodegenerative diseases and certain cancers, in dietary intervention and epidemiological studies.

Additionally, **the frequency of occurrence of pesticide residues was found to be four times higher in conventional crops, which also contained significantly higher concentrations of the toxic metal Cd [cadmium]**....

In conclusion, **organic crops, on average, have higher concentrations of antioxidants, lower concentrations of Cd and a lower incidence of pesticide residues than the non-organic comparators across regions and production seasons** (Barański).

The consumption of organic food has been increasing all over the world. Due to this fact, there are growing numbers of scientific studies examining the nutritional value of organic food. The aim of this review is to provide an overall picture of the beneficial and harmful nutritional content of organically and conventionally produced crops based on existing international comparative surveys. Furthermore, the authors attempt to define the relationship between organic and conventional food production systems and the nutritional value of food products as well as the consumption of organic and conventional diets which have important human health implications.

Organic crops contain a significantly higher amount of certain antioxidants (vitamin C, polyphenols and flavonoids) and minerals, as well as have higher dry matter content than conventional ones. Moreover, there is a lower level of pesticide residues, nitrate and some heavy metal contaminations in organic crops compared to conventional ones.

There is a relationship between the different fertilisation and plant protection methods of these two plant production systems and the nutritional composition of crops. Consequently, it can be concluded that **organically produced plant derived food products have a higher nutritional value, including antioxidants than conventional ones. Furthermore, due to the fact that there is a lower level of contamination in organic crops, the risk of diseases caused by contaminated food is significantly reduced** (Györéné).

Given that organic plant foods are more natural, more Biblical, and probably more nutritious than commercial produce, organic plant foods would fit best with a Creationist Diet. However, the greater cost can be a hindrance to some. As such, it will not be said you have to consume organic plant foods to follow a Creationist Diet. In regards to fruits and vegetables, whether organic or commercial, they are incredibly healthy and should be consumed in copious amounts. It is just that organic produce is more so. It is thus strongly encouraged if you can afford it.

It should also be noted that pesticide residues do not reside on just the outside of the fruit or vegetable but within it. This is due to the roots of the plant or tree drawing up pesticides from the soil into the produce, just as the roots do with minerals. Thus washing produce, though something that should be done, is not a substitute for buying organic.

Finally, pesticide residues are greater with fruits and vegetables than with other plant foods. As such, it is not as important to purchase organic grains, nuts, seeds, and legumes, as it is to purchase organic produce. But there is another consideration for these foods.

Genetically Modified Organisms

A Genetically Modified Organism is, "An organism whose genetic characteristics have been altered by the insertion of a modified gene or a gene from another organism using the techniques of genetic engineering" (YourDictoinary.com). Such organisms are best known by the acronym GMO. The term "Genetic Engineering" (GE) is also used.

Genetic engineering can be done with plants, animals, or bacteria and other very small organisms. Genetic engineering allows scientists to move desired genes from one plant or animal into another. Genes can also be moved from an animal to a plant or vice versa. Another name for this is genetically modified organisms, or GMOs.

The process to create GE foods is different than selective breeding. This involves selecting plants or animals with desired traits and breeding them. Over time, this results in offspring with those desired traits.

One of the problems with selective breeding is that it can also result in traits that are not desired. **Genetic engineering allows scientists to select one specific gene to implant**. This avoids introducing other genes with undesirable traits. **Genetic engineering also helps speed up the process of creating new foods with desired traits** (UMMC).

Selective breeding has been practiced for millennia. In fact, Jacob used this practice to alter the color of the sheep in Laban's flock:

[31]And Laban said to him, "What will I give you?" But Jacob said to him, "You will not give me anything; if you shall do this thing for me, I will again tend your sheep and keep [them]. [32]Let all your sheep pass by today, and **separate from there every gray sheep among the lambs, and every one [that is] speckled and spotted among the goats, [this] will be my wage**. [33]And my righteousness shall listen to me on the day of tomorrow, for it is my wage before you; all which shall not

141

be spotted and speckled among the goats, and gray among the lambs, it will be having been stolen [if] with me." [34]So Laban said to him, "Let it be according to your word." ...

[40]Then Jacob separated the lambs, and set before the sheep a speckled ram, and every variegated one among the lambs, and **he separated flocks for himself, and did not mingle them with the sheep of Laban. [41]So it happened in the time which the sheep [were having] in [the] womb [fig., became pregnant], Jacob having taken, placed the rods before the sheep in the troughs, [for] them to conceive by the rods**. [42]But whenever the sheep gave birth, he was not placing them [indiscriminately]. **So the unmarked ones [were] Laban's, but the marked ones were Jacob's**. [Heb., So the feebler would be Laban's, and the stronger Jacob's]. [43]**And the man [became] exceedingly exceedingly [fig., extremely] rich**, and became to him many livestock and oxen and male bond-servants and female bond-servants and camels and donkeys (Genesis 30:31-34,40-43).

It is not clear exactly how Jacob conducted this selective breading, but it is clear that it worked. More speckled and spotted sheep were born than white ones, and Jacob grew richer as a result, but Laban poorer.

However, this alteration of an organism via selective breeding is far less efficient and far less reaching than using genetic engineering. And it is that potential for great alterations of the food supply that has many concerned. But to date, studies have not proven any adverse effects. There are also potential benefits of GMOs. But there is much debate in this regard. However, one thing is certain—the use of GMOs is widespread, especially in the USA:

> **Nearly 90 percent of all the crops grown in the United States have been touched by science**. Genetically modified organisms, or GMOs, are plants that have had their genes manipulated. They give the crops new characteristics, like **insect resistance, larger yields, and faster growing traits**. The use of GMOs is hardly new, but many believe that **sufficient research on the long term effects has not been conducted** (Next Galaxy).

If you've eaten anything today, chances are you've snacked on GMOs. GMO stands for genetically modified organism. **Genetically modified (GM)** foods are made from soy, corn, or other crops grown from seeds with genetically engineered DNA.

According to the U.S. Department of Agriculture (USDA), **GM seeds are used to plant more than 90 percent of corn, soybeans, and cotton grown in the United States.** Unless you consciously avoid them, GM foods likely find their way into many of your snacks and meals.

Some people believe GM foods are safe, healthy, and sustainable, while others claim the opposite (Healthline. GMOs).

Some people have expressed concerns about GE foods, such as:

- Creating foods that can cause an allergic reaction or that are toxic
- Unexpected or harmful genetic changes
- Genes moving from one GM plant or animal to another plant or animal that is not genetically engineered
- Foods that are less nutritious

These concerns have proven to be unfounded. None of the GE foods used today have caused any of these problems. The US Food and Drug Administration (FDA) assesses all GE foods to make sure they are safe before allowing them to be sold. In addition to the FDA, the US Environmental Protection Agency (EPA) and the US Department of Agriculture (USDA) regulate bioengineered plants and animals. **They assess the safety of GE foods to humans, animals, plants, and the environment** (UMMC).

So what are the benefits of GMOs? According to the Office of Science at the U.S. Department of Energy, **one of the pros of genetically modified crops is a better taste, increased**

nutrients, resistance to disease and pests, and faster output of crops.

The Food and Agriculture Organization of the United Nations also says that **farmers can grow more food on less land with genetically modified crops....**

But what happens to these plants and animals that have been genetically modified? What happens when we eat these foods? Unfortunately, **no one knows for sure what happens,** though **evidence is mounting that genetic modification may not be a good thing....**

The Office of Science at the U.S. Department of Energy also lists some of the controversies associated with genetically modified foods. One of these controversies are the **potential health risks, including allergies, antibiotic resistance, and unknown effects.** Other negatives that stem from GMOs is that scientists are **tampering with nature** by mixing genes and no one knows what this is doing to the animals or the environment.

Phil Damery and colleagues at Iowa State University describe the risks of genetically modified foods to humans in their paper, "The Debate on Labeling Genetically Modified Foods." Damery says that the agricultural food industry claims that GM foods are tested rigorously, but **the food companies conduct all their own testing.** The U.S. Food and Drug Administration never reviews the studies, just the conclusions that agricultural food companies provide to the FDA. Damery states that, **when studies were conducted by non-agricultural food organizations, they found serious health risks with GM foods and the way they tested for safety** (Decoded).

The wheat of today has nearly 30 percent less minerals. Why is the wheat we eat today less nutritious than before? **Because of GMOs.** Researchers believe that the significant **increase in number of individuals with celiac disease and gluten intolerance is a result of nutritionally bankrupt wheat,** as well as the dramatic increase in its consumption...

Genetically modified foods are literally everywhere in our grocery stores — in raw foods, oils, processed foods and more. **Contrary to what Monsanto tells the public, this**

genetic modification does harm the food quality and nutrition, and puts other crops at risk of contamination. To make matters worse, **the Food and Drug Administration does not require that genetically modified foods to be labeled as such...**

Over 60 countries currently regulate, or ban GMOs, and in this regard, the U.S. desperately lags behind. Genetic modification started under the guise to increase yields, make crops more drought- and disease-tolerant, and enhance nutrition. **While GMOs may increase yields and create more uniform fruits and vegetables, nutrition values and taste dramatically decreased.** In fact, the next time you see an organic "heirloom" tomato in the market, and you dismiss it because it's shaped funny or not bright red, buy one, and just try it. That is the way a tomato is supposed to taste!

Here are percentages of the most common GMO foods today:

Corn: 90 percent GMO
Soy: 94 percent GMO
Canola: 90 percent GMO
Hawaiian papaya: 90 percent GMO
Sugar beets: 95 percent GMO (Dr. Axe).

On July 29, [2016] President Barack Obama signed a bill into law requiring the labeling of food containing genetically modified ingredients, following a drawn-out battle between the food industry and pro-labeling groups on the issue.

As much as 75 percent of the food Americans get at their local supermarket includes genetically modified ingredients, so no matter if you're anti-GMO, pro-GMO, or aren't really sure where you stand on the issue, you'll be affected by the new law in some way....

The USDA has two years to finalize the regulations. The law isn't specific about how long food companies have to start labeling their products after the regulations are finalized, but small producers—defined by the FDA as having less than 500 employees—will have one year longer than larger companies, like, say, Nestle. **Tiny food companies—defined as making less than $1 million in sales per year from human food—will be completely exempt, as will food served in restaurants and other food establishments**, based on the law's language (Modern Farmer. What).

There is obviously a great debate about GMOs that we will not be able to settle here. But a couple of things are certain. First, the alternations in foods via genetic engineering goes far beyond what was possible via selective breeding in Bible times, so GMOs are not natural and would not fully fit with a Creationist Diet.

Second, the use of GMOs is widespread. As such, if you wish to avoid them, you must make a conscious effort to do so.

Third, GMO foods do not currently need to be labeled, though that will change in the near future. In the meantime, by definition, foods labeled "organic" cannot contain GMOs. Thus even for foods that tend not to have much pesticide residue but are generally GMO, like grains, buying organic would still be a good idea.

> **The use of genetic engineering, or genetically modified organisms (GMOs), is prohibited in organic products**. This means an organic farmer can't plant GMO seeds, an organic cow can't eat GMO alfalfa or corn, and an organic soup producer can't use any GMO ingredients.
>
> To meet the USDA organic regulations, farmers and processors must show they aren't using GMOs and that they are protecting their products from contact with prohibited substances from farm to table (USDA; Can GMOs).

There are also "Non-GMO Project Verified" or "Certified Non-GE" labels seen on many foods, whether organic or not. Any of these labels would mean the food does not contain any GMOs.

> **Your best bet right now is to look for foods that carry labels from the Non-GMO Project, A Greener World's Certified Non-GE, or USDA organic labels**. (Modern Farmer. What).

146

Non-GMO Project Verified remains the market leader for GMO avoidance and one of the fastest growing labels in the retail sector. We offer North America's most trusted third-party verification for non-GMO food and products (Non-GMO).

... **A Greener World**—the folks behind the Animal Welfare Approved program, which certifies farms that adhere to strict codes for farm animal welfare, outdoor access, and sustainability—**launched a new non-GMO certification program earlier this month called Certified Non-GE**. The company is joining the space shared by the Non-GMO Project and the USDA's "USDA Process Verified" label, which can include a statement that the product isn't made with GM ingredients. **The USDA organic label also certifies these products are made without GMOs** (Modern Farmer. New).

So look for the USDA Organic, Non-GMO Project Verified, or Certified Non-GE labels when shopping for plant foods. Only foods with at least one of these labels would fully fit with a Creationist Diet.

Bibliography:

Barański, M, et. Al. *British Journal of Nutrition*. 2014 Sep 14;112(5):794-811. doi: 10.1017/S0007114514001366. Epub 2014 Jun 26. Higher antioxidant and lower cadmium concentrations and lower incidence of pesticide residues in organically grown crops: a systematic literature review and meta-analyses.
https://www.ncbi.nlm.nih.gov/pubmed/24968103

Crinnion, Walter J. *Alternative Medicine Review*. "Organic Foods Contain Higher Levels of Certain Nutrients, Lower Levels of Pesticides, and May Provide Health Benefits for the Consumer.
https://www.ncbi.nlm.nih.gov/pubmed/20359265

Decoded Science. Genetically Modified Organisms: Pros and Cons of GMO Food.
https://www.decodedscience.org/gmo-food-pro-and-con/23179

Dr. Axe. 9 Charts That Show Why America is Fat, Sick & Tired.
https://draxe.com/charts-american-diet/

Creationist Diet

Györéné KG, Varga A, Lugasi A *Orv Hetil.* 2006 Oct 29;147(43):2081-90. [A comparison of chemical composition and nutritional value of organically and conventionally grown plant derived foods].
https://www.ncbi.nlm.nih.gov/pubmed/17297755

Healthline. GMOs: Pros and Cons.
http://www.healthline.com/health/gmos-pros-and-cons#Overview1

Modern Farmer. New Non-GMO Label Joins the Fray.
http://modernfarmer.com/2016/05/new-gmo-free-label/

Modern Farmer. What You Need To Know About the New GMO Labeling Law.
http://modernfarmer.com/2016/08/gmo-labeling-law/

Next Galaxy. Disadvantages and Advantages of Genetically Modified Crops.
http://thenextgalaxy.com/disadvantages-and-advantages-of-genetically-modified-crops/

Non-GMO Project. About.
http://www.nongmoproject.org/about/

UMMC (University of Maryland Medical Center). Genetically engineered foods.
http://umm.edu/health/medical/ency/articles/genetically-engineered-foods

USDA. Can GMOs Be Used in Organic Products?
https://www.ams.usda.gov/publications/content/can-gmos-be-used-organic-products

Section Two
Animal Foods

Chapter Six:
Pros and Cons of Meat Eating

As indicated in previous chapters of this book, God initially only gave plant foods to human beings for food. But after the Flood, in the same manner as plant foods, animal foods were given to human beings for food.

Decree About Animal Foods

After the Flood, in Genesis 9:3, God told Noah and his family:

3"And every reptile [or, quadruped] which is living [Heb., **Every moving thing that lives] will be to you* for food. Just as [the] vegetables of vegetation**, I have given all [things] to you*" (ALT).

3"**Every moving thing that lives shall be food for you.** I have given you all things, **even as the green herbs**" (NKJV).

Thus after the Flood, God definitely gives "every moving thing that lives" to humans for food. And it should be noted, this is not a mere "permission" as many try to say. God "gives" animal foods to humans for food in the same manner in which He gave us plant foods. Therefore, just as God intended for human belong to eat plant foods, He now also intends for us to eat animal foods. This intention will be referred to as the Noahic Decree.

What this decree means is, a believer in the Bible cannot say it is wrong to eat animal foods. In order to do so, you would have to say it is also wrong eat plant foods, as God gives the exact same directive for the one as for the other.

To put it another way, if you claim to be a Christian but maintain that it is wrong to eat animal foods, then you are getting your ethics from somewhere other than the Bible. But this writer accepts that:

> The Holy Scriptures, both Old and New Testaments, to be the inspired Word of God, without error in the original manuscripts, the complete revelation of His will for our

151

salvation and the Divine and final authority for all Christian faith and life (Tenet #1 on the Confession of Faith for the author's Darkness to Light ministry).

As such, it cannot be said it is inherently wrong on ethical, spiritual, moral, or health reasons to meat. In other words, if it were immoral or unethical to kill and eat animals, God would not have given animal foods to humans for food, "Just as [the] vegetables of vegetation." If you could attain a higher spiritual state by following a vegan diet, God would not have put animal foods alongside of plant foods as food for humans. And if it were unhealthy to eat animal foods, God would not have told us to eat them, as He only want the best for us.

[11]For I know the thoughts that I think toward you, says the LORD, **thoughts of peace and not of evil, to give you a future and a hope** (Jer. 29:11; NKJV).

Moreover, if eating animal foods were intrinsically wrong, then the following would not have happened in Old Testament times:

[1]Then **GOD appeared to him [Abraham]** by the oak of Mambre, he sitting by himself by the door of his tent at noon. [2]So he lifted up his eyes to see. And look! **Three men had stood above him**; and having seen [them] he ran to a meeting with them from the door of his tent, and prostrated himself in reverence [or, worship] upon the ground. [3]And he said, "Lord, if indeed I found grace in Your sight, You shall not pass by Your bond-servant. [4]Let water now be brought, and let them wash your* feet, and you* refresh [yourselves] under the tree. [5]And I will obtain bread, and you* will eat, and after this you* will pass by on your* journey, on account of which [refreshment] you* have turned aside to your* bond-servant. And they said, "So do, just as you have said."

[6]And Abraham hurried to the tent to Sarah and said to her, "Hurry, and knead three measures of fine wheat flour, and make loaves. [7]**And Abraham ran to the herd, and took a young calf, tender and good, and gave it to his bond-servant, and he quickly made [or, prepared] it. Then he took butter and milk, and the calf which he had made [or, prepared]; and he set [them] before them, and they ate**, but he stood by them under the tree (Gen 18:1-5).

152

The "the three men" are the LORD and two angels (see Genesis 18:33; 19:1). Thus the LORD Himself and these two angels eat butter, milk, and calf meat (beef).

Then Jesus Christ, the Sinless One, eats animal foods and gives it to others to eat. It was prophesied in the Old Testament about the Messiah "Butter and honey He will eat" (Isaiah 7:15). Then in the New Testament, it is recorded that Jesus partook of the Jewish Passover meal, which must include lamb (Exod 12:1-8; Matt 26:17). Jesus multiplied fish for people to eat (Matt 14:17-21; 15:34-39). Jesus ate fish and honey after His resurrection (Luke 24:42), and He cooked and gave fish to His disciples to eat (John 20:13).

Moreover, meat is mentioned 47 times in the Bible and fish 56 times. Various game and domesticated animals are also mentioned, such as lamb 95 times, cattle 59 times, goat 48 times, goats 88 times, gazelle 12 times, antelope twice, and deer 16 times. The context of many of these references are as food (e.g. Deut 12:15-25). Thus food animals have a prominent place in the Bible.

As such, there is no cause for vegetarians to think they are "better" than non-vegetarians. But at the same time, there is no cause for carnivores to think they are better than vegetarians. As Paul writes:

[1]Now be receiving the one being weak in the faith, not for disputes over opinions. [2]One believes [it is permissible] to eat all [things], but the one being weak eats [only] vegetables. [3]**Stop letting the one eating despise [or, look down on] the one not eating; and stop letting the one not eating judge the one eating, for God [has] accepted him**....

[16]So stop letting your good be slandered [or, be spoken of as evil]. [17]**For the kingdom of God is not eating and drinking, but righteousness and peace and joy in [the] Holy Spirit** (Rom 14:1-3,16).

[8]But food does not present [or, commend] us to God, for **neither if we eat do we excel [or, are we better off]; nor if we do not eat do we fall short [or, are we inferior]** (1Cor 8:8).

And the writer to the Hebrews says:

[9]"Stop being carried away by varied and strange teachings, for [it is] good [for] the heart to continue **being established by grace, not by foods**, in which the ones having been walking about [in] [fig., having been occupied with] were not benefited" (Heb 13:9).

The point is, what someone eats or does not eat in no way makes them a better person than someone else who does the opposite. I say all of this as very often vegans and vegetarians have an arrogant attitude, thinking they are superior morally, ethically, or spiritually than non-vegetarians, but such attitudes are unbiblically and should not characterize a Christian.

However, despite this clear Biblical evidence, today's vegetarians try to make a case for avoiding animal foods based on differences between how animals are treated and how animal foods are produced today versus in Biblical times. As Dr. Russell writes, "Preparation and contamination of meat, however, present real problems for the meat eater today" (p.34).

Before continuing, it would be good to define some terms that will be important as we proceed.

Terminology

The term "factory farm" is defined as, "a large industrialized farm; especially: a farm on which large numbers of livestock are raised indoors in conditions intended to maximize production at minimal cost" (Merriam Webster).

In other words, this term refers to the modern-day method of raising farm animals. Usually, animals like cattle are kept indoors, in stalls, with little or no room to move around, and are fed soy, corn, or other grains. Animals like chicken or turkeys are kept in cages, with no room to roam, and are fed a purely vegetarian diet of soy, corn, and other grains. Animal foods derived from such farming methods will be referred to as "factory farm" or "commercial" meats, dairy, or eggs.

This is contrasted with what will be called "old-fashioned farming." With this farming method, weather permitting, cattle are kept outdoors, with room to roam and graze on their natural diet of grasses and other greens. Chicken or turkeys have room to roam and have access to the ground, so that they can peck at the ground as they eat, consuming their natural diet of plant based foods mixed with bugs. Meats and other animal foods derived from such farming methods will be referred to "old-fashioned" or "traditional" meats, dairy, or eggs. As we will see, these could also be called Biblical or God-given animal foods.

The import of this distinction between factory farms and the animal foods derived therefrom and old-fashioned farms and their products will be seen as we proceed. I will first present the arguments of vegans and vegetarians against animal foods based on factory farming. I will then discuss how old-fashioned farming would alleviate these concerns. Along the way, I will also point out other fallacies in vegan arguments.

Note: In this chapter, only whole meats, meaning steak, roast, whole chicken pieces, and the like, will be under discussion. Other forms of meats will be addressed in Chapter Eight.

Health Considerations

Animals in factory farms are fattened today in ways that would exceed even the "fatted calf" of Biblical times. And it should be noted that the fatted calf was only eaten on "special" occasions (see Luke 15:23,24). But today, such fatty meat is available on a regular basis.

Dr. Russell writes in this regard:

Unfortunately, the fact that consumers in the past seemed to like and want more fat in their meat promoted the meat industry to use such methods as selective breeding, overfeeding, and chemical stimulation (hormones) to make animals grow bigger and faster.

Overfeeding results in excessively fat animals. If pen raised, an animal's fat content raises considerably. Wild turkeys contain 3 to 5 percent fat, versus 30 to 40 percent in domesticated turkey. Pen-fed cattle contain 40 percentage fat, versus 5 to 8 percentage in grass-fed longhorn and some other breeds of cattle.

Moreover, concerns could be raised about hormones and antibiotics given to livestock. The former is linked to earlier onset of menstruation among girls, and the latter to increased resistance to antibiotics in bacteria, and increased allergic reactions to drugs in humans (Russell, p.75).

155

In the last paragraph, Dr. Russell raises the concern about toxic residues found in factory farm animal foods today. Note the statement about hormones given to animals causing "earlier onset of menstruation among girls." Girls used to start menstruating when they were around 14-16 years old. Now, it is more like 10-12, or even younger. And this earlier sexual maturity among girls is having profound societal implications when these young girls with women's bodies get pregnant.

An article in the June 2006 issue of *Earth Save News* is titled, "How foul is fowl?" It states:

> **The fat and protein content of a bird depends in large part upon its diet and activity level**. (Heard that one before?) Wild birds are generally much leaner, and therefore, lower in fat and higher in protein. Meat breeds are chickens developed for their quick growth—heavy with fat and muscle—they are mass produced specifically to be eaten. The fat and cholesterol in fowl permeate its flesh; they cannot be cut away. Birds and bird parts with a lower fat content are by nature higher in protein. **Excess protein is as damaging to health as is excess fat—causing kidney stones, loss of kidney function, osteoporosis, and cancers** (lymphomas). **You will hardly find a "micro-spec" of dietary fiber or carbohydrate in a bird carcass** (p.3).

Comments about the fat and cholesterol content of factory farm poultry will be made shortly. But here, notice how this article repeats the myth that a high protein diet is damaging to the kidney and bones and causes cancer. The previous chapter warned that such myths are still being repeated by vegan advocates, even though they have been disproved.

Otherwise, of course, there is not fiber or carbohydrates in chicken. But that is why the Creationist Diet includes copious amounts of fruits, vegetable, and other plant foods that contain such. Again, you do not need to be a vegetarian to consume copious amounts of vegetables and other plant foods. As for toxic residues:

The different types of drug residues found in beef can be broken down into five general categories: antimicrobials (antibiotics and sulfonamides), anti-inflammatories, growth promotants, anti-parasitic and insecticides, and analgesics and tranquilizers. According to a survey of members of the American Association of Bovine Practitioners (AABP), the drugs most commonly used by practitioners for dairy cows were antibiotics, followed by anti-inflammatories, tranquilizers and analgesics....

Drugs used for growth promotion are another source of residues in meat and poultry....

Non-steroidal anti-inflammatories (NSAID), such as aspirin, dipyrone, flunixin, phenylbutazone, are commonly used drags which can be found as residues in foods of animal origin....

Dewormers and other antiparasitic drags have also been found as residues in animal foods....

Insecticides may enter food animals either intentionally or unintentionally. According to the results of surveys on feeds, pesticide residues do inadvertently get into forages (14) and feeds (41), and can bioaccumulate when consumed.

Residues have many implications for public health: there is the possibility of direct reaction to the residues (toxic, anaphylaxic, etc.); there is the likelihood of developing drug-resistant strains of bacteria both in the food supply and in the gut; and the presence of residues in the human body may have legal as well as physical implications (Kaneene).

Thus factory farm animals foods can be a source of toxic residues, and these residues can have adverse effects on those who eat these foods and on society in general.

On another issue, the Center for Science in the Public Interest claimed back in 1999:

Keep in mind that **animal foods account for the lion's share of food poisoning**. That means you have to handle raw meat, seafood, poultry, and eggs as though they were contaminated (*Nutrition Action*, October, 1999, p.3).

This might have been the case back before the turn of the century, and the first well-publicized case of food poisoning I remember was in 1993 involving Jack in the Box ground meat. And that is still considered to be one of the "Worst Foodborne Illness Outbreaks in U.S. History." Since then, other animal foods on the list of worse foodborne illnesses include cheese, milk, turkey, and ground turkey. But also on the list are events involving jalapeño peppers, three bean salad, strawberries, green onions, baby spinach, lettuce, tomatoes, and peppers. Deaths were reported in many of these cases (Healthline; Worst).

What this means is, any food can be contaminated with food borne illnesses, and that includes both plant and animal foods. Thus the advice to handle all raw animal foods as if it is contaminated would also apply to plant foods. All vegetables and other produce should be thoroughly washed. But to use the possibility of food poisoning as an argument against eating animal foods is disingenuous. Such an argument could just as easily be used against eating raw produce.

Health Care Costs

Vegans claim there are health care costs associated with the eating of animal foods. For instance, a study using 1992 dollars quantified these costs for the USA:

Direct health care costs attributable to meat consumption are estimated to be +2.8-8.5 billion for **hypertension**, +9.5 billion for **heart disease**, +0-16.5 billion for **cancer**, +14.0-17.1 billion for **diabetes**, +0.2-2.4 billion for **gallbladder disease**, +1.9 billion for **obesity-related musculoskeletal disorders**, and +0.2-5.5 billion for **foodborne illness. The total direct medical costs attributable to meat consumption for 1992 are estimated at +28.6-61.4 billion** (Barnard ND, Nicholson A, Howard JL).

An article in the *New York Times* back in 1995 discussed this study. It was titled, "Health Cost of Meat Diet Is Billions, Study Says." The article went on to claim:

A GROUP of doctors, after reviewing earlier studies of meat consumption and disease, has published a report arguing that the yearly national health care costs of eating meat are comparable to the estimated **$50 billion spent each year** to treat illnesses related to smoking.

Given the increased health risks associated with eating the type of meat produced today, there are quantifiable, financial health care costs to individuals and society from meat eating....

The authors of the analysis, Dr. Neal D. Barnard, Dr. Andrew Nicholson and Jo Lil Howard, are all members of the Physicians Committee for Responsible Medicine, **an organization in Washington that promotes vegetarianism**. They linked regular consumption of red meat and poultry, in particular, to significant increases in the risks of developing high blood pressure, heart disease, diabetes, gallbladder disease, overweight and resulting osteoarthritis, food poisoning and cancers of the colon, lung, ovary and prostate (Brody).

The article goes on to detail that the authors mainly looked at studies involving Mormons and Seventh Day Adventists, comparing those who eat meat with those that don't, and they tried to account for confounding factors like exercise and smoking. But it is impossible to account for all such factors. This is why the article also states, "A spokesman for the American Medical Association, however, said he had 'very serious reservations' about the methods used to come to those conclusions.

The point being, each one of the claimed health effects would need to be investigated one by one, and all possible confounding factors allotted for. And that is very difficult to do.

Dr. Roy M. Schwarz, group vice president for professional standards of the American Medical Association, said **the study did not specify whether factors like age, sex and genetic** history of the people covered in the studies had been taken into account. All such factors could affect health.

"I just have a very difficult time believing that they have controlled for all these different factors," Dr. Schwarz said, adding that he could not reach the same conclusions as the authors of the paper on the basis of evidence they had presented (Brody).

And this author would add additional confounding factors, such as have been mentioned previously and will be discussed shortly. The point is, even though this is an old article, vegetarians continue to make these same types of claims. For instance, an article titled "The Cost of Eating Animals" and published January 6th, 2014 claims:

In the U.S. and other developed countries, eating animals is one of the most significant risk factors found in nearly all of the most common diseases. It is, therefore, heavily implicated in rising health care costs, health insurance premiums, foods prices, and even labor costs for businesses. Those who eat animals are driving up all these costs while driving down productivity.

More than $3 trillion dollars were spent on health care in 2012 ($2.83 trillion in 2009, growing at 6 percent per year) in the U.S.

Of that, minimally $130 billion dollars spent were due to dietary choices related to livestock. I believe this figure is quite conservative and could be as high as $350 billion due to eating animals (Oppenlander).

But in making such claims, vegetarians are making many assumptions that might not be true, and they are not controlling for all possible confounding factors.

Ethical Considerations

The next concern is the treatment of animals in factory farms. John Robbins writes on EarthSave's website:

Factory farms were conceived with the express purpose of producing the most meat, milk and eggs as quickly and cheaply as possible, in the smallest amount of space possible with as little labor as possible. In this pursuit, animals are treated as simple units of production, and are physically and genetically manipulated to accelerate and maximize yield. Turkeys are now so top-heavy they can hardly stand. Pigs are too long to support their own weight. Chickens have their beaks seared off with hot blades so they don't slay their cage-mates. Dairy cows are impregnated repeatedly to keep the milk flowing. **To stave off illness and hasten growth, animals are dosed with a pharmacopoeia of drugs** (*Factory Farm Alarm*).

Another article in the June 2006 issue of *Earth Save News* is titled, "Meat-industrial complex: How factory farms undercut public health." It states:

Drive through Don Oppliger's Feed Yard in Clovis, New Mexico, and you'll see 35,000 head of beef cattle confined to pens that stretch across the flat, barren landscape. **The constant shuffling of hooves raises a bacteria-laden dust cloud that's carried by the prevailing winds into west Texas**, where it joins the plumes of hundreds of other feedlots. At one end of the complex sits **a giant lagoon that catches the operation's chemicals, urine, antibiotics and other effluvia**. In the narrow strip of land that separates the fencing from the road lie the carcasses of dead cows (a.k.a. "downers"), eyes bugged out, tongues dangling and bellies bloated in the summer heat.

Moving from bovine to porcine, **factory hog farms generate an odor so intense** it would knock a buzzard off a #$%@wagon. In cramped warehouse structures, as many as 20,000 hogs are confined for their entire lives. After five months, the mature hogs are sent off to the slaughterhouse to have their throats slit and carcasses dipped in chemical vats to loosen their skins. According to Anita Poole, legal counsel for the Oklahoma-based Kerr Center, which has fought that state's takeover by the hog industry, "The average Joe Blow who

161

might stumble into a hog facility would never want to eat pork again" (p.1).

This is obviously very inflammatory language, designed to turn people off of eating meat. I even had to delete out the foul language. But it does make a point. The lives of animals in factory farms is not very pleasant, to say the least.

Environmental Considerations

There are also environmental problems associated with factory farms. Of particular concern is the pollution created by the large amount of waste produced by farm animals.

John Robbins gives the following statistics:
- **Huge livestock farms are generating an estimated five tons of animal manure for every person in the US**, says Iowa Senator Tom Harkin.
- In one day, a single **hog farm** produces the raw waste of a city of 12,000 people. In 1997, North Carolina's hogs are expected to produce as much waste as roughly five times the state's human population.
- In one year, **a massive egg farm** yields enough manure to fill 1,400 dump trucks.
- **Poultry farms** in Arkansas alone produce 5,100 tons of manure each day.
- The 1,600 **dairy farms** in California's Central Valley generate more waste than 21 million people (*Factory Farm Alarm*).

An article on Farm Sanctuary states:
With over nine billion animals raised and slaughtered for human consumption each year in the U.S. alone, **modern animal agriculture puts an incredible strain on natural resources like land, water, and fossil fuel**. Factory farms yield a relatively small amount of meat, dairy, and eggs for this input, and in return **produce staggering quantities of**

waste and greenhouse gases, polluting our land, air, and water and contributing to climate change.

In the U.S. alone, animals raised on **factory farms generate more than 1 million tons of manure per day** — three times the amount generated by the country's human population.

Factory farms typically store animal waste in huge, open-air lagoons, often as big as several football fields, which are prone to leaks and spills....

During digestion, ruminants like cattle, sheep, and goats emit methane, an infamous "greenhouse gas" and key contributor to global warming....

In order to prevent the spread of disease in the crowded, filthy conditions of confinement operations, and to promote faster growth, producers feed farm animals a number of antibiotics. Upwards of 75 percent of the antibiotics fed to farm animals end up undigested in their urine and manure. **Through this waste, the antibiotics may contaminate crops and waterways and ultimately be ingested by humans** (Farm Sanctuary).

There are thus real concerns about the environmental impact of factory farms.

World Hunger

Vegetarians claim that not eating animal foods will eliminate world hunger. An article on Down to Earth is titled, "World Hunger Can Be Solved with Vegetarian Diet." It states:

> **Simply put, the more people eat meat, the fewer people can be fed. For example, over 10 pounds of plant protein are used to produce one pound of beef protein.** If these grains were fed to humans instead of animals, more food would be available for the **925 million people in chronic hunger worldwide**. Research from Cornell University, of the United States, found that **the grain used to feed livestock in the United States alone could feed 800 million people**....

There is more than enough food in the world to feed the entire human population. So, why are more than one billion people still going hungry every day? **The meat-based diet is largely to blame.** We cycle huge amounts of grain, soybeans, and corn through animals killed for food rather than directly feed starving people. If we stopped intensively breeding farmed animals and grew crops to feed people instead, we could easily feed everyone on the planet with healthy and affordable vegetarian foods.

Similarly, an article on Gentle World titled "Could Veganism End World Hunger?" states:

It is estimated that **a staggering 925 million humans around the world are suffering from the effects of hunger** (mostly in the poor and underdeveloped countries of Asia and Africa), and out of that original number, 870 million arc affected with malnutrition…. Every year, starvation claims the lives of over 2.5 million children under the age of five….

Cows (and the other animals we eat) are poor converters when it comes to turning food into energy and muscle, which is why **it takes anywhere from 13 to 20 pounds of grain-fed to a cow to produce just 1 pound of muscle mass, i.e. beef.** This means that 13-20 times as many people could be fed if those grains were simply eaten by humans. Likewise, **it takes around seven pounds of grain to produce one pound of pork, and 4.5 pounds of grain to produce one pound of chicken**….

These arguments sound logical. And in fact, it was arguments like this that led this writer to cease to consume red meat back in college. But at that time the statistic was that it takes 16 pounds of plant foods to produce one pound of beef, but only three pounds of plant foods to produce one pound of chicken, so I continued to eat chicken.

However, what I didn't realize back then was this line of reasoning presents a very naïve attitude towards the world hunger problem. Both of these articles admit, "it has been proven that there is enough food on earth to feed every last man, woman, and child" (Gentle). But the conclusions they draw from this fact are fallacious. The world hunger problem is not due to a massive amount of food being fed to animals but due to the affluent overconsuming and wasting food.

At stake are also tenacious problems of overconsumption and the inequitable commandeering of global resources, neither of which will be solved merely by passing the braised tofu.
In the name of "growth," that capitalist holy cow, **a smaller number of people consume far more than their share of essential resources.** Wealth concentration generates disparate purchasing power that allows **richer nations as well as the better-off in every nation to consume – and waste – a disproportionate share of food, fuel, water and other resources.** Arable land itself is put towards profit through speculation, mining and logging, rather than feeding people. The predictable argument that overpopulation is the main problem remains a red herring. **When one person can consume or waste between two and five people's share at a time when per-capita food production has increased, inequity, not human numbers, and the richer, not the poorer, are still the problem.**
Overconsumption and the corporatisation of food supply chains also underwrite the factory farming responsible for unconscionable levels of animal suffering and the depletion of marine ecosystems. **When they can afford to do so at all, the poor have eaten meat sustainably and relatively humanely through small numbers of livestock or by fishing in limited quantities** (Guardian).

This writer disagrees with the anti-capitalistic attitude of this article, and elsewhere it recommends a near vegetarian diet. But it does make a good point—the world food problem is one of distribution, not of eating meat or of an inadequate production of food. As such, the solutions lie in the affluent not overconsuming and wasting food and in improving the economic lot of those in poor countries.
On the first point of the affluent overconsuming food, that should be obvious to anyone who just looks at a crowd of Americans. Two-thirds are overweight or obese.

On the second point, consider the following:

With **an estimated 70 billion pounds of food waste in America each year**, we must work together to capture more of this valuable resource for the **nearly 42 million people in the United States who feel the effects of food insecurity**.

Food Waste Statistics:

- An estimated **25 – 40% of food grown, processed and transported in the US will never be consumed**.
- **When food is disposed in a landfill it rots and becomes a significant source of methane - a potent greenhouse gas** with 21 times the global warming potential of carbon dioxide.
- **More food reaches landfills and incinerators than any other single material in municipal solid waste** (Feeding America).

This report provides the latest estimates by USDA's Economic Research Service (ERS) on **the amount and value of food loss in the United States**. These estimates are for more than 200 individual foods using ERS's Loss-Adjusted Food Availability data. In 2010, **an estimated 31 percent or 133 billion pounds of the 430 billion pounds of food produced was not available for human consumption at the retail and consumer levels**. This amount of loss totaled an estimated $161.6 billion, as purchased at retail prices. For the first time, ERS estimates of the calories associated with food loss are presented in this report. **An estimated 141 trillion calories per year, or 1,249 calories per capita per day, in the food supply in 2010 went uneaten**. The top three food groups in terms of share of total value of food loss are meat, poultry, and fish (30 percent); vegetables (19 percent); and dairy products (17 percent). The report also provides a brief discussion of the economic issues behind postharvest food loss (USDA; Estimated).

Americans waste an unfathomable amount of food. In fact, according to a Guardian report released this week, roughly

50 percent of all produce in the United States is thrown away—some 60 million tons (or $160 billion) worth of produce annually, an amount constituting "one third of all foodstuffs." **Wasted food is also the single biggest occupant in American landfills**, the Environmental Protection Agency has found.

What causes this? **A major reason is that food is cheaper in the United States than nearly anywhere else in the world, aided (controversially) by subsidies to corn, wheat, milk, and soybeans**. But the great American squandering of produce appears to be a cultural dynamic as well, **enabled in large part by a national obsession with the aesthetic quality of food**. Fruits and vegetables, in addition to generally being healthful, have a tendency to bruise, brown, wilt, oxidize, ding, or discolor and that is apparently something American shoppers will not abide. **For an American family of four, the average value of discarded produce is nearly $1,600 annually**. (Globally, the United Nations Food and Agriculture Organization estimates that **one-third of all food grown is lost or wasted**, an amount valued at nearly $3 trillion.) (Atlantic).

To comment, note in the first quote that not only is wasted food contributing to world hunger, but it is contributing to global warming.

On the last quote, note the mention of subsidies. In some cases, these subsidies are to pay farmers to not to grow crops. Yes, the US government pays farmers to not to grow corn, wheat, and the like. This is done to keep the prices of these grains from falling too low. But what it means is that we are capable of producing far more food than we already are.

Note also the reference to aesthetics. Americans will not buy or eat food that does not look good, even though it is perfectly fine to eat. And that simple aversion leads to great food losses. But there are ways to solve this problem.

A staggering 30-to-40 percent of the United States food supply goes to waste and nearly half of it is household food that end up in landfills.

Although most people are aware of the issues of food waste, we fall short with impactful solutions. **Individuals and**

families can make a difference by making choices that reduce waste at home. Plan meals ahead of time and grocery shop for only what you will need and use. Prepare perishable foods soon after buying. Store foods properly to prevent them from spoiling too soon. These are just a few strategies to reduce your own food waste.

Considering the mounting issue of food waste, some innovative companies are creating unique solutions to combat the challenge of food waste in business and on farms. Zero Percent makes it easy for the food service industry to donate surplus foods. Imperfect Produce is a produce home delivery service that sells fruits and vegetables that don't meet grocery stores' cosmetic standards and are totally fine to eat, but would otherwise be thrown out (Los Angeles).

Finally, the problem of poor countries not being able to produce sufficient food for themselves is best solved through capitalism. When their economic states improve, they will be able to improve their own food situation through improved food production methods.

Bottom line of all of this is this—eating a vege-burger rather than a hamburger might make you feel better, but it will not help to feed a single hungry person. Such is a case of "symbolism over substance." If you are truly concerned about world hunger, it will take getting involved on your part to help to solve it.

Donating your time and money to local food bank would be a good place to start. Or better, start a business and employ unemployed poor people. They will then have the money to purchase their own food.

Globally, about 800 million people suffer malnourishment. That's a staggering figure. But only ten years ago the total was almost 1 billion. **A drop of nearly 200 million in the number of chronically hungry people should encourage anyone committed to ending global hunger. It can be done**....

Global hunger is a "wicked problem." It cannot be easily solved. **No one solution works in every instance. It is connected to many other complex problems such as poverty, inequality, conflict, poor health and so on. Ending hunger is not all about providing more food** (CRS).

This article on the website for Catholic Relief Services goes on to outline the various activities they are involved in to try to end world hunger. The subtitles are: Agriculture, Microfinance, Education, Partnership, Peacebuilding. All of these and many other areas need to be addressed, while not eating meat will do nothing to solve the crisis.

The Old-Fashioned Farm Alterative

As can be seen, many of the arguments by vegetarians as to why we should all become vegetarians do not hold water. But I left some of their claims un-responded to so I could respond to them together here.

The response was hinted at in the First Edition of this book when I quoted Rex Russell, MD as saying:

> Therefore, **I recommend eating only meat from cattle that are raised without hormones, antibiotics, or pesticides.** This means we don't need to eat meat to survive; but if we do eat meat, it would be better if it were **range-fed, organic, chemical free-meat** (p.75).

However, I went on to say, "The problem is, of course, finding such meat." I said that as back in 2000, I was not aware of anywhere to purchase such meats in the Pittsburgh, PA area where I live. But since then I have found out there are many such places, as there is in just about anywhere else in the USA.

The first such place I discovered was Pounds' Turkey Farm, located in Leechburg, PA, which also sells beef and chicken. The home page of their website (www.poundsturkeyfarm.com) states:

> Nestled in the northern-most tip of Westmoreland County (PA), at Pounds' Turkey Farm **we've been offering Farm Fresh Thanksgiving and Christmas turkeys for 80 years**. While the fresh turkeys remain a local favorite, we have also developed an extensive line of turkey products made right at the farm. … Our year 'round market also offers Chicken, Our Own Beef & more.

Notice that they have been in business for 80 years. Therefore, it was due to my ignorance that I did not know about this source for old-fashioned meats back in 2000. Their "About the Farm" page states:

> **Specializing in raising turkeys the old fashioned way**, we provide delicious farm fresh turkeys for the Thanksgiving and Christmas holidays… In addition to our holiday turkeys, we make more than 60 turkey products here on the farm….
>
> **A herd of 35 Angus cattle and their yearly offspring provide our customers with tender and delicious all natural beef**. We have recently improved our grazing system, pastures, fencing and watering systems.

Note the phrase "the old-fashioned way." How they raise their animals is nothing new—it is how humans raised animals ever since animals were first domesticated by humans, which started with Abel (Gen 4:2), up until the rise of factory farms in the 1950s. That is why the term "old-fashioned" is being in used this book to refer to such farms and their products.

Then an article titled "A Brief Overview of Our Farming Philosophy & Practices – Re: Turkey Flocks" describes how Pounds' turkeys are treated.

> **Our flocks are raised in large open air coops, with daily access to fresh air, sunshine, cool water and feed**. They are however protected from severe weather and natural predators. We clean the coops, including our feed and water systems frequently, and Tim & Rick Pounds, along with **our employees are in the coops observing and managing the flocks for hours each day**…
>
> **Our turkeys have all the benefits of the outdoors, from wind to bugs to rain, but are safe and sound in their spacious coops**….
>
> Our All-Natural Turkey label indicates that **our flocks have been raised with no antibiotics and no growth promotants**.

Several points should be noted in this paragraph. First, note their animals have access to "fresh air, sunshine, cool water and feed" but are protected from the weather and predators. They are thus better off than wild turkeys. Second, the open-air coops are large, so the turkeys have room to roam.

Third, and because of point two, with the room to roam, the animals do not become unnaturally fat. And the avoidance of growth promotants also prevents the birds from becoming unnaturally fat. Consequently, the meat is low in fat. Maybe not as low as wild turkeys, but that is only because of the hard life wild turkeys lead.

Fourth, and also because of point two, the turkeys are raised without antibiotics. I say this as the reason antibiotics are routinely given to factory farm raised animals is because of the way they are packed in, but if they are not so packed in, then widespread use of antibiotics is not needed.

To explain, due to the very close living quarters in factory farms, if one animal gets sick, the disease will spread quickly throughout the flock or herd. This could easily happen before the initial sick animal is detected, as the crowded conditions and massive flocks or herds make monitoring each animal nearly impossible. As a result, antibiotics are given proactively to prevent an epidemic.

One of the major reasons farmers are using more antibiotics is that demand for meat is going up, and **animals are being confined in smaller and smaller living quarters, which can increase the spread of disease**. Antibiotic resistance not only applies to the animals, but it can affect the humans eating the meat (Eat Wild; Notes).

But in small operations like Pounds', the animals are not so cramped together. Therefore, a disease is not likely to spread quickly through the flock or herd, and a sick animal can be detected and removed before it infects the others. This possibility of detection is indicated by Pound's saying their employers are "observing and managing the flocks for hours each day."

What this means is, if you see the phrase "antibiotic-free" on the label of an animal food, that is an indication the animal was raised humanly. And that eliminates two of the objections of vegetarians to animal foods, that of toxic residues and that of the mistreatment of farm animals.

171

Finally, the turkeys are not given growth hormones, thus further eliminating the objections of toxic residues.

I also purchase meats and dairy products at Pittsburgh's East End Food Co-op (www.eastendfood.coop). All animal products it sells are from small, local farms in which the animals are pasture raised and/ or grass-fed. I learned how cattle are raised in such farms from watching the former TV show *Living Beyond Organic* on TBN.

The practice is as follows: the farmer's field is divided into three parts by fencing. Let's label them Field A, Field B, and Field C for convenience. Weather permitting, the cattle are kept outside in Field A. They have access to fresh air and sunshine and room to roam, but most of all, to their natural diet of grasses and other greens.

The pasture area is fenced in to keep the cattle from roaming off and to protect them from predators. Again, their life is better than what it would be in the wild.

However, by restricting the pasture area somewhat, the cows get the impression that their grazing area is limited. They thus eat faster, fearing the cow next to them will eat their portion, so this is a natural way of fattening up cattle, with no growth hormones needed. But the cattle are not so packed together as to cause a need for proactive antibiotics or to cause them to become overly fat, which in turn keeps the meat relatively lean. Again, not as lean as in wild animals, but not near as fatty as factory farm meat.

As the cattle graze, they leave droppings, which is to say manure. But unlike factory farms where manure is considered a waste product that must be removed and dumped elsewhere, causing environmental damage, here the manure is left on the ground as natural fertilizer.

Once the cattle have eaten the grass to the round in Field A, they are moved to Field B. Then Field A is left fallow, allowing the grass to grow back being naturally fertilized by the manure, with no artificial fertilizer necessary. The land is watered naturally by rain or irrigation. Therefore, it is a self-contained ecosystem, with no outside intervention needed.

When the cattle graze the grass to the ground in Field B, they are moved to Field C. By the time that field is grazed to the ground, the grass in Field A has grown back. The cattle are then moved back to that field, and the process repeats.

This process is not new; it is how cattle were raised for millennia, before the invention of factory farms. And with this old-fashioned method, there is no need for antibiotics, growth hormones, or the use of grains that humans consume. There are no waste products that need to be discarded. The animals are humanely raised, and the land is used in a productive manner.

In addition, due to the consumption of their natural diet of grasses and other greens, the cattle do not emit as much methane gas as they do in factory farms. The reason for that problem is the cattle in factory farms are being fed an unnatural diet of grains that their digestive systems were not designed to digest. But worse, grains are not the only unnatural items fed to factory farm animals.

Fresh pasture and dried grasses are the natural diet of all ruminant animals. In factory farms, animals are switched to an unnatural diet based on corn and soy. But corn and soy are not the only ingredients in their "balanced rations." **Many large-scale dairy farmers and feedlot operators save money by feeding the cows "by-product feedstuffs" as well**. In general, this means waste products from the manufacture of human food. In particular, it can mean **sterilized city garbage, candy, bubble gum, floor sweepings from plants that manufacture animal food, bakery, potato wastes or a scientific blend of pasta and candy** (Eat Wild. Notes).

This source also notes that often the candy and bakery items are fed to the animals still wrapped. Needless to say, God did not design cattle to eat such "by-product feedstuffs." As a result, the cattle burp and fart a lot, emitting lots of methane gas.

Conversely, with the consumption of their natural diet of greens, the burping and farting is kept to a minimum and thus so is the methane emissions. As a result, there is minimal environmental damage from old-fashioned farms. In fact, old-fashioned farms can actually be good for the environment:

- **Organic grassfed beef production creates far fewer GHG (greenhouse gas) emissions** than conventional/feedlot beef production.

- Skilled management of cattle on grass can **draw CO2 (carbon dioxide) down from the atmosphere** and deposit it in pastures as (SOC) soil organic carbon....

Although all cattle produce greenhouse gasses, the UCS (Union for Concerned Scientists) has determined that **a well-maintained pasture and careful management of the grazing animals can draw greenhouse gasses out of the air and store them in the soil where they fuel plant growth**. The overall impact is positive. Feedlots [in factory farms] have no living plants – just bare dirt and manure; instead of absorbing greenhouse gasses, they emit them (Eat Wild Notes).

Lastly, a study by Consumer Report's found a significant difference between factory farm and grass-fed beef in regards to food poisoning. Note that "conventionally raised" means in a factory farm.

A landmark, October 2015 study by Consumer Reports is the largest study to date showing that **choosing grass-fed meat over conventional meat will reduce your risk of food poisoning and result in fewer antibiotic-resistant bacteria**.

They tested 300 samples of beef purchased at stores across the United States and determined that **beef from conventionally raised cows was three times as likely as grass-fed beef to contain bacteria resistant to multiple antibiotics**, posing a food poisoning threat.

"One of the most significant findings of our research," declared Consumer Reports, "is that beef from conventionally raised cows was more likely to have bacteria overall, as well as bacteria that are resistant to antibiotics, than beef from sustainably raised cows" (Eat Wild. Notes).

All of this together means the objections of vegetarians to the consumption of meats and other animals foods simply do not apply to old-fashioned farms.

And such farms are not unique. They are very common and getting more so every day. A database on Eat Wild's website will enable the reader to find such a farm in your area (www.eatwild.com). A similar source for animal products from animals raised in a humane manner is Humaneitarian's website (www.humaneitarian.org).

The second site lists other label terms to look for in addition to "Antibiotic-free" that indicate the animal was raised in a humane manner. They are: Grass-fed, Pasture-raised, Free-range, Pastured, Certified Humane, and Organic. There are technical distinctions between these terms, with some having more definitive definitions than others:

Grass-fed:

The American Grassfed Association defines grassfed products from ruminants, including cattle, bison, goats and sheep, as those food products from animals that **have eaten nothing but their mother's milk and fresh grass or grass-type hay from birth to harvest** – all their lives. They are also **raised with no confinement and no antibiotics or hormones**, and must be born and raised in the U.S.

For grassfed non-ruminants, including pigs and poultry, grass is a significant part of their diets, but not the entirety of their diets, since these animals may need to consume something other than forage. **The USDA defines grassfed as ruminant animals fed solely on grass and forage from weaning to harvest with no confinement during the growing season.** AGA has developed a certification program and our own set of stringent grassfed standards (American Grassfed).

Pasture-raised:

Pasture-raised animals receive a significant portion of their nutrition from organically managed pasture and stored dried forages. Unlike 100% grass-fed cows, pasture-raised cows may receive supplemental organic grains, both during the grazing season and into winter months. Our co-op wide pasture requirements specify that all cows must have a minimum of 120 days on pasture during the grazing season, and they must have outdoor access to pasture year-round. **They may be brought indoors because of severe weather and for the daily milking.**

175

Supplemental organic grains can include any of the following: corn, soy, oats, barley, triticale and other small grains. Animals also receive necessary mineral supplements that sometimes include non-iodized salt (Organic Valley).

Free Range:

"Free range" does have an official definition: "Producers must demonstrate to the Agency that the poultry has been allowed access to the outside."

The definition of "outside," though, is shaky; does that mean there's a window chickens could theoretically squeeze through? Do the birds actually go through it? And **outside could be a gorgeous rolling hill or it could be ... a parking lot**. Some producers include a fenced-in section of open concrete in their grow-out houses, with enough room for maybe 5 percent of the thousands of chickens in that house, and this may technically satisfy the term. (Although Mr. Kastel is seeing indications that the Obama administration may crack down on this.)

Chef Schneller noted, though, that **not all operations are cynical. "The chickens might have more space, access to sunshine**. They won't be foraging, though, so it's not a taste or nutrition issue. It might be more humane" (Salon, ellipse in original).

Pastured:

What some producers and farmers call "pastured" chicken is much more in line what with many people think they're getting with free range. This means that the birds are actually kept in coops at night, but are **left to forage on grass, seeds, worms, etc., during the day**. They might be fed grain as well, but they have access to a greater variety of food in their diet, and **the result is much more richly flavored meat and eggs — and a much more humane life for the birds**. It's also much more expensive to raise chickens this way, because of the amount of space required and how that limits how many chickens you might be able to raise at a time. What's more, chickens can quickly turn a field into a moonscape with their pecking, so **true pastured chickens will often be moved around a very large pasture as areas they've torn up need time to regrow.**

Unfortunately, "pastured" isn't a legal term yet, so consumers have to do their own research on the brands that use this label (Salon).

Certified Humane:

The Certified Humane Raised and Handled® label assures consumers that:

- The producer meets our Animal Care Standards and applies them to farm animals, from birth through slaughter.
- **Animals are never kept in cages, crates, or tie stalls. Animals must be free to do what comes naturally.** For example, chickens must be able to flap their wings and dust bathe, and pigs must have space to move around and root.
- **Animals be fed a diet of quality feed, without animal by-products, antibiotics or growth hormones.**
- Producers must comply with food safety and environmental regulations. Processors must comply with the American Meat Institute Standards (AMI), a slaughter standard written by Dr. Temple Grandin, a member of HFAC's Scientific Committee (Certified Humane).

Organic:

The USDA National Organic Program (NOP) defines organic as follows:

Organic food is produced by farmers who emphasize the use of renewable resources and the conservation of soil and water to enhance environmental quality for future generations. Organic meat, poultry, eggs, and dairy products come from animals that are given **no antibiotics or growth hormones.** Organic food is produced without using most conventional pesticides; fertilizers made with synthetic ingredients or sewage sludge; bioengineering; or ionizing radiation. Before a product can be labeled "organic," a Government-approved certifier inspects the farm where the food is grown to make sure the farmer is following all the rules

177

necessary to meet USDA organic standards. Companies that handle or process organic food before it gets to your local supermarket or restaurant must be certified, too (Organic.org).

Thus, any of these terms will tell you the animal was not raised in a factory farm under inhumane conditions. But there are differences. And it is these differences that obstinate vegans will latch onto to claim such labels cannot be trusted. As one vegan writer states, "today's meat industry has animals locked and caged inside warehouses (yes, some of which are labeled 'organic', 'free-range' and 'grass-fed')" (Peaceful Dumpling).

Now it is true the term "free-range" has no legal definition, that is why Pounds' Turkey Farm does not label their meats as such, even though they raise their animals in a manner that would be consistent with people's image of what this means, that of animals being outside (weather permitting), with room to roam and access to the ground. And their meats arc not fully grass-fcd, as during the winter months when the animals must be kept indoor, they are fed grains. But here in the Pittsburgh area with our cold winters, that is the best that can be done.

It is also true that technically an animal could be considered to be grass-fed if it were kept inside in cages 100% of the time but fed cut grass (hay) rather than grains. But such simply is not the usual practice. Farms that keep animals indoors in cages almost always feed them grains, while those that are so conscientious as to feed their animals grasses due so by keeping them outside and letting them graze for it. They are only moved inside and fed hay during inclement weather.

But to know for sure, you would need to find out from the farm itself. Information on how animals are raised and fed can be found on the websites of such farms (such as the preceding quotes from Pounds' demonstrate) or even at the point of sale.

During my most recent trip to the Co-op, I noticed there were little signs on the coolers for the meats with the names of each of the farms on them that the meats were from. Each sign indicated what the farm fed the animals and how they were raised. I took pictures of the signs, so I could record their contents here. Following is the text of each sign:

Dormel Farms. Located in Somerset County, PA. Owned and operated by the Arnold family since the 1960s. The beef is organic and grass-fed and finished. It is also extra lean (approximately 92% lean).

Kananga Farm. Located in Ligoneer, PA. Owned and Operated by Dianne and Kim Miller for more than 20 years. Beef is bred, fed, and finished on local grasses. The Millers utilize mob grazing methods, which is designed to leave the land more fertile every time it is grazed.

North Woods Ranch. 100% Grass-fed Cattle. Locally & naturally raised. Scottish Highland beef, 100% grass-fed. Age 21+ days and Berkshire Pork, pasture raised, non-GMO/ soy. Family owned and operated in Northern Allegheny County. www.nwoodsranch.com
Our animals are cared for with the utmost respect and kindness. The animal is a fellow worker on the ranch, actively working to restore the lands and increase the biological worth in a completely natural manner.

Friendship Farms. Located in the Laurel Highlands, PA. Owned and Operated by the Costello family since the 1960s. Angus cattle are bred for quality and nurtured with care as they are rotated around the farm on pastures of alfalfa, clover, and orchard grass. Pastures are fertilized naturally and weeds are mown not sprayed. The cattle are never treated with hormones or artificially derived feeds. The Costello's farm also features homemade breads and a plant nursery.

Ron Gargasz Farms. Located in Volant, PA. Owned and Operated by the Gargasz family since the 1940s. Gargasz farm raises organic beef that is grass-fed and grass finished. Ron also grows many other things besides beef which are sold on his farm and occasionally through a distributer.... "My farm operation is relatively small and is nourished predominately by my footsteps and my love of nature. The beef and grains are raised by the most sustainable production methods."

Jamison Lamb. Located in Latrobe, PA. Owned and operated by John and Sukey Jamison since the 1970s. Lamb is all grass-fed using intensive rotation grazing methods. The Jamisons also own and operate the processing facility, so they control the lamb from birth until it arrives here.

Providence Acres Farm. Located in the Laurel Highlands. Owned and operated by the Kelly family. Lamb, beef, and pork are all pasture raised and the farm is Certified Humanly Grown (CHG).

Thus some of the preceding terms are used to make it clear how the animals are raised and fed. The point of "grass finished" is that some farms that usually feed their cattle grasses will feed their cattle grains shortly before slaughter. This is because what cattle eat shortly before slaughter determines the taste of the meat, and most people are used to the taste of grain-fed rather than grass-fed meat. The "rotated around the farm" and "mob grazing methods" statements refer to the previously mentioned practice of keeping the cattle in a penned off field to encourage more aggressive grazing, then moving them to another field to allow the grass to regrow in the first field.

You could also contact a given farm and ask. I have done so with Pounds' a couple of times. Even though the first time was during their busy holiday season, the owner nicely took the time to answer my questions. I called them again while working on this chapter to get some further details, and the owner again took the time to answer my questions. Some old-fashioned farms will even invite people to tour their farms. Such would never happen with factory farms.

However, even with all of this, such old-fashioned farms still do not satisfy the die-hard vegetarian. The afore-quoted article on Gentle World states:

However, **this is not to say that grass-fed beef is a viable alternative**. Livestock grazing threatens native and endangered species through habitat destruction and displacement, and causes soil erosion, which in turn can transform fertile farmland into deserts (a process known as desertification).

But a conscientious farmer, which a farmer has to be to stay in business, will take steps to prevent such problems. By fencing in the herds, they will not endanger other species, just as the herd will not be endangered by predators. And soil erosion would ruin the farm, so steps are taken to prevent that. Such steps are alluded in the afore-quoted signs from the Co-op.

Only three vegetarian arguments are left. The first is that humans should just leave the land alone. But we were given dominion over the earth, not to destroy it, but to keep it (Gen 1:26-29). As such, that is not a viable position for a Bible-believing Christian

The second argument is that this grazing land could be used for grains that would then feed people, alleviating world hunger. But we already saw that the world hunger problem is not due to a lack of food production but due to economic and other factors.

And in regards to both of these points, consider the following:

- **Grazing animals eat plants that cannot be digested by humans**.
- Meat from grass-fed animals requires only one calorie of fossil fuel to produce two calories of food. Many grain and vegetable crops require from 5 to 10 calories of fossil-fuel for every calorie of food or fiber produced.
- Well-managed pasture absorbs far more rain water than most other land uses.
- **Grazed lands help slow global warming by removing carbon dioxide from the air**. Grazing land in the Great Plains contain over 40 tons of carbon per acre. Cultivated soils contain about 26 tons.
- **Well-managed grazing lands provide much-needed habit for wildlife, reduce water runoff, and provide cleaner, more abundant water for wildlife and human use.**
- Grazing lands are among our most picturesque landscapes (Eat Wild. Notes).

The final vegetarian argument is it is simply wrong for human beings to kill and eat animals. But as we have already seen, such a stance is untenable for the Bible-believing Christian. The Bible is clear from

181

Genesis Chapter Nine on that God intends for human beings to eat meat in this day and age. This is clear from the Noahic Decree and the example of the LORD Himself in the Old Testament and Jesus Himself in the New Testament.

I say "this day and age" as vegetarians often emphasize that Adam and Eve were vegans, as were all antediluvians. They will further claim that in the millennium or in eternity (depending one's view of the end times) all people will be vegans. As such, they claim we should all be vegans now. But we today are not living in the Garden of Eden nor in the final state. We are living in the time period between the Fall and the awaited Second Coming of Christ. And the Bible is clear that during this time period God intends for us to eat meat.

Further and extensive Biblical proof of this point, along with rebuttals of Biblical counter-arguments by vegetarians, is found in this writer's other book on nutrition and the Bible, *God-given Foods Eating Plan* (see Appendix One). That extensive discussion will not be repeated here. But even a non-believer in the Bible should consider the following:

> I believe that people who choose to be strict vegans for the welfare of animals need to consider this question: **is promoting a 100 percent vegan diet for the welfare of animals a correct moral path if it leads to significant health problems for humans?** Personally, I feel bad about an animal being killed to be my food. But if there were no fishermen or farmers around, I believe that **I would gratefully sacrifice an animal with my own hands since I believe that the health of my family requires eating small amounts of animal foods** (Chet Day's; Vegan).

> I've watched "Animal Planet" and other TV shows and documentaries about how wild carnivorous animals obtain their meals in their natural habitats, and it's not humane AT ALL. Its ghastly.
>
> Lions and other big cats, wolves, hyenas, orca whales, coyotes, crocodiles... are all carnivorous predators, and **their prey usually dies a hideously gruesome, terrifying, painful**

death. Prey animals are often torn to pieces, gutted and devoured while still *alive and screaming.*

Even pet cats will torture mice or birds they catch, often breaking their legs/wings first or puncturing them so they can't get away, then bat them around like cat-toys before eating them. Orca whales "play" with seals, breaking their spines as they toss their "toy" into the air and catch it with their teeth, or toss the seal back and forth to each other like a ball, before eating it.

Surely we already show more kindness to our food animals than a hyena, a cat, or a boa constrictor does? And we can do even better (anonymous comment on Psychology Today; 84%, emphases except bolding in original).

Animals in the wild are also always at risk of starvation and disease, both of which are slow and painful ways to die. Animals on factory farms might not do much better, but animals raised on old-fashioned farms live a much better life and are killed more humanely than how the animals would live and die in the wild.

Hunting

Before proceeding, it would be good to mention hunting. Such is how animal foods were initially derived after the Noahic Decree. This is known as shortly after that decree, it is said:

[8]Now Cush fathered Nimrod [LXX, Nebrod]: he began to be a giant [Heb., mighty one] upon the earth. [9]**He was a giant [Heb., mighty] hunter** before the LORD God; because of this, they say, "As Nimrod [the] **giant hunter** before the LORD" (Gen 10:8f).

Then somewhat later:
[27]So the boys grew. And **Esau was a man having known [how] to be hunting [or, skilled in hunting]**, dwelling in the country, but Jacob was a natural [or, simple] man, dwelling in a house. [28]Now **Isaac loved Esau, because his game was his food**, but Rebecca was loving Jacob (Gen 25:27f).

[1]Now it happened after Isaac grew old, and [fig., that] his eyes were [too] dimmed [for him] to be seeing; and he called Esau, his elder son, and said to him, "My son;" and he said, "Listen! I [am here]." [2]And he said, "Listen! I have grown old, and do not know the day of my death. [3]Now then **take your vessels [fig., weapons], both quiver and bow, and go into the plain, and hunt game for me, [4]and make me meats, as I like, and bring to me that I shall eat,** that my soul shall bless you, before I die." [5]But Rebecca heard Isaac speaking to Esau his son. So **Esau went into the plain to hunt game for his father** (Gen 27:1-5).

These verses show hunting became important to humans shortly after the Noahic Decree. And game meat is similar to old-fashioned farm meat in not being tainted by all of the problems of factory farm meats, and much of what was said about animals raised on old-fashioned farms apply to wild animals—no antibiotics, no growth hormones, no restricted movement, not overly fat, so the meat is low in fat, even lower than pasture-raised cattle, no environmental damage, and a natural diet. But they would be worse off than old-fashioned farm animals in having to deal with predators, starvation, and disease that old-fashioned farm animals are protected from. But the resultant meats would be similar and would provide the same benefits. To that point we now turn.

Benefits of Old-fashioned Meats

Not only is not wrong in any respect to consume old-fashioned meats or game meats, but there are even health benefits from doing so. The home page for the aforementioned Eat Wild website states:

> Eatwild was founded in 2001. Its mission was to promote **the benefits—to consumers, farmers, animals, and the planet—of choosing meat, eggs, and dairy products from 100% grass-fed animals or other non-ruminant animals fed their natural diets**....
>
> Today, Eatwild.com provides research-based information about "eating on the wild side." This means choosing present-day foods that approach the nutritional content of wild plants and game—our original diet. **Evidence is growing on an almost daily basis that these wholesome foods give us more**

of the nutrients we need to fight disease and enjoy optimum health. Few of us will go back to foraging in the wild for our food, but we can learn to forage in our supermarkets, farmers markets, and from local farmers to select the most nutritious and delicious foods available.

To comment, notice that Eat Wild was founded in 2001. As such, I cannot fault myself for not knowing about it and its extensive database of old-fashioned farms back in 2000 when the First Edition of this book was published, but it would now be disingenuous for anyone to claim they cannot find a local source of old-fashioned meats.

But for this section, what concerns us is Eat Wild's page detailing the benefits of eating old-fashioned meats, or as they call it, grass-fed products. The page is titled, "Health Benefits of Grass-Fed Products." It begins:

> **Meat, eggs, and dairy products from pastured animals are ideal for your health**. Compared with commercial products, **they offer you more "good" fats, and fewer "bad" fats. They are richer in antioxidants**; including vitamins E, beta-carotene, and vitamin C. Furthermore, **they do not contain traces of added hormones, antibiotics or other drugs**.
>
> Below is a summary of these important benefits. Following the summary is a list of news bulletins that provide additional reasons for finding a local provider of grass-fed food.

What follows is an extensive discussion of the benefits of grass-fed products. It is so extensive, I can only quote a few highlights. But I encourage the reader to pursue this webpage for further details.

> **There are a number of nutritional differences between the meat of pasture-raised and feedlot-raised animals. To begin with, meat from grass-fed cattle, sheep, and bison is lower in total fat....**
>
> Because meat from grass-fed animals is lower in fat than meat from grain-fed animals, **it is also lower in calories**....

Extra Omega-3s. **Meat from grass-fed animals has two to four times more omega-3 fatty acids than meat from grain-fed animals**. Omega-3s are called "good fats" because they play a vital role in every cell and system in your body. For example, of all the fats, they are the most heart-friendly. People who have ample amounts of omega-3s in their diet are less likely to have high blood pressure or an irregular heartbeat. Remarkably, they are 50 percent less likely to suffer a heart attack....

The CLA Bonus. **Meat and dairy products from grass-fed ruminants are the richest known source of another type of good fat called "conjugated linoleic acid" or CLA**.... CLA may be one of our most potent defenses against cancer.... In a Finnish study, women who had the highest levels of CLA in their diet, had a 60 percent lower risk of breast cancer than those with the lowest levels. Switching from grain-fed to grassfed meat and dairy products places women in this lowest risk category....

Vitamin E. In addition to being higher in omega-3s and CLA, **meat from grassfed animals is also higher in vitamin E**.... In humans, vitamin E is linked with a lower risk of heart disease and cancer. This potent antioxidant may also have anti-aging properties. Most Americans are deficient in vitamin E.

It was previously indicated that vegetarians claim meat eating increases the risk of heart disease and cancer, but with its low fat content and elevated levels of omega 3s, CLA, and vitamin E, grass-fed meats would actually decrease one's risk of these degenerative diseases. These claims are verified by independent scientific studies:

Chemical and mineral composition and the intramuscular fatty acid (IMF) profile of the Longissimus dorsi muscle (LM) of 60 purebred Hereford, 1/4 Braford and 3/8 Braford steers **finished either in a feedlot or on improved pastures of the Pampa biome were evaluated**. Pastures were improved with the introduction of Lolium multiflorum, Trifolium repens, and Lotus corniculatus. On average, beef from pasture-fed steers presented higher concentrations of the fatty acids C18:3n-3

(P<0.001), C20:3n-3 (P=0.035), total n-3 (P<0.001) and lower n-6/n-3 ratio (P<0.001) in the IMF, and higher Mg and lower K content in muscle relative to those finished in the feedlot.... **beef produced exclusively on improved pastures presented higher concentration of components that are considered beneficial to human health, such as n-3 fatty acids [omega 3s], and a lower n-6/n-3 [omega 6/ omega 3] ratio** (Freitas).

The objective of this study was to compare fatty acid weight percentages and cholesterol concentrations of longissimus dorsi (LD), semitendinosus (ST), and supraspinatus (SS) muscles (n = 10 for each) of range bison (31 mo of age), feedlot-finished bison (18 mo of age), range beef cows (4 to 7 yr of age), feedlot steers (18 mo of age), free-ranging cow elk (3 to 5 yr of age), and chicken breast.... **Range-fed animals had higher (P < 0.01) n-3 fatty acids than feedlot-fed animals or chicken breast....**

Conjugated linoleic acid (CLA, 18:2cis-9, trans-11) in LD was greatest (P < 0.01) for range beef cows (0.4%), and lowest for chicken breast and elk (mean = 0.1%). **In ST, CLA was greatest (P < 0.01) for range and feedlot bison and range beef cows** (mean = 0.4%) and lowest for elk and chicken breast (mean = 0.1%). **Also, SS CLA was greatest (P < 0.01) for range beef cows** (0.5%) and lowest for chicken breast (0.1%). **Mean total fatty acid concentration (g/100 g tissue) for all muscles was highest (P < 0.01) for feedlot bison and feedlot cattle and lowest (P < 0.01) for range bison, range beef cows, elk, and chicken.** ...

We conclude that lipid composition of bison muscle varies with feeding regimen, and **range-fed bison had muscle lipid composition similar to that of forage-fed beef cows and wild elk** (Rule).

Growing consumer interest in grass-fed beef products has raised a number of questions with regard to the perceived differences in nutritional quality between grass-fed and grain-fed cattle. Research spanning three decades suggests that **grass-based diets can significantly improve the fatty acid (FA)**

composition and antioxidant content of beef, albeit with variable impacts on overall palatability. **Grass-based diets have been shown to enhance total conjugated linoleic acid (CLA) (C18:2) isomers, trans vaccenic acid (TVA) (C18:1 t11), a precursor to CLA, and omega-3 (n-3) FAs** on a g/g fat basis. While the overall concentration of total SFAs is not different between feeding regimens, grass-finished beef tends toward a higher proportion of cholesterol neutral stearic FA (C18:0), and **less cholesterol-elevating SFAs** such as myristic (C14:0) and palmitic (C16:0) FAs.

Several studies suggest that grass-based diets elevate precursors for Vitamin A and E, as well as cancer fighting antioxidants such as glutathione (GT) and superoxide dismutase (SOD) activity as compared to grain-fed contemporaries. Fat conscious consumers will also prefer the **overall lower fat content of a grass-fed beef product**. However, consumers should be aware that the differences in FA content will also give **grass-fed beef a distinct grass flavor and unique cooking qualities** that should be considered when making the transition from grain-fed beef. In addition, **the fat from grass-finished beef may have a yellowish appearance from the elevated carotenoid content (precursor to Vitamin A)** (Daley).

What all of this means is, there is a clear nutritional difference between grain-fed and grass-fed beef, and these nutritional differences should lead to differing effects on the health of those eating each type of meat. Unfortunately, to date, there have not been any studies comparing the long-term health effects of people consuming grain-fed meats versus those consuming grass-fed meats. But given the stark nutritional differences, it is logical to assume there would be significant health effects. This supposition needs to be kept in mind when hearing about yet one more study that claims meat has deleterious health effects.

For instance, when I was working on the first draft of this chapter, an article on my Google News page was titled, "High dietary red meat intake linked to common bowel condition diverticulitis."

The article was dated January 11, 2017 and appeared in *Science Daily*. It stated:

A high dietary intake of red meat, particularly of the unprocessed variety, is linked to a heightened risk of developing the common inflammatory bowel condition, diverticulitis, reveals research published online in the journal *Gut*.

Diverticulitis occurs when the small pockets or bulges lining the intestine (diverticula) become inflamed. It is relatively common, accounting for more than 200,000 hospital admissions every year in the US at an annual cost of $US 2 billion....

Insufficient dietary fibre intake is also thought to have a role, but few other dietary factors have been explored in any detail.

In a bid to rectify this, the research team assessed the potential impact of total dietary red meat, poultry, and fish intake on the risk of developing diverticulitis in nearly 46,500 men, taking part in the Health Professionals Follow up Study....

Those who ate higher quantities of red meat tended to use common anti-inflammatory drugs and painkillers more often; they smoked more; and they were less likely to exercise vigorously. Their fibre intake was also lower.

Those who ate more poultry and fish were more likely to exercise vigorously, take aspirin, and to smoke less.

But after taking account of these potentially influential factors, total red meat intake was associated with heightened diverticulitis risk.

Compared with the lowest levels of consumption, the highest level of red meat intake was associated with a 58% heightened risk of developing diverticulitis, with each daily serving associated with an 18% increased risk. However, risk peaked at six servings a week.

First, note the confounding factors. Red meat eaters smoked more, exercised less, and consumed less fiber. But there is no logical connection between eating red meat and these three factors. Red meat eaters could not smoke, exercise, and eat vegetables and other fiber containing foods just as much as anyone else. The researchers claim to have accounted for these confounding factors, but that is not so easy to do. Such confounding factors render the results questionable.

But what is interesting is the increased use of anti-inflammatory drugs and painkillers among meat-eaters. There might be a connection here. The article goes on to state:

> Exactly how red meat intake might affect diverticulitis risk is not clear, and further research is required. But **higher red meat consumption has been linked to the presence of inflammatory chemicals, such as C reactive protein and ferritin**, as well as heart disease/stroke and diabetes, explain the researchers.

Note the mentioned of "the presence of inflammatory chemicals." That is probably why heavy meat-eaters feel a need to take anti-inflammatories. However:

> Research shows that **omega-3 fatty acids reduce inflammation** and may help lower risk of chronic diseases such as heart disease, cancer, and arthritis… People with diabetes often have high triglyceride and low HDL levels. Omega-3 fatty acids from fish oil can help lower triglycerides and apoproteins (markers of diabetes), and raise HDL (UMMC).

We have just seen that grass-fed beef contains significant amounts of Omega 3s. These omega 3s would counteract the inclination of meat to elevate inflammation, so it is be logical to assume the consumption of grass-fed beef does not increase the risk of diverticulitis, nor of heart disease, stroke, and diabetes. And this is not just theory:

> Eating moderate amounts of grass-fed meat for only 4 weeks will give you healthier levels of essential fats, according to a 2011 study in the *British Journal of Nutrition*.
>
> The British research showed that **healthy volunteers who ate grass-fed meat increased their blood levels of omega-3 fatty acids and decreased their level of pro-inflammatory omega-6 fatty acids**. These changes are linked with a lower

risk of a host of disorders, including cancer, cardiovascular disease, depression, and inflammatory disease.

Interestingly, **volunteers who consumed conventional, grain-fed meat ended up with lower levels of omega-3s and higher levels of omega-6s** than they had at the beginning of the study, suggesting that eating conventional meat had been detrimental to their health (Eat Wild. Notes).

The point is, any study claiming deleterious effects of red meat that does not indicate if the beef is grain-fed or grass-fed is meaningless. But most studies do not make this distinction.

It is most unfortunate that people believe the misinformation about animal products taught by George Malkmus: that meat is a killer food and is the cause of 90% of mankind's health woes. Granted, **much of the meat available in the grocery stores these days is in fact junk meat**. Animals are often fed a contaminated diet, and meat is often processed using harmful preservatives and chemicals; **but this is no reason to assail "clean" meats freely given to us by God**. To claim that God gave us meat to shorten our days, make us sick, and kill us *betrays the true character of God*.

As we explained in our "FAQ's About Meat and Your Health" videos·, **virtually every single study "proving" the harmful effects of meat eating is flawed for at least two reasons**:

No study has ever been done on people who were eating Biblically approved meats from animals that were properly grown and fed. All studies have either used highly modified "protein" such as milk casein OR standard junk meats including luncheon meats, hot dogs and the like.

In virtually every study, including The China Project, **the people who ate meat also ate junk food**....

This also means that the previous **claims about meat consumption increasing health care costs is also not true. The opposite is probably the case when grass-fed beef is consumed—it would decrease health care costs. All of this must be remembered whenever confronted with claims of**

191

the deleterious effects of meat-eating (Chet Day's; italics in original).

These differences could be why one study found, "The association between unprocessed red meat consumption and mortality risk was found in the US populations, but not in European or Asian populations" (Wang. Red.). This is significant as factory farms are more common in the USA than in Europe or Asia. Thus most Americans eat factory farm meat while most Europeans and Asians do not.

Cost

There is a clear-cut difference between factory farm meats and old-fashioned meats in regards to nutrient content and the ethical and environmental issue surrounding meat-eating. But there is also another clear-cut difference, that of cost.

The reason factory farms were invented was to provide a steady stream of cheap meat to fast food restaurants, as detailed in the movie *Food Inc.* But old-fashioned meats can cost two to three times as much as factory farm meats.

For instance, this past Thanksgiving I did some price comparisons. Giant Eagle is the largest traditional supermarket chain in the Pittsburgh area. Turkeys could be purchased at my local Giant Eagle for as little as $0.89/ pound. But at Pounds' Turkey Farm they were $2.99/ pound, while at the Co-op, organic, free range turkeys were $5.99/ pound. For a 20 pound turkey, this comes to $29.40 for a Giant Eagle turkey, $59.80 for a Pounds' turkey, and $119.80 for an organic, free range turkey at the Co-op. That is a significant difference.

However, other meats are not quite as significant. Ground meat costs as little as $2.50/ pound at Giant Eagle, $2.89/ pound at Pounds', and from $5.99-9.99/ pound at the Co-op. The costs of steaks vary based on the cut, but they are in the low tens/ pound at Giant Eagle and Pounds' and in the mid-tens/ pound at the Co-op.

The reason Pounds' meats are in-between the other two is their meats are not fully grass-fed, as indicated previously. They are also not fully organic, as the grains fed to the animals in winter months have been sprayed with "a limited amount of pesticides" (as the owner explained it to me). But their meats are still healthier and more humanly

192

produced and better for the environment than factory farm meats, though probably not quite as good as the meats at the Co-op.

The point is, as the saying goes, "You get what you pay for." Given the great nutritional, ethical, and environmental differences between factory farm meats and old-fashioned meats, for those who are concerned about such issues, then old-fashioned meats are worth the cost. But it does mean you might not be able to consume as much meat as you are used to. But that is okay. As previously indicated, even limited amounts of animal foods can alleviate the potential problems of vegan diets, while providing the potential benefits. A dietary approach of a mostly plant-based diet but with some animal foods also fits better with the overall principle of the Creationist Diet.

Conclusion on Pros and Cons of Meat-Eating

Many testimonials can be found on the Internet of people who formerly followed a vegan diet but ran into problems with it. These problems were resolved when they began including at least limited amounts of animal foods in their diet. But just as many testimonials can be found of the exact opposite, of former carnivores who say their health improved as a result of switching to a vegan diet. But then those same carnivores-turned-vegans might later give opposite testimonials of how their health began to fail after a few years on the vegan diet but then improved when they added meat back into their diets.

The reason for this apparent contradictory phenomenon should be obvious at this point. Plant foods contain nutrients that animal foods do not, and vice-a-versa. Thus when someone who has developed nutrient deficiencies from following one diet switches to the opposite one, these nutrient deficiencies are quickly resolved. But it takes time for new nutrient deficiencies to develop on the new diet. But when they do, switching to the opposite diet will resolve them.

Of course, all of this switching back and forth could be avoided simply by including healthy versions of both plant foods and animal foods in one's diet.

There are also psychological factors at play here. Changing one's diet is not easy, as longtime habits are hard to break. A such, when people do successfully change their diets, they convince themselves it has positive effects. This is especially the case with new vegans, who along with convincing themselves they have done something good for their own bodies, think they have done something good for the welfare of animals and even for the entire planet.

Even when health problems develop, such psychological effects can be so strong that the person deludes themselves that all is well or that it cannot possibly be their "ideal" diet. But such self-delusion can only last so long. Eventually, the truth breaks through, and the person changes their diet, only to as strongly proclaim the reverse diet is the best. Hopefully, this book will enable the reader to avoid all of this experimenting and switching back and forth of eating plans.

Yes, there are sound health reasons to include copious amounts of whole, natural plant foods in one's diet. But doing so does not require eliminating all animal foods from the diet.

Moreover, yes, there are sound health, ethical, and environmental reasons for avoiding factory farm meats. But old-fashioned meats offer an alternative that is not tainted with any of these concerns. Such meats arc expensive, but the inclusion of limited amounts will go a long way in avoiding the problems associated with longtime vegan diets, while providing health benefits.

Putting all of this information together, can meats be included in a Creationist Diet? Answer: Yes. Meats are God-given foods. And there are some sound nutritional reasons for including meats in the diet. But the reader must carefully consider the pros and cons of meat eating and decide for yourself whether to consume meat or not, "be letting each be fully convinced in his own mind" (Romans 14:5).

But since God gave meats to humans later than plant foods, if meats are consumed, they should have a lesser place in a Creationist Diet as compared to plant foods. And since it was to Noah that the decree about eating meats was given, then a good name for a mostly plant-based diet but one that includes meat would be the "Noahic Diet."

However, if you decide to include meat in your diet, the Bible gives limitations that need to be considered. These will be discussed in Chapter Eight. But first, one important class of meats will be addressed separately in the next chapter, as the issues surrounding it are so complicated it requires a whole chapter to fully cover.

But this chapter will close will with a quote from noted preacher C.H. Spurgeon, "Before he sinned man did not kill animals, but lived on fruits; every meal of flesh should remind us of our fall" (p.4).

Bibliography:

Atlantic, The. Why Americans Lead the World in Food Waste. https://www.theatlantic.com/business/archive/2016/07/american-food-waste/491513/

American Grassfed. Frequently Asked Questions. http://www.americangrassfed.org/about-us/faq/

Barnard ND, Nicholson A, Howard JL. *Preventative Medicine.* 1995 Nov;24(6):646-55. *The medical costs attributable to meat consumption.*

Brody, Jane E. *New York Times.* Health Cost of Meat Diet Is Billions, Study Says. Published: November 21, 1995. http://www.nytimes.com/1995/11/21/science/health-cost-of-meat-diet-is-billions-study-says.html?pagewanted=all

Catholic Relief Services. Hunger. http://www.crs.org/get-involved/learn/hunger?gclid=Cj0KEQiAzNfDBRD2xK1O4pSmiOkBE iQAbzzeQUC3k-AL_Ucn6krbWHw1Y2oV6ZirVVYtjzkhdXAak_8aAsUT8P8HAQ

Certified Humane. Overview. http://certifiedhumane.org/how-we-work/overview/

Chet Day's Tips. Hallelujah Acres Research Cast Doubt On "Ideal Diet. By Greg Westbrook. http://www.chetday.com/hallelujah-diet-dangers.htm

Chet Day's Tips. Vegan Diet: Recipe for Disaster? Dr. Ben Kim. http://www.chetday.com/strictvegandiet.htm

Daley, CA, et. al., *Nutrition Journal.* 2010 Mar 10;9:10. doi: 10.1186/1475-2891-9-10. A review of fatty acid profiles and antioxidant content in grass-fed and grain-fed beef. https://www.ncbi.nlm.nih.gov/pubmed/20219103

Down to Earth. World Hunger Can Be Solved with Vegetarian Diet. https://www.downtoearth.org/blogs/2012-05/world-hunger-can-be-solved-vegetarian-diet

Earth Save News. Vol. 17. No. 2. June 2006. http://www.earthsave.org/news/ES06_june.pdf

Eat Wild. Home Page. http://www.eatwild.com/

Eat Wild. Health Benefits of Grass-Fed Products. http://www.eatwild.com/healthbenefits.htm

Eat Wild; Notes & News. http://www.eatwild.com/news.html

Farley, Dixie. *Vegetarian Diets: The Plusses and the Pitfalls*. US Food and Drug Administration – http://www.fda.gov/bbs/topics/CONSUMER/CON00138.html

Farm Sanctuary. Factory Farming and the Environment. https://www.farmsanctuary.org/learn/factory-farming/factory-farming-and-the-environment/

Feeding America. Food Waste in America. http://www.feedingamerica.org/about-us/how-we-work/securing-meals/reducing-food-waste.html?referrer=https://www.google.com/

Freitas, AK, et. al. *Meat Science*. 2014 Jan;96(1):353-60. doi: 10.1016/j.meatsci.2013.07.021. Epub 2013 Jul 19. Nutritional composition of the meat of Hereford and Braford steers finished on pastures or in a feedlot in southern Brazil. https://www.ncbi.nlm.nih.gov/pubmed/23954275

Guardian. Turning vegetarian will not solve the food crisis. https://www.theguardian.com/commentisfree/2012/aug/28/vegetarian-food-security-hunger

Gentle World. Could Veganism End World Hunger? http://gentleworld.org/could-veganism-end-world-hunger/

Healthline. Worst Foodborne Illness Outbreaks in U.S. History. http://www.healthline.com/health-slideshow/worst-foodborne-illness-outbreaks#6

Jacobson, Michael, et al., *Safe Food Eating Wisely in a Risky World*, Living Planet Press, 1991. Quoted in John Robbins. *Fish: What's the Catch?* - http://www.earthsave.org/news/fishwhat.htm

Kaneene, J.B. & R. Miller. *Review of Science Technology*. Off. int. Epiz., 1997,16 (2), 694-708. Problems associated with drug residues in beef from feeds and therapy.

Klaper, Michael, M.D. *The 'Blood Type Diet:' Fact or Fiction?* - http://www.earthsave.org/news/bloodtyp.htm

Los Angeles Daily News. Ways to help the Earth with your choices of what to eat. http://www.dailynews.com/lifestyle/20170417/nutrition-ways-to-help-the-earth-with-your-choices-of-what-to-eat

Marcus, Erik. *Mad Cow Right Now: Some Answers About Britain's Perils—and Our Own—Seem Finally to be at Hand:* http://www.vegan.com/issues/1999/feb99/bse.htm

Mayell, Mark . *52 Simple Steps to Natural Health*. New York: Pocket Books, 1995.

http://www.oie.int/doc/ged/D9384.PDF

Nutrition Action. Vol. 26, No. 8, October 1999, "Food Safety Guide," pp.1,3-9.

Organic.org. FAQ. http://www.organic.org/home/faq

Organic Valley. What does pasture raised mean? http://organicvalley.custhelp.com/app/answers/detail/a_id/22/~/what-does-pasture-raised-mean%3F

Peaceful Dumpling. Eat Your Dirt: Vitamin B12. http://www.peacefuldumpling.com/vitamin-b12-eat-your-dirt

Pound's Turkey Farm. http://www.poundsturkeyfarm.com

Oppenlander, Dr. Richard. The Cost of Eating Animals. http://plantbaseddietitian.com/cost-of-eating-animals/

Psychology Today. 84% of Vegetarians and Vegans Return to Meat. https://www.psychologytoday.com/blog/animals-and-us/201412/84-vegetarians-and-vegans-return-meat-why

Psychology Today. Why Do Most Vegetarians Go Back To Eating Meat? https://www.psychologytoday.com/blog/animals-and-us/201106/why-do-most-vegetarians-go-back-eating-meat

Rauma AL, Torronen R, Hanninen O, Mykkanen H. *Journal of Nutrition*. 1995 Oct;125(10):2511-5. *Vitamin B-12 status of long-term adherents of a strict uncooked vegan diet ("living food diet") is compromised.*

Robbins, John. *Factory Farm Alarm:* http://www.earthsave.org/news/factfarm.htm

Fish: What's the Catch? http://www.earthsave.org/news/fishwhat.htm

Frequently Asked Questions: http://www.earthsave.org/faq.htm

Rule DC, et.al. *Journal of Animal Science*. 2002 May;80(5):1202-11. Comparison of muscle fatty acid profiles and cholesterol concentrations of bison, beef cattle, elk, and chicken.

Russell, Rex MD. *What the Bible Says about Healthy Living*. Grand Rapids, MI: Baker Book House, 1999.

Salon. What do "free range," "organic" and other chicken labels really mean?
http://www.salon.com/2011/01/20/what_chicken_labels_really_mean/

Science Daily. High dietary red meat intake linked to common bowel condition diverticulitis.
https://www.sciencedaily.com/releases/2017/01/170111122833.htm

Schecter A, Cramer P, Boggess K, Stanley J, Olson JR. *Chemosphere.* 1997 Mar-Apr;34(5-7):1437-47. *Levels of dioxins, dibenzofurans, PCB and DDE congeners in pooled food samples collected in 1995 at supermarkets across the United States.*

Shark Attack Files on the *Discovery Channel.* March 1, 2000.

Simon, Michele, JD, MPH. *Hog Factory Farming: Lagoons or Environmental Menace? -*
http://www.vegan.com/issues/1999/nov99/lagoon.htm

Spurgeon, C.H. *Spurgeon's Devotional Bible.* Grand Rapids, MI: Baker Book House, reprinted 1987.

UMMC. University of Maryland Medical Center. Omega-3 fatty acids.
http://umm.edu/health/medical/altmed/supplement/omega3-fatty-acids

USDA. Estimated Amount, Value, and Calories of Postharvest Food Losses at the Retail and Consumer Levels in the United States. Jean C. Buzby, Hodan F. Wells, and Jeffrey Hyman.
http://www.endhunger.org/PDFs/2014/USDA-FoodLoss-2014.pdf

Vegetarian Pages Web site. *How to win an argument with a meat eater* –
http://www.veg.org/veg/FAQ/extinction.html

Wang X, et. al. *Public Health Nutrition.* 2016 Apr;19(5):893-905. Red and processed meat consumption and mortality: dose-response meta-analysis of prospective cohort studies.
https://www.ncbi.nlm.nih.gov/pubmed/26143683

Chapter Seven:
Pros and Cons of
Fish Consumption

This chapter will look at an important class of meats, that of fish.

Fish and Fishing in the Bible

The word fish appears 61 times in the Bible. The first is in Genesis 1:26, when God gives dominion over the earth to human beings:

[26]And God said, "Let Us make humanity according to Our image and according to [Our] likeness, and let them be ruling [over] **the fish of the sea** and the birds [or, flying creatures] of heaven and the livestock and all the earth and all the reptiles [or, quadrupeds], the ones walking upon the earth."

Given the proximity of the nation Israel to the Mediterranean Sea, and with the Sea of Galilee within its borders, fishing was an important source of income and food in ancient Israel. This is seen in many of the judgements upon Israel being upon their waters and fish:

[1]Thus says the LORD, "Of what kind [is] the scroll [or, certificate] of divorce of your* mother, by which I sent her away? Or to which debtor have I sold you*? Listen! You* were sold for your* sins, and for your* iniquities I sent your* mother away. [2]For why did I come, and there was no person? I called, and there was not the one obeying? My hand is strong to redeem, is it not? Or I am able to deliver, am I not? Listen! **By My threat I make the sea destitute and will make rivers a desert, and their fish will be dried up from [there] not being water and will die by thirst**. [3]And I will clothe the sky [with] darkness and will make its covering as sackcloth" (Isaiah 50:1-3; see also Ezek 29:4f; Hos 4:3; Zeph 1:3).

The importance of fish to the economy and diet of Israel can be seen in one of the gates of the wall of Jerusalem being called the "Fish Gate" (2Chr 33:14; Neh 3:3; Zeph 9:10).

But it is in the New Testament that the importance of fish is really seen. In fact, a simple outline of a fish was one of the earliest symbol of the Christians faith, for two reasons. First, the Greek word fish (*Ichthus*) forms an acronym in Greek that translated means, "Jesus Christ, God's Son, Savior." Second, fish are mentioned quite often in the Gospels.

Some of the apostles were fishermen to begin with, and they even went fishing after Jesus' resurrection (Matt 4:18-22; John 21:1-6). Jesus used fish in illustrations (Matt 7:10; Luke 11:11). Jesus multiplied fish (and loaves of bread) on two occasions, feeding multitudes with them (Matt 14:13-21; 15:29-.38). And Jesus Himself ate fish (Luke 24:42) and cooked it for the apostles to eat (John 21:9f). Paul also used fish in an illustration (1Cor 15:39).

All of this means fish is clearly a Biblical food. Next to Jesus and the apostles eating fish, the most important reference is the following:

[11]"Now which father [among] you*, [if] his son will ask [for] a loaf of bread, he will not give to him a stone, will he? Or also [if he asks for] **a fish**, he will not give to him a serpent instead of a fish, will he? [12]Or also if he asks [for] an egg, he will not give to him a scorpion, will he? [13]If you* then being evil know [how] to be giving **good gifts** to your* children, how much more will the Father of heaven [fig., your* heavenly Father] give [the] Holy Spirit to the ones asking Him?" (Luke 11:11-13).

Thus Jesus specifically calls "a fish" a "good gift." With this statement and His example of eating and serving fish, it can be said that God intends for human beings to eat fish. Therefore, it is no surprise that fish is a very nutritious food, with there being many health benefits to eating fish.

Nutritional Content of Fish

Fish is among the healthiest foods on the planet. It is loaded with important nutrients, such as protein and vitamin D. Fish is also the world's best source of omega-3 fatty acids, which are incredibly important for your body and brain...

Fish is high in many important nutrients, including high-quality protein, iodine and various vitamins and minerals. Fatty types of fish are also high in omega-3 fatty acids and vitamin D (Authority; 11).

Seafood is a high-protein food that is low in calories, total fat, and saturated fat. High in vitamins and minerals...

Seafood is generally considered to be **a low-calorie protein source**.... A 3-ounce serving of most fish and shellfish provides about 30-40% of the average daily recommended amount of protein. The protein in seafood is easier to digest because seafood has less connective tissue than red meats and poultry....

Seafood is generally considered to be **low in total fat and saturated fat**. Most fish and shellfish contain less than 5 percent total fat, and even the fattiest fish, such as mackerel and king salmon, have no more than 15 percent fat. A large proportion of the fat in seafood is polyunsaturated, including **omega-3 fatty acids, which have added health benefits**....

Almost all fish and shellfish contain well **under 100 mg of cholesterol** per 3-ounce cooked serving, and many of the leaner types of fish have less than 60 mg....

Fish is a natural source of **B-complex vitamins, vitamin D and vitamin A** (especially oily fish)....

Fish is also a good source of minerals such as **selenium, zinc, iodine and iron**.... Small fish eaten whole, such as sardines and anchovies, are an important source of **calcium** needed for bone development (Seafood Health Facts).

The mention of vitamin D deserves special notice. The best way to attain vitamin D is through sunlight. But that is not always possible, especially for those of us living in northern climates. But fish is the only good natural dietary source of this essential vitamin. "Fatty fish is an excellent source of vitamin D, an important nutrient that over 40% of people may be deficient in" (Authority; 11).

That said; fish is a very nutritious food, packed with many essential nutrients, and it is low in saturated fat and cholesterol. But it is fish's omega 3 fatty acid content that is its claim to fame, so to speak. Omega 3s were already mentioned in the previous chapter as being present in grass-fed animal meats and as being especially beneficial. But fish contains far more omega 3s than even grass-fed land animals, so a closer look at omega 3s would be appropriate here.

Omega 3s

When it comes to fat, there's one type you don't want to cut back on: **omega-3 fatty acids**. Two crucial ones -- **EPA and DHA -- are primarily found in certain fish. ALA (alpha-linolenic acid), another omega-3 fatty acid, is found in plant sources such as nuts and seeds**. Not only does your body need these fatty acids to function, but also they deliver some big health benefits (WebMD; Facts).

Omega-3 fatty acids are considered essential fatty acids. They are necessary for human health, but **the body can't make them**. You have to get them through food. Omega-3 fatty acids are found in fish, such as salmon, tuna, and halibut, other seafoods including algae and krill, some plants, and nut oils. Also known as polyunsaturated fatty acids (PUFAs), **omega-3 fatty acids play a crucial role in brain function, as well as normal growth and development** (UMMC).

The human body can make most of the types of fats it needs from other fats or raw materials. That isn't the case for omega-3 fatty acids (also called omega-3 fats and n-3 fats). These are essential fats—the body can't make them from scratch but must get them from food. **Foods high in Omega-3 include fish, vegetable oils, nuts (especially walnuts), flax seeds, flaxseed oil, and leafy vegetables.**

What makes omega-3 fats special? They are **an integral part of cell membranes** throughout the body and affect the function of the cell receptors in these membranes. They provide the starting point for **making hormones** that regulate blood clotting, contraction and relaxation of artery walls, and inflammation. They also bind to receptors in cells that **regulate genetic function** (Harvard).

Omega 3 fatty acids are thus very important to human health, and they must be attained through the diet. And fish is by far the best source of omega 3s in the human diet.

A couple of these quotes mention ALA, which is found in some plant foods. ALA is not an omega 3 *per se*, but the human body converts it into omega 3s, specifically DHA. But it is not an efficient conversion.

... **the conversion efficiency from ALA to DHA is very limited in healthy individuals**; furthermore, the apparent inefficiency of the conversion from ALA to DHA is markedly variable between individuals within different sectors of the populations such that **the lack of sufficient dietary DHA could compromise optimal health** in those with very minimal conversion capacities (DHA).

Thus while the consumption of plant based sources of ALA can contribute to one's omega 3 intake, it is minimal as compared to that which can be attained by eating fish. However, there is some evidence that in vegans, this conversion rate is improved.

The conversion of the plant-based omega-3 ALA to the long-chain EPA and DHA **may be increased in vegans and vegetarians** who do not eat fish, suggest results from the European Prospective Investigation into Cancer and Nutrition (EPIC). (Daniells).

But note the "may." The evidence in this regard is shaky. The strongest evidence still supports fish as being the best source for omega 3s, and this is yet one more evidence that a vegan diet is not ideal.

The health effects of omega-3 fatty acids come mostly from EPA and DHA. ALA from flax and other vegetarian sources needs to be converted in the body to EPA and DHA. However, **many people's bodies do not make these conversions very effectively**. This remains an ongoing debate in the nutrition community; fish and sea vegetable sources of EPA and DHA versus vegetarian sources of ALA (UMMC).

That said; being such a rich source of so many nutrients, especially of omega 3s, it is of no surprise that the consumption of fish has been associated with many health benefits.

Health Benefits to Eating Fish

Many studies have been done on the health benefits of eating fish. Below are highlights of the results of these studies.

Eating at least one serving of fish per week has been linked to **reduced risk of heart attacks and strokes**, two of the world's biggest killers....

Fish consumption is linked to **reduced decline in brain function in old age**. People who eat fish regularly also have more grey matter in the brain centers that control memory and emotion....

Eating fish has been linked to **reduced risk of type 1 diabetes** and several other autoimmune diseases....

Some studies show that children who eat more fish have a **lower risk of developing asthma**....

People who eat more fish have a **much lower risk of developing macular degeneration**, a leading cause of vision impairment and blindness....

There is preliminary evidence that eating fatty fish like salmon **may lead to improved sleep** (Authority; 11).

Omega-3 fatty acids are found in fish—especially oily fish such as salmon, sardines, and herring. These omega-3 fatty acids can help **lower your blood pressure, lower your heart rate, and improve other cardiovascular risk factors**.

Eating fish **reduces the risk of death from heart disease**, the leading cause of death in both men and women. Fish intake has also been linked to **a lower risk of stroke, depression, and mental decline with age**.

For pregnant women, mothers who are breastfeeding, and women of childbearing age, fish intake is important because it supplies DHA, a specific omega-3 fatty acid that is **beneficial for the brain development of infants** (JAMA; Eating Fish).

Following is supporting evidence for each of these benefits.

While marine omega-3 fatty acids have been associated with a lower mortality in heart failure patients, data on omega-3 and incident heart failure are inconsistent. **We systematically reviewed the evidence on the association of omega-3 fatty acids and fish intake with the incidence of heart failure in this meta-analysis**....

A total of 176,441 subjects and 5480 incident cases of heart failure from 7 prospective studies were included in this analysis....

This meta-analysis is consistent with **a lower risk of heart failure with intake of marine omega-3 fatty acids** (Djoussé).

Marine omega-3 fatty acids have beneficial effects on cardiovascular risk factors. Consumption of fatty fish and marine omega-3 has been associated with lower rates of cardiovascular diseases. We examined the association of fatty fish and marine omega-3 with **heart failure (HF)** in a population of middle-aged and older women....

Participants in the Swedish Mammography Cohort aged 48-83 years completed 96-item food-frequency questionnaires...

Moderate consumption of fatty fish (1-2 servings per week) and marine omega-3 fatty acids were associated with a lower rate of first HF hospitalization or death in this population (Levitan).

Specific dietary patterns, including the Mediterranean diet, have been associated with stroke prevention. Our aim was to investigate whether adherence to a healthy **Nordic diet, including fish, apples and pears, cabbages, root vegetables, rye bread, and oatmeal, was associated with risk of stroke**....

During a median follow-up of 13.5 years, 2283 cases of incident stroke were verified, including 1879 ischemic strokes. **Adherence to a healthy Nordic diet**, as reflected by a higher Healthy Nordic Food Index score, **was associated with a lower risk of stroke**. The hazards ratio comparing an index score of 4 to 6 (high adherence) with an index score of 0 to 1 (low adherence) was 0.86 (95% confidence interval 0.76-0.98) for total stroke. Inverse associations were observed for ischemic stroke, including large-artery atherosclerosis. No trend was observed for hemorrhagic stroke; however, a statistically insignificant trend was observed for intracerebral hemorrhage....

Our findings suggest that **a healthy Nordic diet may be recommended for the prevention of stroke** (Hansen, Anita).

We systematically reviewed the association of omega-3 fatty acids intake with the incidence of dementia and Alzheimer's disease (AD) in this meta-analysis of prospective cohort studies, as evidence from previous studies suggests inconsistent results....

We identified relevant studies by searching PubMed, EmBase, and Web of Science databases up to June 2013. Prospective cohort studies reporting on associations of dietary **intake of long-chain omega-3 fatty acids or fish** with the incidence of dementia and AD were eligible....

A higher intake of fish was associated with a lower risk of AD. However, there was no statistical evidence for similar inverse association between long-chain omega-3 fatty acids intake and risk of dementia or AD, nor was there inverse association between fish intake and risk of dementia (Wu; Omega-3).

Note: The omega 3 intake included that from supplements and ALA from plant foods. For those, there was no benefit, but there was for fish.

It has been suggested that intake of fatty fish may protect against both type 1 and type 2 diabetes. Hypotheses rest on the high marine omega-3 fatty acid eicosapentaenoic acid+docosahexaenoic acid (EPA+DHA) and vitamin D contents, with possible beneficial effects on immune function and glucose metabolism. Our aim was to investigate, for the first time, **fatty fish consumption in relation to the risk of latent autoimmune diabetes in adults (LADA)**....

Weekly fatty fish consumption ($\geq$1 vs <1 serving per week), was associated with a reduced risk of LADA but not type 2 diabetes (OR 0.51, 95% CI 0.30–0.87, and 1.01, 95% CI 0.74–1.39, respectively). Similar associations were seen for estimated intake of n-3 PUFA ($\geq$0.3 g per day; LADA: OR 0.60, 95% CI 0.35–1.03, type 2 diabetes: OR 1.14, 95% CI 0.79–1.58) and fish oil supplementation (LADA: OR 0.47, 95% CI 0.19–1.12, type 2 diabetes: OR 1.58, 95% CI 1.08–2.31).

Conclusions:

Our findings suggest that **fatty fish consumption may reduce the risk of LADA**, possibly through effects of marine-originated omega-3 fatty acids (Löfvenborg).

The association between fish consumption and risk of **age-related macular degeneration (AMD)** is still unclear. The aim of the current meta-analysis and systematic review was to quantitatively evaluate findings from observational studies on fish consumption and the risk of AMD. ... A total of 4202 cases with 128,988 individuals from eight cohort studies were identified in the current meta-analysis.

The meta-analyzed RR was 0.76 (95% CI, 0.65-0.90) when any AMD was considered. Subgroup analyses by AMD stages showed that **fish consumption would reduce the risk of both early (RR, 0.83; 95% CI, 0.72-0.96) and late (RR; 0.76; 95% CI, 0.60-0.97) AMD**. When stratified by the follow-up duration, fish consumption was **a protective factor of AMD in both over 10 years** (n = 5; RR, 0.81; 95% CI, 0.67-0.97) **and less than 10 years** (n = 3; RR, 0.70; 95% CI, 0.51 to 0.97) follow-up duration. Stratified analyses by fish type demonstrated that **dark meat fish** (RR, 0.68, 95% CI, 0.46-0.99), **especially tuna fish** (RR, 0.58; 95% CI, 95% CI, 0.47-0.71) **intake was associated with reduced AMD risk.**

Evidence of a linear association between dose of fish consumption and risk of AMD was demonstrated. The results of this meta-analysis demonstrated that fish consumption can reduce AMD risk (Zhu).

Several studies have investigated the potential health benefits, including those associated with neurological function, of the n-3 fatty acid DHA. This has arisen in part because of the association between higher intakes of fish, which is a major dietary source of DHA, and reduced disease risk. **In addition to DHA, fish also provides choline and vitamin D.** The objective of the present study was to assess whether women in the first half of pregnancy with low fish intake also had low blood concentrations of vitamin D, choline and DHA. A total of 222 pregnant women at 16 weeks of gestation were examined for dietary intake, erythrocyte (phosphatidylethanolamine PE) DIIA, plasma frcc cholinc and 25-hydroxyvitamin D (25(OH)D).

Women who consumed ≤ 75 g fish/week (n 56) compared to ≥ 150 g fish/week (n 116) had lower dietary intake of DHA, total choline and vitamin D (P< 0·001), and lower erythrocyte PE DHA (5·25 (sd 1·27), 6·83 (sd 1·62) g/100 g total fatty acid, respectively, P< 0·01), plasma free choline (6·59 (sd 1·65), 7·40 (sd 2·05) µmol/l, respectively, P= 0·023) and 25(OH)D (50·3 (sd 20·0), 62·5 (sd 29·8) nmol/l, respectively, P< 0·01). DHA intake was positively related to the intake of vitamin D from foods (ρ 0·47, P< 0·001) and total choline (ρ 0·32, P< 0·001).

Dietary intakes and biomarkers of DHA, choline and vitamin D status were assessed to be linked. This raises the possibility that **unidentified concurrent nutrient inadequacies might have an impact on the results of studies addressing the benefits of supplemental DHA** (Wu; Lower Fish).

The point for this study is that it might not be just the omega 3s in fish that are responsible for the benefits of eating fish but also other nutrients that fish contains that are found little elsewhere, like vitamin D and choline. That is why fish consumption is a much better way to attaining omega 3s than supplements. Supplements only contains omega 3s without the other beneficial nutrients in fish.

This study investigated the **effects of fatty fish on sleep, daily functioning** and biomarkers such as **heart rate variability (HRV)**, vitamin D status (serum 25-hydroxyvitamin D (25OHD), and eicosapentaenoic acid (EPA, 20:5n-3) + docosahexaenoic acid (DHA, 22:6n-3) in red blood cells. Moreover **the relationship among sleep, daily functioning, HRV, vitamin D status, and levels of EPA+DHA was investigated**....

Ninety-five male forensic patients from a secure forensic inpatient facility in the USA were randomly assigned into a Fish or a Control group. The Fish group received **Atlantic salmon three times per week** from September to February, and the **Control group was provided an alternative meal** (e.g., chicken, pork, beef), but with the same nutritional value as their habitual diet, three times per week during the same period. Sleep (sleep latency, sleep efficiency, actual sleep time, and actual wake time), self-perceived sleep quality and daily functioning, as well as vitamin D status, EPA+DHA, and HRV, were assessed pre- and post-intervention period.

There was **a significant increase in sleep latency from pre- to post-test in the Control group. The Fish group reported better daily functioning than the Control group during post-test**. Fish consumption throughout the wintertime had also **an effect on resting HRV and EPA+DHA**, but not on vitamin D status. However, at post-test, **the vitamin D status in the Fish group was still closer to the level regarded as optimal compared to the Control group**. Vitamin D status correlated negatively with actual wake time and positively with sleep efficiency during pre-test, as well as positively with daily functioning and sleep quality during post-test. Finally, HRV correlated negatively with sleep latency and positively with daily functioning.

Fish consumption seemed to have a positive impact on sleep in general and also on daily functioning, which may be related to vitamin D status and HRV. (Hansen, CP).

Scientific literature is increasingly reporting on dietary deficiencies in many populations of some nutrients critical for **foetal and infant brain development and function**. Purpose: To highlight the potential benefits of maternal supplementation with docosahexaenoic acid (DHA) and other important complimentary nutrients, including vitamin D, folic acid and iodine during pregnancy and/or breast feeding for foetal and/or infant brain development and/or function.

Methods: English language systematic reviews, meta-analyses, randomised controlled trials, cohort studies, cross-sectional and case-control studies were obtained through searches on MEDLINE and the Cochrane Register of Controlled Trials from January 2000 through to February 2012 and reference lists of retrieved articles. Reports were selected if they included benefits and harms of maternal supplementation of DHA, vitamin D, folic acid or iodine supplementation during pregnancy and/or lactation.

Maternal DHA intake during pregnancy and/or lactation can prolong high risk pregnancies, increase birth weight, head circumference and birth length, and can enhance visual acuity, hand and eye co-ordination, attention, problem solving and information processing. Vitamin D helps maintain pregnancy and promotes normal skeletal and brain development. Folic acid is necessary for normal foetal spine, brain and skull development. **Iodine is essential for thyroid hormone production necessary for normal brain and nervous system development during gestation that impacts childhood function.**

Maternal supplementation within recommended safe intakes in populations with dietary deficiencies may prevent many brain and central nervous system malfunctions and even enhance brain development and function in their offspring (Morse).

Note that fish is an excellent source of all of the nutrients mentioned here, except for folic acid.

Fibromyalgia (FM) is a complex multidimensional disorder with pain as its main symptom. Fibromyalgia imposes a psychosocial burden on individuals that negatively impacts quality of life. The relationship of dietary habits with these psychosocial aspects is still unclear....

The purpose of this cross-sectional study was to assess dietary habits in a representative sample of women with FM and to explore their association **with mental health, depression, and optimism** in this population....

A daily or almost-daily consumption of fruit and vegetables and a moderate consumption of fish (2 to 5 servings per week) were associated with higher scores in

mental health (P<0.001, P<0.05, and P<0.001, respectively) and lower levels of depression (P<0.001, P<0.01, and P<0.01, respectively). A **daily or almost-daily consumption of vegetables and a moderate consumption of dairy products and fish were associated with higher levels of optimism** (P<0.05, P<0.05, and P<0.001, respectively). A **daily or almost-daily consumption of cured meats and sweetened beverages were associated with higher levels of depression and lower levels of optimism,** respectively (both P<0.05).

The results this study suggest that a daily or almost-daily intake of fruit and vegetables and a moderate intake of fish may be associated with more favorable psychosocial outcomes in women with FM. Conversely, excessive intake of cured meats and sweetened beverages was related to worse scores in optimism and depression outcomes (Ruiz-Cabello).

I read this last study with particular interest, as I was diagnosed with fibromyalgia back on August 27, 2001. Since then, I have found that a careful attention to my diet makes a huge difference in how well I handle my symptoms, so I would concur with this study in that regard.

That said; notice that yet one more benefit is being attributed to fruits and vegetables. It should be obvious at this point that the single best thing you can do diet-wise for your health is to eat more fruits and vegetables. It will be see in the next chapter that processed meats would not fit God's decree about animal foods, and it can be seen here that they can be problematic, as are "sweetened beverages" such as soda. Dairy will be discussed later, but here, notice the beneficial effect of it.

But in regards to the subject of this chapter, notice that fish consumption is associated with reduced rates of depression and higher levels of optimism. That is truly a powerful effect.

There is also evidence that fish is protective against cancer.

OBJECTIVE: We investigated the association between **fish and n-3 PUFA consumption and pancreatic cancer risk** in a population-based, prospective study in Japanese men and women....

CONCLUSION: **High n-3 PUFA, especially marine n-3 PUFAs, and DHA consumption was associated with a lower risk of pancreatic cancer** in a population with a large variation in fish consumption, although the data apply to only a portion of the JPHC study subjects (Hidaka).

All in all, there is much evidence that fish is one of the healthiest foods you can consume. It is packed with nutrients that are hard to find elsewhere, namely Omega 3s, vitamin D, choline, and iodine. As a result, its consumption is associated with health improvements in many areas. Add in the prominent place fish holds in the Bible, especially in the Gospels, and it is clear God intends for human beings to eat fish.

But the title of this chapter is "Pros *and Cons* of Fish Consumption." We will shortly turn to the "Cons" part of the tile, but a look at which form of fish is best will be a good lead in to that subject.

Farm-Raised vs. Wild Caught Fish and Potential Problems with Fish

Which is better, farm raised or wild caught fish? On this question, there is much debate. The following are comments in this regard:

> While eating more fatty fish is a good idea, **some are likely to have higher levels of mercury, PCBs, or other toxins**. These include mackerel, wild swordfish, tilefish, and shark.
> **Farm-raised fish of any type may also have higher levels of contaminants**. Children and pregnant women should avoid these fish entirely. Everyone else should eat no more than 7 ounces of these fish a week. **Fish like wild trout and wild salmon are safer** (WebMD; Facts).

> It used to be that wild-caught fish were considered healthy. Over the past several decades, however, **concerns have arisen about the effects heavy metal contaminants (such as mercury), pollutants (such as polychlorinated biphenyls, PCBs), pesticides, fertilizers and even trash have on the safety of water and fish**. The demand for certain types of fish and some fishing practices, such as bottom trolling, have **taken their toll on the environment and the availability of fish**....
> Although **modern-day fish farming** is designed to address safety concerns, it also **has drawbacks**. Some pens built in open water can be at the expense of the surrounding ecosystems, such as coastlines, underwater reefs, trees and swamps, and the wildlife that depend on them. Fish that are raised in areas where they're not normally found may escape and breed or compete with local fish — resulting in decreases in the wild species. **Fish farms** — including those in contained

reservoirs — **create enormous quantities of organic waste (feces)** that can contaminate water in the surrounding environment if not handled properly.

At this time there's no easy answer when it comes to what type of fish to choose — wild-caught or farm-raised. However, to help you navigate the farm versus wild dilemma, here are a few tips:...

Know which fish are overfished and avoid them....

Buy U.S. fish. The U.S. has strict environmental and food safety laws governing farmed and wild-caught fish. Purchasing U.S. fish is one way you can help ensure safety and sustainability (Mayo; Which).

Wild-caught trout have more calcium and iron. Farmed-raised trout have more vitamin A and selenium. But for the most part, they are nutritionally equivalent.

One of the main reasons we eat fish, of course, is that they are a uniquely potent source for long-chain **omega-3 fatty acids**. And here, **farmed fish often have the advantage**. Today's farmed Atlantic salmon provide significantly more omega-3 fats than wild-caught Atlantic salmon, for example....

In 2004, a widely-cited study found the levels of **PCBs, a potentially carcinogenic chemical, to be ten times higher in farmed fish than in wild-caught fish. That sounds pretty scary, but the amount of PCBs in the farmed fish was still less than 2% of the amount that would be considered dangerous**. The differences may also have been exaggerated. Subsequent studies found **PCB levels in farmed fish to be similar to those of wild fish**....

U.S. regulations prohibit the use of hormones or antibiotics to promote growth in farmed fish. This is not necessarily the case in other countries....

There are currently no genetically modified fish for sale in the U.S. At least, not as food. You can buy genetically modified fish for your tropical fish tank that glow in the dark, thanks to some genes borrowed from iridescent coral....

Wild-caught fish are sometimes harvested using practices that do a lot of collateral damage to the ecosystem and other fish. Fish-farming practices, on the other hand, can pollute the water and threaten local flora and fauna. Once again, it depends a lot on who is doing the fishing and/or farming.

Here in the U.S., for example, the National Oceanic and Atmospheric Administration [NOAA] regulates wild-catch fishing, setting, and enforcing standards that protect the marine environment and fish populations. **Fish farming operations in the U.S. are also strictly regulated.... Unfortunately, this is not the case everywhere** (Quick).

Several points are being raised in this quotes. First, fish can be contaminated with PCBs, mercury, and other contaminants. That is true whether the fish is wild caught or farm-raised. But in either case, the amount of contaminants is well below the level considered to be dangerous. As such, this issue is not as serious as many make it out to be. Evidence for this is the aforementioned health benefits of fish. It would seem that the good qualities of fish far outweigh any negative effects from contaminates. Moreover, in the next chapter we will see a way to avoid the most contaminated fish.

Second is the nutrient content of fish. It does vary between wild caught or farm-raised, but there is not a clear-cut advantage to one over the other.

Third, note that in the USA, fish cannot be given hormones or antibiotics, and there are no edible genetically modified fish. This is important as vegetarians often claim otherwise and use such claims to scare people off of eating fish.

Fourth, there is possible environmental damage from either form of fishing. But only wild caught fish has the problem of overfishing. But that can be avoided by not eating such fish. A database in this regard is available at Seafood Watch (www.seafoodwatch.org). And it is possible to harvest fish in a manner that is not damaging. For example, on this website are details of Alaska's salmon harvesting practices. It states:

> **Pacific salmon in Alaska are among the most intensively managed species in the world, with excellent monitoring of fish populations and the fishery itself....**
>
> **Alaskan fishery managers have taken the long view**, limiting the entry of new fishermen and boats, and monitoring salmon populations to ensure they remain large enough to reproduce naturally....
>
> The comparatively healthy river systems in Alaska, combined with precautionary fishery management, have **resulted in salmon runs that are more resilient**. Over the past 10 years, **Alaska has landed roughly 20 times as much salmon as California, Oregon and Washington combined**. The current health of Alaskan salmon populations and their

habitat reflects the success of the state's management practices (Overfishing).

Thus Alaskan salmon would be the best choice for this type of fish. And salmon just happens to be one of the healthiest fish there is. To know it is from Alaska and harvested in a sustainable manner, look on the label for "From an ASMI certified sustainable fishery." ASMI stands for "Alaska Seafood Marketing Institute."

Another label to look for is "MSC." The Seafood Watch website explains what it means and the implications.

Marine Stewardship Council (MSC) has developed standards for sustainably managed and traceable wild-caught seafood. The number of fisheries that meet MSC ecolabel standards has steadily increased.

Today, 231 fisheries are MSC-certified, representing more than 8.8 million tons of seafood, and more than 26,000 seafood products bear the blue MSC ecolabel. Additionally, **over 88 fisheries are engaged in the assessment process to become MSC-certified** (Illegal).

But any fish that is caught or farmed under US regulations would be better than fish caught under the regulations of other countries. Thus buying USA would also be a good step in avoiding all of these problems.

However, personally, I think a better solution than government regulation would be to let the free market handle things by devising a system by which certain fishers own the fish in a certain area. In that way, it would be to their long-term economic advantage to ensure the fish population remains prosperous. This is one of the reason for fish farms, where the fish can be fenced off and owned by a particular fisher.

Forward-thinking fish eaters realize that aquaculture is the way of the future. Today, 50 percent of the world's fish is raised on farms. Some are gargantuan pens in open water, some are plastic tubs in Iowa barns, some are tightly integrated and sustainable ecosystems. Aquaculture is a fledgling, imperfect industry, but **farmed fish are better at converting feed to meat than any other animal and will be the protein source of earth's future** (Munchies).

In other words, the reason fish get overfished in the high seas is no one owns them. As a result, each fisher is competing against other fishers for the same fish, so they take as much as they can when they can and small fish along with large fish. But if certain fishers owned the fish, then they would not feel the need to harvest before the other guy, and they could throw smaller fish back, knowing they would be able to catch them again when they get larger, when the same fish will bring a larger profit. But whether government regulation or the free market, there are possible solutions to the overfishing problem.

The Seafood Watch website presents possible solutions to other problems associated with large-scale fishing. Separate pages present current problems, but also solutions, with a "Story of Hope" demonstrating that the proposed solutions do in fact work.

But "ethical vegans" will still argue that fish feel pain and thus should not be killed. But consider the following:

Suffering (related to but different from pain), depends on a degree of self-awareness that fish likely don't have. To oversimplify, a fish would have to think, "Well, this sucks for me to experience suffering" and the evidence just isn't there. Instead, **think of a fish as computers that react to a constant stream of stimuli in specific ways.**

Essentially, fish are "other." Not animals exactly, not self-conscious, and incapable of pain. It's an argument with historical roots: **Both Judaism and Catholicism regulate fish separately from "meat."** (It's cream cheese and lox, not cream cheese and roast beef.) By classifying them separately from animals, **pescetarians [vegetarians who eat fish] argue that killing a fish is more ethical than killing, say, a chicken** (Munchies).

Fish do not feel pain the way humans do, according to a team of neurobiologists, behavioral ecologists and fishery scientists. The researchers conclude that fish do not have the neuro-physiological capacity for a conscious awareness of pain....

The current overview-study raises the complaint that a great majority of all published studies evaluate a fish's reaction to a seemingly painful impulse - such as rubbing the injured body part against an object or the discontinuation of the feed intake - as an indication of pain. However, this methodology does not prove verifiably whether the reaction was due to a conscious sensation of pain or an unconscious impulse perception by means of nociception, or a combination of the two. Basically, **it is very difficult to deduct underlying emotional states based on behavioural responses**. Moreover, fish often show only minor or no reactions at all to interventions which would be extremely painful to us and to other mammals.

Pain killers such as morphine that are effective for humans were either ineffective in fish or were only effective in astronomically high doses that, for small mammals, would have meant immediate death from shock. **These findings suggest that fish either have absolutely no awareness of pain in human terms or they react completely different to pain**. By and large, it is absolutely not advisable to interpret the behaviour of fish from a human perspective....

However, at a legal and moral level, the recently published doubts regarding the awareness of pain in fish **do not release anybody from their responsibility of having to justify all uses of fishes in a socially acceptable way and to minimise any form of stress and damage to the fish when interacting with it** (Science Daily).

On the last point, even if fish do feel pain, they can be killed in a manner that significantly reduces it.

> Both percussive and electrical stunning and killing systems, if applied correctly, can induce immediate and irreversible insensibility, thereby **subjecting the animals to less pain, stress, and undue suffering as compared with other methods**...
>
> Innovations may offer alternatives, including combining methods in order **to stun and kill quickly, efficiently, and without causing undue suffering**. In Norway, for example, a system is reportedly in development whereby salmon are electrically stunned and, before they can regain consciousness, are quickly subjected to percussive stunning after which they undergo exsanguination by gill-cutting. Prototype equipment for percussive and electrical stunning systems has recently become available, and some salmon processors, after performing trials, believe it to be economically feasible for large producers (Humane Society).

Thus again, there are possible solutions to problems that vegetarians raise. Each problem can be solved with old-fashioned human ingenuity. God gave us brains, and when we put our minds to it, we can solve problems. Given how incredibly healthy fish is for us to eat, it is to our advantage to do so.

Complaints of Vegans

However, vegans, vegetarians, and animal rights advocates are not looking for solutions, other than to tell people to not eat fish (or any other animal foods). And they will use scare tactics and false information to do so.

What's wrong with eating fish? Consuming fish not only **entails animal cruelty**, but it is also bad for the ocean and potentially detrimental to your health.

There is persuasive evidence that **fish can feel pain** and can even show fear....

Apart from the **undeniable animal suffering involved, fishing is a global environmental menace that threatens our oceans....**

Farmed fish do not offer greater sustainability than wild-caught fish. **Many farmed fish are genetically modified, and are fed diets laced with high doses of antibiotics.** As a result of their crowded undersea cages, fish farms are often rife opportunistic parasites like sea lice.

Eating fish of any sort is accompanied by worrisome health risks. **Fish can accumulate high levels of mercury and carcinogens like PCBs.** As the world's oceans become increasingly polluted, eating fish becomes fraught with ever-increasing health concerns (Vegan.com).

This chapter has demonstrated that each of these claims is false or there are potential solutions to them. But such websites do not mention such. Moreover, there are numerous health benefits to eating fish, and this is due to fish containing nutrients that are hard to attain elsewhere. Vegans try to claim the benefits of fish can be attained elsewhere, but again, this chapter has demonstrated that is not true.

By trying to scare people into not eating fish, the vegan/ vegetarian/ animal rights advocates are putting the lives of fish above that of human beings. And that is a decidedly unbiblical attitude:

[26]**And God said, "Let Us make humanity according to Our image and according to [Our] likeness, and let them be ruling [over] the fish of the sea** and the birds [or, flying creatures] of heaven and the livestock and all the earth and all the reptiles [or, quadrupeds], the ones walking upon the earth." [27]And God made humanity, according to [the] image of God, He made him, male and female He made them. [cp. Matt

19:4] [28]And God blessed them, saying, "Be increasing, and be being multiplied, and fill the earth and exercise lordship over [or, subdue] it, and **rule [over] the fish of the seas** and the birds [or, flying creatures] of heaven and all the livestock and all of the earth and all the reptiles [or, quadrupeds] walking upon the earth" (Gen 1:26-28).

Maybe all of the information in this chapter is why there are many people who call themselves vegetarians but who eat fish. The technical term for someone following such a diet would be "pescetarian," though it has also been dubbed a "seagan" diet, meaning a diet that is wholly plant-based, except to include seafood.

Such a diet does make sense. Including fish in an otherwise vegan diet would avoid the potential drawbacks of a full vegan diet, while providing the benefits of fish consumption. Thus some longtime vegans, are advocating such a diet, "so long as they stick to sustainably-fished, low-mercury seafood" (Huffington Post; Seagan).

All that is left is for vegetarians to argue that it is ethically wrong to kill and eat animals, whether they feel pain or not. But as was stated in the previous chapter, such is an untenable position for the Bible-believing Christian. God gave "every moving thing that lives" to us for food, and that includes fish. Fish is in fact, one of the healthiest foods you can eat.

Bibliography:

Authority Nutrition. 11 Evidence-Based Health Benefits of Eating Fish.
https://authoritynutrition.com/11-health-benefits-of-fish/

DHA-EPA Institute. Conversion efficiency of ALA to DHA in Humans.
http://www.dhaomega3.org/Overview/Conversion-Efficiency-of-ALA-to-DHA-in-Humans

Daniells, Stephen. Omega-3: ALA intakes enough for EPA/DPA levels for non-fish eaters?
http://www.nutraingredients-usa.com/Research/Omega-3-ALA-intakes-enough-for-EPA-DPA-levels-for-non-fish-eaters

Djoussé L, et. al., *Clinical Nutrition*. 2012 Dec;31(6):846-53. Fish consumption, omega-3 fatty acids and risk of heart failure: a meta-analysis.
https://www.ncbi.nlm.nih.gov/pubmed/22682084/

Hansen, CP, et. al. *Stroke*. 2017 Jan 3. pii: *STROKEAHA*. Adherence to a Healthy Nordic Diet and Risk of Stroke: A Danish Cohort Study.
https://www.ncbi.nlm.nih.gov/pubmed/28049735

Hansen, Anita L, Ph.D. et. al., Fish Consumption, Sleep, Daily Functioning, and Heart Rate Variability *Journal of Clinical Sleep Medicine.* 2014 May 15; 10(5): 567–575. Published online 2014 May 15.
https://www.ncbi.nlm.nih.gov/pmc/articles/PMC4013386/

Harvard School of Public Health. Omega-3 Fatty Acids: An Essential Contribution.
https://www.hsph.harvard.edu/nutritionsource/omega-3-fats/

Hidaka A, et. al. *American Journal of Clinical Nutrition.* 2015 Dec;102(6):1490-7. Fish, n-3 PUFA consumption, and pancreatic cancer risk in Japanese: a large, population-based, prospective cohort study. https://www.ncbi.nlm.nih.gov/pubmed/26537936

Huffington Post. 'Seagan' Diet Suggests It's Not A Crazy Idea For Vegans To Eat Seafood.
http://www.huffingtonpost.com/entry/seagan-diet-vegans-eating-seafood_us_57879151e4b08608d333169c

Humane Society. An HSUS Report: The Welfare of Farmed Fish at Slaughter. Stephanie Yue, Ph.D.
http://www.humanesociety.org/assets/pdfs/farm/hsus-the-welfare-of-farmed-fish-at-slaughter.pdf

JAMA (*Journal of the American Medical Association*). Eating Fish: Health Benefits and Risks.
http://jamanetwork.com/journals/jama/fullarticle/203693

Levitan EB, et. al. *European Journal of Clinical Nutrition.* 2010 Jun;64(6):587-94. doi: 10.1038/ejcn.2010.50. Epub 2010 Mar 24. Fatty fish, marine omega-3 fatty acids and incidence of heart failure. https://www.ncbi.nlm.nih.gov/pubmed/20332801

Seafood Health Facts. Seafood Nutrition Overview.
http://www.seafoodhealthfacts.org/seafood-nutrition/healthcare-professionals/seafood-nutrition-overview

Löfvenborg JE, et. al., *Nutrition and Diabetes.* 2014 Oct 20;4:e139. doi: 10.1038/nutd.2014.36. Fatty fish consumption and risk of latent autoimmune diabetes in adults.
https://www.ncbi.nlm.nih.gov/pmc/articles/PMC4216999/

Munchies. Vegetarians Who Eat Fish Are Actually Onto Something.
https://munchies.vice.com/en/articles/vegetarians-who-eat-fish-are-actually-onto-something

Morse, Nancy L. *Nutrients.* 2012 Jul; 4(7): 799–840. Published online 2012 Jul 24. Benefits of Docosahexaenoic Acid, Folic Acid, Vitamin D and Iodine on Foetal and Infant Brain Development and Function Following Maternal Supplementation during Pregnancy and Lactation.

Creationist Diet

https://www.ncbi.nlm.nih.gov/pmc/articles/PMC3407995/

Quick and Dirty Tips. Farm-Raised vs. Wild-Caught Fish. By Monica Reinagel, MS, LD/N, CNS, Nutrition Diva. March 5, 2014 1056 78 41.

http://www.quickanddirtytips.com/health-fitness/healthy-eating/farm-raised-vs-wild-caught-fish

Ruiz-Cabello P, *Journal of Academic Nutrition and Diet*. 2016 Nov 24. pii: S2212-2672(16)31190-X. doi: 10.1016/j.jand.2016.09.023. Association of Dietary Habits with Psychosocial Outcomes in Women with Fibromyalgia: The al-Ándalus Project.

https://www.ncbi.nlm.nih.gov/pubmed/27890478

Seafood Watch. Overfishing.

http://www.seafoodwatch.org/ocean-issues/wild-seafood/overfishing

Seafood Watch. Illegal Fishing.

http://www.seafoodwatch.org/ocean-issues/wild-seafood/illegal-fishing

Science Daily. Do fish feel pain? Not as humans do, study suggests.

https://www.sciencedaily.com/releases/2013/08/130808123719.htm

UMMC. University of Maryland Medical Center. Omega-3 fatty acids.

http://umm.edu/health/medical/altmed/supplement/omega3-fatty-acids

Vegan.com. Vegan Fish.

http://www.vegan.com/fish/

WebMD. The Facts on Omega-3 Fatty Acids.

http://www.webmd.com/healthy-aging/omega-3-fatty-acids-fact-sheet

Wu BT, et. al. British Journal of Nutrition. 2013 Mar 14;109(5):936-43. Low fish intake is associated with low blood concentrations of vitamin D, choline and n-3 DHA in pregnant women.

https://www.ncbi.nlm.nih.gov/pubmed/22691303

Wu S, et. al. *Neuroscience Biobehavior Review*. 2015 Jan;48:1-9. doi: 10.1016/j.neubiorev.2014.11.008. Epub 2014 Nov 21. Omega-3 fatty acids intake and risks of dementia and Alzheimer's disease: a meta-analysis.

https://www.ncbi.nlm.nih.gov/pubmed/25446949

Zhu W, et. al. *Nutrients*. 2016 Nov 22;8(11). pii: E743. Fish Consumption and Age-Related Macular Degeneration Incidence: A Meta-Analysis and Systematic Review of Prospective Cohort Studies.

https://www.ncbi.nlm.nih.gov/pubmed/27879656

Chapter Eight:
Restrictions on Meat Eating

Biblical limitations and guidelines on meat eating will be discussed in this chapter.

Clean vs. Unclean Meats in the Bible

The first issue to be discussed is the distinction between clean and unclean animals.

The Noahic Covenant:

Before the Flood, God told Noah:

[1]And the LORD God said to Noah, "<u>You</u> enter and all your house [fig., family] into the ark, for have I seen you righteous before Me in this generation. [2]Now **from the animals, the clean ones**, take in to you **seven [by] seven**, male and female, but from the animals, **the not clean ones two [by] two**, male and female. [3]And **from the birds** [or, flying creatures] of the sky, **the clean ones, seven [by] seven**, male and female, and from the birds [or, flying creatures], **the not clean ones, two [by] two**, male and female, to sustain continually seed on all the earth. [4]For yet seven days <u>I</u> bring rain upon the earth forty days and forty nights, and I will blot out every rising up [fig., offspring] which I made from [the] face of the earth."

[5]And Noah did all, as many [things] as the LORD God commanded him. [6]Now Noah was six hundred years old and the cataclysmic flood [of] water became upon the earth (Gen 7:2).

Then after the Flood:

[20]And Noah built an altar to God, and he took **from all the animals, the clean ones**, and **from all the birds, the clean ones**, and offered a whole burnt-offering upon the altar. (Gen 8:20).

What this means is, God must have explained to Noah distinctions between clean and unclean animals, and Noah knew that only clean animals were to be used for sacrifice. That is why seven of each clean animal were taken, but only two of each unclean animal. Thus all the storybooks you've seen with the animals lined up in two's are wrong. There was actually seven of each of the clean animals.

Moreover, if Noah sacrificed one each of the clean animals, this would have left three pairs of each of them to re-populate the earth, while there was only one pair of each unclean animal. As a result, the clean animals would flourish faster than the unclean ones. Thus God was setting things up so that the people would have sufficient animals for sacrifice and for food after the Flood.

In addition, if Noah had sacrificed or eaten one of the unclean animals, then that species would have become extinct. As such, Noah must have abided by the distinction between clean and unclean animals in his own diet.

The point of all of this is that the distinction between clean and unclean animals did not originate with the Mosaic Law. It was a part of the Noahic Covenant. As such, as with the decree about eating meat, the distinction between clean and unclean animals would be for all peoples, "for eternal generations" (see Gen 9:12).

Leviticus 11:

This distinction between clean and unclean meats is repeated to Moses, which he records in Leviticus 11. The chapter begins:

¹And the LORD spoke to Moses and Aaron, saying, ²"Speak to the sons [and daughters] of Israel, saying, '**These [are] the animals which you* will eat** from all the animals upon the earth (Lev 11:1f).

Let's pause and notice how this is worded: "These [are] the animals which you* **will** eat." The NKJV has, "These are the animals which you **may** eat." But the form of the Hebrew verb used here is a *qal*, imperfect. This is the same form in which verbs appear in the Ten Commandments (Exod 20:1ff). In the Greek Septuagint, a future tense is used here, just as in the Ten Commandments.

The point is, the text is reinforcing that God did not just give "permission" to human beings to eat meat in Genesis 9. He gave meats to use to eat, and He intends that we eat them. We **will** eat them, not we **may** eat them. That said; the text continues:

[3]Every animal **parting [the] hoof and making divisions of two hooves, and taking up, chews the cud [or, ruminates]** among the animals, **these you* will eat.**

[4]"**However, of these you* will not eat**, from the ones taking up, chews the cud, and from the ones parting the hooves and dividing [the] hooves: the camel, because it **chews the cud, but does not divide the hoof, this [is] unclean to you***. [5]And the rough-foot [i.e., maybe a rabbit or rock badger], because it chews the cud, but does not divide the hoof, this [is] unclean to you*. [6]And the rabbit [or, hare], because it chews the cud, but does not divide the hoof, this [is] unclean to you*. [7]And **the swine [or, pig], because this [animal] divides the hoof, and makes division of [the] hoof, but it does not chew the cud, this [is] unclean to you***. [8]You* will not eat of their flesh, and you* will not touch their carcasses; these [are] unclean to you* (Lev 11:3-8).

Thus Moses first gives a method by which to identify which animals are clean and which are unclean and then gives specific examples. Note that "chew the cud" means "ruminate" (as the ALT indicates). "What is a ruminant animal" you might ask? An Internet article by this title answer this question.

> Many different species of ruminant animals are found around the world. **Ruminants include cattle, sheep, goats, buffalo, deer, elk, giraffes and camels**. These animals all have a digestive system that is uniquely different from our own.
>
> **Instead of one compartment to the stomach they have four.** Of the four compartments the rumen is the largest section and the main digestive centre. **The rumen is filled with billions of tiny microorganisms that are able to break down grass and other coarse vegetation that animals with one stomach (including humans, chickens and pigs) cannot digest**.
>
> Ruminant animals do not completely chew the grass or vegetation they eat. The partially chewed grass goes into the large rumen where it is stored and broken down into balls of "cud." **When the animal has eaten its fill, it will rest and "chew its cud." The cud is then swallowed once again where it will pass into the next three compartments**—the reticulum, the omasum and the true stomach, the abomasum.

223

Many of the plants that grow on earth cannot be used directly by humans as food. Over 50 percent of the energy in cereal crops that are grown for food is inedible to humans. **Ruminants have the ability to convert these plants and residues into high quality protein in the form of meat and milk** (Ruminants).

Thus God has nicely designed a system by which we humans can derive nourishment from plants that we would not otherwise be able to digest. This quote mentions cereal crops, but the same would be true for grasses. We cannot digest them, but cattle and other ruminants can.

This relates back to the discussion in Chapter Five about world hunger. Since grasses can grow in places that edible grains cannot, the consumption of meats and dairy increases the human food supply by enabling us to derive nutrition from these otherwise inedible plants.

That said; for an animal to be clean, it must both chew the cud and have divided hoofs. If it only does one or the other, it is unclean. And note the strong language used for unclean animals, "You* will not eat of their flesh, and you* will not touch their carcasses." Thus God is in no uncertain terms warning us against unclean animals. And note the specific mention of swine (or pig). That will be important later.

The characteristics by which to identify clean versus unclean seafood is given next:

[9]"And these [are] what **you* will eat from all the [creatures] in the waters**: all, as many as are to them [fig., **have] fins and scales** in the waters and in the seas and in the brooks, these **you* will eat**. [10]But all, as many as are not to them [fig. **do not have] fins or scales** in the water, or in the seas, and in the brooks, from all which the waters produce, and of every soul living in the water, **are an abomination**. [11]And they will be abominations to you*. **You* will not eat from their flesh, and you* will abhor their carcasses**. [12]And **all, as many as are not to them [fig. do not have] fins and scales of the [creatures] in the water, these are an abomination to you*** (Lev 11:9-12).

Thus clean seafood must have both fins and scales. This makes for an easy way to identify which is which. Shellfish have neither, so they are unclean, while marine mammals do not have scales, so they also are unclean. But many fish have both, as we will see shortly.

But first, note again the strong language used here. Unclean sea creatures are "an abomination," and we are to "abhor their carcasses."

Next are birds. Here only unclean birds are listed:

¹³'And **these you* will abhor of the birds, and they will not be consumed, they are an abomination**: the **eagle** and the ossifrage [i.e., a large bird of prey], and the sea-eagle, ¹⁴and the **vulture**, and [the] kite [i.e., a small hawk], **and the like to it**; ¹⁵and [the] crow [or, raven] and the like to it; ¹⁶and [the] **ostrich**, and [the] owl, and [the] sea-gull, and the like it, and [the] hawk **and the like to it**, ¹⁷and [the] night-raven and the cormorant [i.e., a large ocean bird] and [the] ibis [i.e., an Egyptian bird], ¹⁸and [the] water-hen, and [the] pelican, [the] and **swan**, ¹⁹and [the] owl and [the] heron [i.e., a freshwater wading bird], and [the] curlew [i.e., a yellowish bird dwelling in clefts] and **the like to it**, and [the] hoopoe [i.e., native to Europe, Asia, Africa] and [the] bat. ²⁰And **all winged creatures [that] creep, which go upon four [feet], are abominations to you*** (Lev 11:13-20).

Note the repeated phrase, "and the like to it." What these birds have in common is they are either birds of prey or scavengers. Since only unclean birds are listed, it is assumed that birds that do not fit these descriptions are clean. And note again the strong language. Such birds are an abomination and are to be abhorred. Next are insects:

²¹'But these you* will eat from the **creeping winged animals**, which go upon four [feet], which have legs above their feet, to be leaping with them on the earth. ²²And these of them you* will eat: the **devouring locust** and like to it, and the **cricket** and the like to it, and the **migratory locust** and the like to it, and the **grasshopper** and the like to it. ²³Every creeping thing from among the winged creatures, which is [fig., **has] four feet is an abomination to you*** (Lev 11:21-23).

Note that devouring locusts, crickets, migratory locusts, grasshoppers, "and the like to it" are mentioned as being clean. But any insect not like these four or which have four feet are "an abomination to you." Next are some related laws:

24'And **by these you* will be defiled**; every one touching their carcasses will be unclean until the evening. 25And **every one taking of their dead bodies will wash his garments** and will be unclean until the evening. 26Among all the animals which is dividing the hoof and makes claws, and does not chew the cud, will be unclean to you*; **every one touching their dead bodies will be unclean until evening** (Lev 11:24-26.

The carcasses of animals should not be touched, and a person must wash himself if he does. Knowing what we know today about germs and the spread of disease, this seems basic. But it was actually quite earthshaking at the time. Therefore, God revealed to Moses ways for the Israelites to avoid the spread of disease that was not common practice at the time. And in the same way, the distinction between clean and unclean animals was given for health reasons, as we will see shortly. But to continue with the text:

27'And all which **moves upon its forefeet** among all the wild beasts **which moves upon four [paws], will be unclean to you***; everyone touching their dead bodies will be unclean until evening. 28And **the one taking of their dead bodies will wash his garments** and will be unclean until evening: these are unclean to you* (Lev 11:27f).

Note the mention of moving upon its forefeet and four paws. Such animals are unclean and would include dogs and cats. And note again the regulations regarding touching dead animals.

29'And these [are] **unclean to you* from the creeping things**, the ones creeping upon the earth: the weasel, and the **mouse**, and the lizard [or, land crocodile], 30[the] ferret [or, field mouse], and [the] chameleon, and [the] spotted lizard, and [the] newt, and [the] mole. 31These [are] unclean to you* from all the creeping things upon the earth; everyone touching [them] having died will be unclean until evening (Lev 11:29-31).

Here we have additional unclean animals listed. And note that they are not to be touched. Knowing what we do now about how mice and other rodents can carry diseases, not touching them makes sense. But such was not known back then. However, God gave these instructions to protect His people from disease, just as He did the distinction between clean and unclean animals. It needs to be noted how these regulations are interspersed. This is seen in how the text continues.

[32]'And **anything on which shall fall from them having died it will be unclean**; from every wooden vessel, or garment, or skin, or sack, every vessel in which work should be done in it, **will be dipped in water**, and will be unclean until evening; then it will be clean. [33]And every clay vessel into which from these will fall, as many things as shall be inside, will be unclean, and **it will be broken**. [34]And all food being eaten, on which water will come [from such a vessel] upon it, will be unclean; and every beverage which is drunk in any [such] vessel, will be unclean. [35]And everything on which there shall fall from their dead bodies will be unclean; ovens and stands for jars will be broken down. These are unclean, and they will be unclean to you* (Lev 11:32-35).

Of course you would wash or pitch anything upon which a dead animal fell, and you would not drink from a vessel into which a dead animal had fallen. But again, such was not common practice at the time.

[36]'However, [if the water be] of fountains of water, or a pond, or a gathering of water, it will be clean; but the one touching their carcasses will be unclean. [37]And if [one] of their carcasses should fall upon any sowing seed which will be sown, it will be clean. [38]But if water be poured on any seed, and [one] of their dead bodies fall upon it, it is unclean to you. [39]And **if [one] of the animals die, which it is [intended] for you* to eat, the one touching their carcasses will be unclean until evening**. [40]And the one eating from their carcasses will wash his garments, and will be unclean until evening; and **the one carrying their carcasses will wash his garments, and bathe himself in water, and will be unclean until evening** (Lev 11:36-40).

The important point here is that touching even dead clean animals makes a person unclean. Again, we know why today, but they didn't

227

back then. And immediately after these regulations which were given to protect the Israelites from disease, God goes back to discussing clean versus unclean animals:

[41]'And **every creeping thing which creeps upon the earth, this will be an abomination to you***; **it will not be consumed**. [42]And every [animal] **creeping on [its] belly**, and every [animal] going on four [feet] through all [fig., continually], which abounds with feet among all the creeping things creeping upon the earth, you* will not eat it, for it is an abomination to you*. [43]And **by no means shall you* defile your* souls [or, make yourselves abominable] with any of the creeping things**, the ones creeping upon the earth, and you* will not be defiled by them, and you* will not be unclean by them.

Additional unclean animals are indicated here, namely snakes, snails, and the like. And note again the strong language. You will "defile your soul" if you cat any of them.

Leviticus 11 concludes with the reason for all of these regulations:

[44]**"For I am the LORD your* God; and you* will be consecrated, and you* will be holy, because I the LORD your* God am holy; and you* will not defile your* souls** with any of the creeping things, the ones creeping upon the earth. [45]For I am the LORD, the One having brought you* up out of [the] land of Egypt to be your* God; and you* will be holy, **for I the LORD am holy**. [1Pet 1:16] [46]'This [is] the law concerning animals and birds and every soul [or, creature] moving in the water, and every soul [or, creature] creeping on the earth; [47]**to distinguish between the unclean and between the clean; and between the [animals] being alive, being eaten [or, which should be eaten] and between the [animals] being alive, not being eaten [or, which should not be eaten]**'" (Lev 11:44-47)

Many claim the reason for these food regulations was to make a distinction between the Israelites and the surrounding nations, but that is not what the Bible says. The Scriptures teach the reason for these regulations is God is holy, so we should be also. Thus the distinction between clean and unclean animals flows from the nature of God and our need to be like Him in His holiness. They are not arbitrary

228

distinctions. And the eating of unclean meats would detract from our ability to be like Him, as they are defiling, as these verses assert.

In addition, it must be emphasized that the regulations against the eating of unclean meats are interspersed with other regulations that are designed to protect the Israelites from disease. It must follow that the avoiding the eating of unclean meats also protects from disease.

This entire chapter has been quoted and much time and space has been spent on it as most Bible readers just skim over this chapter, thinking it has no relevance to them. But it has great relevance, as we shall see. But first, we need to look at what else the Bible has to say on this subject.

Elsewhere in the Old Testament:

Deuteronomy 14:1-11 repeats much of what is said in Leviticus 11. We will not take the time to review it, but the fact that these regulations are repeated shows how important they are to God. And note that verse 11 says, "You" will eat every clean bird." Thus the previous assumption was correct that in Leviticus 11:13-20 listing unclean birds that should not be eaten, it was assumed clean birds would be eaten.

But it must be asked, did he Israelites take these laws seriously? In a word, "No." But that is because they did not take any of the Law seriously. It was that very disobedience which led to the Northern Kingdom being conquered by the Assyrians in 722 BC and the Southern Kingdom by the Babylonians in 587 BC.

A discussion of those historical events is outside of the scope of this book. But a reading of the Prophetic Books of the Old Testament will show that these catastrophes occurred due to the sins of the Israelites. Foremost among these sins was the worshipping of false gods. But one of their sins was the eating of unclean meats, especially pig meat:

[1]"I became manifest to the [ones] not seeking Me; I was found by the [ones] not questioning Me. I said, 'Listen! I Am,' to the nation who did not call on My name. [2]I stretched out My hands the whole day to a disobeying and being obstinate people, who were not walked in a true way, but after their sins. [3]This [is] **the people provoking Me continually before Me; they sacrifice in the gardens, and they burn incense on the bricks to the demons**, which do not exist. [4]They sleep in the tombs and in the caves because of dreams, **the ones eating pig**

flesh, [cp. Lev 11:7] and [the] broth of sacrifices; all their vessels having been defiled; [5]the ones saying, "[Stay] far from me, do not draw near to me, for I am pure!" This [is the] smoke of My wrath, a fire burns with it all the days [fig., continually] (Isa 65:1-4).

[1]Thus says the LORD, "The heaven [is] a throne to Me and the earth a footstool of My feet; [cp. Matt 5:34-35]; what kind of a house will you* build for Me? [Acts 7:49] Or what kind [is the] place of My rest? [2]For all these [things] My hand made, and all these [things] are Mine," says the LORD. "And upon whom will I look with respect, <u>but</u> upon the humble and tranquil [person] and one trembling [at] My words? [3]But **the lawless [person] sacrificing a calf to Me [is] as the one killing a dog; and the one offering fine wheat flour [is] as pig blood**; the one giving frankincense for a memorial [is] as a blasphemous [person]. Yet they chose their [own] ways, and their abominations which they desired in their soul. [4]And <u>I</u> will choose their mockeries and will repay [their] sins to them; because I called them, and they did not obey Me; I spoke, and they did not hear; and **they did the evil [thing] before Me, and what [things] I did not desire, they chose**" (Isa 66:1-4).

[17]"**The ones** purifying themselves and cleansing themselves in the gardens, and **eating pig flesh in the porches, and the abominations, and the now [Heb., mouse], will be consumed together**," says the LORD. [18]"And <u>I</u> know their works and their thought[s]. I come to gather together all the nations and the tongues [fig., language groups]; and they will come, and see My glory. [19]And I will leave a sign upon them, and I will send out from them ones having been rescued into the nations, to Tarshish, and Phud, and Lud, and Mosoch, and Thobel, and to Greece, and to the islands far away, who have not heard My name, nor have seen My glory; and they will declare My glory among the nations (Isa 66:17-19).

In the first passage, the LORD says that people who eat pig flesh "provoke" Him and are equivalent to those who sacrifice to demons. In the second passage, the LORD says the people are so lawless that their offerings are like dead dogs and pig blood. The point of the comparison is, dead dogs and pig blood are some of the most abominable things there are. In the third passaged, the LORD says people who eat pig and mouse flesh will be consumed. Thus in no uncertain terms, the LORD is declaring the sinfulness of eating pig meat, which is lumped together with dead dogs and mouse flesh. The one is as abominable as the others.

To be clear on terminology about pigs, the following discussion will be helpful:

Ironing out the differences between the **varieties of swine** may seem complicated, because **many pig-related terms are used interchangeably**. We could walk a pig-like animal into a room of people, ask them what the animal is, and get a wide range of responses, including **pig, hog, boar, or swine**. Colloquially speaking, they could all be correct; however, **farmers and hunters tend to use specific terms for swine depending on whether it's domesticated and the animal's stage in life.**

For instance, to farmers, **"swine"** is a generic term for all types of pigs, a **"boar"** is a non-castrated male, a **"hog"** is an older and bigger swine, a **"sow"** is an adult female, and a **"piglet"** is a juvenile swine. Then there are words that further clarify the animal's size or maturity, such as gilt, shoat, weaner, feeder, barrow—the list seems to go on and on.

However, these terms are used a bit differently when discussing swine in the wild. **All wild pigs are known as "boars" or "wild boars," regardless of their gender**. Still, some folks might call them wild hogs, and nobody's going to argue with them about terminology.

But what about domestic pigs that escape and breed in the wild? Well, these are known as feral pigs/hogs and not boars, since, even though they live in the wild (and may have for several generations), they are not true wild boars.

So, how do domestic pigs and wild boars differ genetically and physically? Well, **all swine share a common ancestor — the Eurasian wild boar or *Sus scrofa*** (Knowledge Nuts).

From a Creationist perspective, this all makes sense. God created one pair of *Sus scrofa*, and Noah took one pair of *Sus scrofa* onto the ark. From that one pair, all these different varieties of swine developed.

Creationist Diet

For our purposes, the words swine, hog, and pig will be used interchangeably for the well-known farm animal. The term boar will be used for the wild animal.

That said; there were a few faithful Jews at this time who did follow the laws of God, including worshipping only the LORD and obeying the uncleanliness laws. One of these faithful Jews was Ezekiel:

[9]"And you take to yourself **wheat and barley and bean[s] and lentil[s] and millet and spelt, and you will cast them into one clay vessel, and will make them into loaves of bread for yourself.** And according to [the] number of the days which you lie on your side, a hundred and ninety [Heb., three hundred and ninety] days, you will eat them. [10]And your food which you will eat [will be] by weight, twenty shekels [about 10 ounces or 70 grams] [for] the day; from time until time [fig., at set times] you will eat them. [11]And you will drink water by measure, the sixth of the hin [about 1.5 quarts or liters], from time until time you will drink. [12]**And you will eat them [as] a barley loaf; in filth of human manure you will hide [Heb., bake] them before their eyes**. [13]And you will say, 'Thus says the LORD, the God of Israel: **"Thus will the sons [and daughters] of Israel eat unclean [food] among the nations** [or, Gentiles].""'

[14]Then I said, **"Most certainly not, O LORD, O God of Israel! Listen! My soul has not been defiled with uncleanness; and I have not eaten a carcass [fig., that which died of itself] or a [animal] torn by wild beasts from my generation [or, birth] until now; neither has all [fig., any] corrupt flesh entered into my mouth."** [cp. Acts 10:14] [15]Then He said to me, "Listen! I have given to you manure of oxen instead of human manure, and you will prepare your loaves upon them." [16]And He said to me, "Son of humanity, listen!, **I break [the] support of bread in Jerusalem; and they will eat bread by weight [i.e., in rations] and in want**; and will drink water by measure, and in a vanishing; [17]in order that they shall become needy of bread and water; and a man and his brother will perish, and **they will melt in their iniquities** (Ezekiel 4:9-16).

This whole passage is a bit strange, but I will try to break it down for the reader. The LORD is using Ezekiel as an object lesson to the Jews. He is to lie on each side for a certain number of days to illustrate

232

the amount of time the Jews will be in captivity. To sustain him during this time, the LORD gives a "bread recipe" to Ezekiel. The ingredients mentioned here are all God-given foods and have all already been discussed. But here, note that this passage is the basis for *Ezekiel Bread*. This is a very healthy brand of sprouted grain bread.

However, where an issue arises is when God tells Ezekiel to bake this bread using human manure as the fuel source. Ezekiel recoils from that idea, as human manure is unclean. This is seen in Deuteronomy 23:12f:

[12]"And a place will be to you [fig., you will have a place] **outside of the camp**, and you will go out there outside, [13]and a peg will be to you [fig., you will have a shovel] on your belt; and it will be when you sit down [fig., **relieve yourself**] outside, then you will dig a hole with it and will bring back [the ground and] will cover your excrement with it.

Having a latrine outside of the camp might seem basic to us today, but as with other regulations we have seen designed to protect the Israelites from disease, such a practice was not common at the time. But the important point for our discussion is that relieving oneself outside of the camp was a sign that human manure was unclean (compare Duet 23:10-14). As an aside, this is why Jesus was crucified outside of the city of Jerusalem, as He became "unclean" by taking our sins upon Himself (Heb 13:11-14).

In any case, Ezekiel recoils from the idea of eating something unclean. And in his response, he says he has never eaten an animal that was defiled by dying of itself or by being torn by wild beasts, "neither has any corrupt flesh entered into my mouth." This last statement is most certainly a reference to never having eaten unclean meats.

God graciously gives Ezekiel the alternative of using oxen manure instead of human manure to bake the bread. This might not sound like a pleasant alternative, but remember, the Jews were used to using animal manure as fertilizer, so they were not averse to handling it.

In any case, the whole point of this illustration is as a prophecy of God breaking the food supply of the Israelites, as a punishment upon them for their iniquities. But for our purposes, the important point is that Ezekiel followed Old Testament uncleanliness laws, including not eating unclean meats. This was in contradiction to the sinning Jewish nation, who were not obeying the Law and all of its regulations.

An indication of the importance of this law to God can be seen in the proclamation of an angel of the LORD to the mother of Samson:

[1]And the sons [and daughters] of Israel yet again did the evil before the LORD; and the LORD delivered them into [the] hand of [the] Philistines forty years. [2]And there was one [or, a certain] man of Zorah [LXX, Saraa], from [the] family of [the] kindred of Dan, and his name [was] Manoah, and his wife [was] barren, and did not give birth. [3]And **an angel of the LORD appeared to the woman, and said to her,** "Listen! You [are] barren and have not given birth; yet you will conceive a son. [4]And now be very cautious, and **drink no wine or strong drink, and do not eat any unclean [thing].** [5]For Listen! You have in [your] womb [fig., have conceived], and will give birth to a son; and no razor will come upon his head, for the child will be a Nazirite of God from the womb; and he will begin to deliver Israel from [the] hand of [the] Philistines."

[6]And the woman went in and spoke to her husband, saying, "A man of God came to me! And his appearance [was] like [the] appearance of an angel of God, very dreadful; and I did not ask him from where he is, and he did not tell me his name. [7]And he said to me, 'Listen! You [are] having in [the] womb [fig., have conceived], and will give birth to a son; and now **drink no wine or strong drink, and do not eat any unclean [thing]; for the child will be holy to God from the womb until [the] day of his death.'"**

[8]And Manoah prayed to the LORD and said, "O Lord, my Lord [Gr. and Heb., *Adonai*], [concerning] the man of God whom you sent; let him now come to us once more, and teach us what we shall do to the child being born." [9]And God heard the voice of Manoah, and the angel of God came yet again to the woman; and she sat in a field, and Manoah her husband was not with her. [10]And the woman hurried, and ran, and reported to her husband, and said to him, "Listen! The man who came to me [the other] day has appeared to me!"

[11]And Manoah arose and went after his wife, and came to the man, and said to him, "Are you the man, the one having spoken to the woman?" And the angel said, "I [am]." [12]And Manoah said, "Now will your word come [to pass]! What will be [the] judgment of the child, and

his works?" [13]And the angel of the LORD said to Manoah, "From all [things] [concerning] which I spoke to the woman, she will beware. **[14]From all [things] which comes from [the] vine of wine, she will not eat, and let her not drink wine or strong liquor, and let her not eat anything unclean. All, as many [things] as I commanded her she will observe."** ...

[24]And the woman gave birth to a son, and she called his name Samson [LXX, Sampson]. And the child grew, and the LORD blessed him (Judges 13:1-14,24).

Three times in this passage it is said that Samson's mother is not to drink wine or strong drink or to eat anything unclean. We know today the reason for the alcohol prohibition—drinking alcohol during pregnancy can lead to fetal alcohol syndrome. But notice the reason for the prohibition against eating anything unclean—for the child will be holy to God. It thus follows that eating unclean meats is defiling.

But it is worth noting that if the Jews had been following the regulation against eating unclean meats as a general practice, the angel of the LORD would not have to had made a point about this prohibition. But since the Jews by and large were not, it needed to be noted.

As an aside, rather than "an angel of the LORD," the NKJV has "the Angel of the LORD" throughout this chapter. The definitive article and capital "A" are due to the translators taking this angel as being a pre-incarnate appearance of Jesus. This is based on verse 18, where the angel says his name is "wonderful," and verse 22, where Manoah says they have seen God. That is a possible interpretation. However, in verse 3 where the angel is first mentioned and in verse 6, there is no definitive article in either the Hebrew or Greek text. Therefore, in the ALT, it is rendered as "an angel" rather than "the Angel" as the article would have it. There is a definitive article with "angel" in the rest of the chapter, but that is due to it being an article of previous reference.

In any case, after the Babylonian captivity, the Jews as a whole learned their lesson about breaking God's laws, and since then Jews have been stanch monotheists, only worshipping the LORD, the one true God of the Bible. This can be seen in the post-exilic Old Testament books, where there is no longer mention of Jews committing the sin of worshipping false gods.

In the same way, after the Babylonian captivity, Jews became stanch in obeying other aspects of the Law, including obeying the God-given distinction between clean and unclean meats, with there no longer being mention of Jews committing the sin of eating unclean meats.

Apocryphal/ Deuterocanonical Books:

The "Apocryphal/ Deuterocanonical" books are the "extra" books found in Roman Catholic and Eastern Orthodox Bibles as compared to Jewish and Protestant Bibles. There are debates as to their inspiration. That debate is addressed at length in Volume One of this writer's three volume set, *Why Are These Books in the Bible and Not Others?* (see Appendix One).

But whether inspired or not, these books were all written during the time period between the Old and New Testaments. Therefore, they give us a window into the beliefs and practices of the Jews at that time. And in them, the Jews are still stanch monotheists, refusing to commit the sin of worshipping false gods. And they are also stanch in their refusal to commit the sin of eating pig and other unclean meats.

For instance, in the Book of Judith, the heroine of the story goes undercover and enters the camp of the Babylonians to attempt to deliver Jerusalem from being sacked by Nebuchadnezzar's army. When she does, she takes her own food with her, so she will not have to eat the food of the Babylonians (Judith 10:6).

When Judith arrives at the Babylonian camp, she deceitfully tells the Babylonians how to overtake Jerusalem. Rather than attacking, they should continue to besiege the city. Judith describes what will happen:

[11]"And now, that my lord shall be not be a cast out and ineffectual, even death will fall upon their presence, and **sin overtook them**, in which **they will provoke their God to anger**, on that day they shall do strangeness [fig., what is wrong]. [12]**When the food shall fail them, and all water is scarce, they intended to lay hands on their beasts of burden and all, as many [things] as God commanded to them by His laws not to eat, they decided to consume** (Judith 11:12).

The point is, when the Jews sin against God by eating unclean meats, God will deliver them into the hands of the Babylonians. The story then takes an interesting twist, but I will not spoil it for the person who has not yet read this book.

Then during the Maccabean period of 175-134 BC, Judea is under the control of the Greeks. The Grecian leader Antiochus tries to turn the Jews from their religion. He knowns that if he can get them to eat pig meat, that will be a repudiation of their faith. He therefore tortures them to try to get them to do so. But they resolutely refuse to do so. These events are recorded in the Second Book of Maccabees:

[18]**Eleazar, any [or, one] of the being first [fig., principal] scribes, a** man already having advanced his age and the sight of the face good [fig., of a noble presence], **was being compelled, having opened his mouth, to eat pig meat.** [19]**But he having welcomed a death with good repute rather than life with defilement** was being brought voluntarily to the wooden wheel [of torture], **having spit [the pig meat] out,** [20]and according to which manner it is being necessary to be coming, the ones enduring to defend which [things are] **not right to taste [even] on account of the natural love to be living** (2Macc 6:18-20).

[1]Now it happened also **seven brothers with their mother** having been taken to be constantly **compelled by the king to be grasping from the forbidden pig meats, being maimed with scourges and whips.** [2]But one of them having become spokesman, thus having said, "What do you intend to be asking or to be learning from us? For **we are ready to be dying, rather than to be transgressing the ancestral laws**" (2Macc 7:1f).

Despite being brutally tortured to death, these Jews resolutely refuse to take so much as one bite of pig meat. These same stories are repeated in the Fourth Book of Maccabees:

[1]Indeed, **the tyrant Antiochus,** sitting in public state with his advisors on a certain high place and with the soldiers to him having stood by armed in a circle around [him], [2]was ordering to the spear-bearers to **seize each one of [the] Hebrews and to be compelling [them] to be tasting meats of pigs** and [foods] offered to idols. [3]And **if any would not be willing to eat unclean food, these having tortured on the wheel, to be killed** (4Macc 5:1-3).

[14][In] this manner **being urged to the horrible eating of [pig] flesh by the tyrant, Eleazar asked [to speak] a word.** [15]And having received authority to be speaking, he began thus to be publicly speaking: [16]"We, O Antiochus, having been persuaded to be conducting our lives by Divine Law, **consider no compulsion to be [as] forcible [as] our ready obedience to the Law.** [17]**Therefore indeed we consider [it] not worthy to be acting contrary to the Law [in] any manner.** [18]And yet if (as you suppose) our Law is not by divine truth, but otherwise we are considering it to be divine, not even thus is it being permitted to us to invalidate against honor with godliness. [19]Therefore **you shall not consider [it] to be a small sin if we would eat unclean food.** [20]**For to be acting contrary to the Law over small and great [matters] is of equal value [or, seriousness],** [21]**for through either the Law is likewise treated disdainfully** (4Macc 5:14-20).

This book then goes into graphic descriptions of the tortures these Jews endure. The language is so graphic that I will not repeat it here. Suffice it to say, the tortures are horrendous. But the Jews continue to refuse to eat even taste pig meat, as that is "horrible." It is with that background that we come to the time of the New Testament.

The New Testament:

After the narrative of the birth of Jesus, the New Testament opens with the arrival of John the Baptist. Matthew describes him as follows:

[4]Now John himself was having his clothing [made] from hairs of a camel and a leather belt around his waist, and **his nourishment was migratory locusts and wild honey** (Matt 3:4).

We saw In Leviticus 11:22 that migratory locust are one of just four clean insects, so John's diet might have been weird, but it was in accordance with the Old Testament food laws. As an aside, note that John was not a vegan, as he ate both insects and honey.

Then there is the following heated conversation between Jesus and the Pharisees:

[42]So Jesus said to them, … [46]**"Who out of you* convicts Me concerning sin?** But if I am speaking truth, why are you* not believing Me? [47]The one being from God, the words of God he hears [or, pays attention to]. Because of this, you* do not hear, because you* are not from God."

[48]Then the Jews answered and said to Him, **"We say rightly that You are a Samaritan, and You have a demon, do we not?"** [49]Jesus answered, "I have no demon, but I am honoring My Father, and you* are dishonoring Me" (John 8:42a, 46-49).

Notice that Jesus challenges them to point out to Him just one sin He has committed. But rather than doing so, the Jews make derogatory remarks about Him. The point is, they could not think of a single sin Jesus had committed. But given the background of the Old Testament and Apocryphal/ Deuterocanonical books, if Jesus had ever eaten unclean meats, just one bite of pig meat, you can sure the Jews would have mentioned it. But they did not. Therefore, most certainly Jesus abided by the Old Testament food laws.

However, there are two passages in the New Testament that cause most Christians to think these Old Testament food laws have been overturned and are not applicable to Christians. But before turning to them, think a moment about all that has been covered already.

The distinction between clean and unclean meats was first revealed by God to Noah, way back at the time of the Flood. On a young-earth creationist timescale, that was about 2,400 BC. Then a millennium later, after the Exodus of 1446 BC, God gave specific descriptions and lists of clean versus unclean meats to Moses. It was indicated that these distinctions were an outgrowth of the holiness of God and our need to be like Him in His holiness, while unclean meats are defiling.

The Jews by and large ignored these laws, as they did the other commandments, until the Babylonian captivity in 586 BC. But after that, the Jews stanchly obeyed all Old Testament regulations, including the ones about clean versus unclean meats.

Therefore, the distinction between clean and unclean meats had been in force for millennia, and Jews had been strictly obeying the law against the eating of unclean meats for hundreds of years. With that background, the distinction between clean and unclean meats had been ingrained into the Jewish mindset. Consequently, if after all of this time

239

of these regulations being commanded and being obeyed, they were now no longer applicable, you would think God would be crystal clear in declaring He had changed His mind and His nature and the eating of unclean meats was no longer an offense to His holiness and that we did not need to avoid unclean meats in order to be like Him in His holiness.

But we have no such thing. All we have are two passages that are open to alternative translations and interpretations. The first is Mark 7:18,19. Quoting it first from the NKJV:

[18]So He said to them, "Are you thus without understanding also? Do you not perceive that **whatever enters a man from outside cannot defile him**, [19]because it does not enter his heart but his stomach, and is eliminated, *thus* **purifying all foods?**"

There are two claims about this passage. First it is said Jesus says that what people eat does not defile them, and it is assumed this includes unclean meats. Second, in the final phrase it is said Jesus purifies all foods, by which it is taken to mean, He declares all foods clean. Other versions make this point even clearer by rendering this phrase in just that manner:

(*Thus* He declared all foods clean.) (NASB).
(In saying this, Jesus declared all foods clean.) (NIV).
(Thus he declared all foods clean.) (ESV).

Notice how each of these versions make this phrase a parenthetical comment by Mark rather than the direct words of Jesus. But they are all paraphrases, not literal translations.

In fact, the words "Thus" (or "In saying this"), "He" (or "Jesus"), "declared," and "clean" are not in the Greek text. Only the words "all foods" are, while the word "purifying" (which is in the Greek text) is omitted. The NKJV has the literal rendering, but it should be noted that the word "thus" in the NKJV is in italics, indicating it has been added.

Before giving the literal rendering of the ALT for this passage, it would be helpful to look at the context. It begins all the way back at the beginning of the chapter:

[1]And the Pharisees and some of the scribes, having come from Jerusalem, are gathered together to Him. [2]And **having seen some of His disciples eating loaves of bread with defiled [or, ceremonially unclean] hands**—that is, not [ritually] washed—they found fault. [3]For **the Pharisees and all the Jews, if they do not wash their hands with [the] fist [fig., in a ritualistic manner], do not eat**, **keeping the handed down tradition of the elders**. [4]And [coming] from the marketplace, unless they baptize [or, ceremonially wash] themselves, they do not eat, and many other [traditions there] are which they received [and] are keeping: [like] baptisms [or, ceremonial washings] of cups and pitchers and brazen vessels and cots.

[5]Afterwards the Pharisees and the scribes question Him, "Why do Your disciples not walk about [fig., conduct themselves] according to the handed down tradition of the elders? But **they eat their loaves of bread with [ritually] unwashed hands**" (Mark 7:1-5).

Note the issue at hand. It is not the eating of unclean meats that is being discussed, nor any other Old Testament regulation. What is being discussed is "the handed down tradition of the elders." These would be additions that the Jewish hierarchy had added to what God had said. God's laws themselves are not the issue. This is made clear next:

[6]But answering, He [Jesus] said to them, "Correctly did Isaiah prophesy concerning you*, the hypocrites! As it has been written:

This people honors Me with their lips [fig., *words*]*, but their heart is distant, far away from Me.* [7]*But in vain* [or, *to no purpose*] *do they worship Me,* **teaching [as] teachings [or, doctrines] [the] commandments of people***. [Isaiah 29:13, LXX]

[8]"For **having left behind [or, having neglected] the commandment of God, you* keep the handed down tradition of people**: baptisms [or, ceremonial washings] of pitchers and cups, and many such other similar things you* do."

[9]And He was saying to them, **"[All too] well do you* regard as nothing the commandment of God, so that you* should keep your* handed down tradition"** (Mark 7:6-9).

Thus the issue is that the human traditions of the Jewish hierarchy are taking the place of God's commandments. It is those added traditions that Jesus is repudiating, not any of God's commandments. It is the breaking of these unbiblical traditions that do not defile.

[14]And having summoned all the crowd, He was saying to them, "Be paying attention to Me, all [of you*], and be understanding: [15]There is **nothing from outside the person entering into him which is able to defile him**, but the [things] coming out from him, those are the [things] defiling the person. [16]If anyone has ears to be hearing, let him be hearing [or, be paying attention]" (Mark 7:14-16).

Here, "nothing from outside the person" refers to that which is eaten with ritually unclean hands, not unclean meats, as that has not been mentioned in the conversation. We then come to the main verses:

[17]And when He entered into a house from the crowd, His disciples began questioning Him concerning the parable. [18]And He says to them, "So you* also are without understanding! You* do perceive that nothing from outside entering into the person is able to defile him, do you* not? [19]Because it does not enter into his heart, but into the stomach, **and goes out into the latrine, purifying [or, purging] all the foods.**" [20]But He was saying, "That [which] comes out from the person, that defiles the person. [21]For from within, out of the heart of people, proceed evil thoughts, adulteries, fornications, murders, [22]thefts, covetous desires [or, greed], wicked deeds, deceit [or, treachery], debauchery, an evil eye [fig., envy], blasphemy, arrogance, foolishness. [23]All these evils come out from within and defile the person" (Mark 7:17-23).

The ALT is a literal rendering, so it says simply "purifying all foods." And that is right after the mention of "the latrine." The point of Jesus' statement is the body purifies foods when we relieve ourselves, meaning the waste or non-nutritive parts of foods are eliminated. That's it. The statement is about a basic human bodily function. There is no repudiation of the law against the eating of unclean meats, as such have never been mentioned in the entire discussion.

242

The second passage is Acts chapter 10. In it, Peter is called by the Lord to preach the Gospel to Cornelius, a Gentile. Knowing that Peter would be reluctant to do so, given Jewish prejudice against Gentiles, the Lord uses strong measures to overcome his reluctance and prejudice and gives him the following vision:

⁹Now the next day, as these are traveling and approaching the city, Peter went up on the housetop to pray, about [the] sixth hour [i.e., 12:00 noon]. ¹⁰But he became very hungry and was desiring to eat; but while they [were] preparing [a meal], a trance fell on him, ¹¹and he observes heaven [or, the sky] having been opened, and a certain object like a great sheet descending to him, having been tied at [the] four corners and being lowered on the ground, ¹²in which were **all the four-footed animals of the earth and the wild beasts and the reptiles and the birds of heaven** [or, of the air]. ¹³And a voice came to him: "Having gotten up, Peter, slaughter and eat!" ¹⁴But Peter said, **"No way, Lord! Because never did I eat any[thing] common [fig., ritually impure] or unclean [or, which defiles].**" [cp. Ezek 4:14] ¹⁵And a voice [came] again a second time to him: **"What God [has] cleansed, by all means stop calling common!"** [fig., ritually impure!"] ¹⁶Now this was done three times, and again the object was taken up into heaven (Acts 10:9-15).

Note the mention of "four-footed animals." Such were previously declared to be unclean. That is why Peter exclaims that he never ate such meats. Now, stop and think about that for a moment. This event is occurring several years after Jesus' death and resurrection and after the three and a half years Peter had spent with Jesus during His earthy ministry. During that time, Peter never ate unclean meat. But if in the previous passage from the Gospel of Mark, Jesus had declared unclean meats clean, why not? Why did Peter not begin eating unclean meats at that time? Could it be because Peter did not understand the words of Jesus in that manner?

Then even after Jesus' resurrection and ascension and for several years thereafter, Peter still never ate unclean meats. But if something about Jesus' ministry had overturned the longstanding God-given regulation against the eating of unclean meat, then why not?

But now, after all of this time, Peter is being told to eat unclean meats, and he recoils in horror, even exclaiming "No way, Lord!" That

243

is what is to be expected from someone who had it ingrained in him that eating unclean meats was a sin but is now being told to eat them. But does Peter take this vision to mean it is now okay to eat unclean meats? He gives us his interpretation of this vision later in the chapter:

³⁴Then Peter having opened his mouth, said, "Truly, **I comprehend that God is not One to accept faces [fig., to be prejudice]**, [cp. Eph 6:9; James 2:1] ³⁵**but in every nation the one fearing Him and working righteousness is acceptable to Him** (Acts 10:34).

Thus the point of the vision was that Peter must get over his prejudice and realize that any person who fears God is acceptable to Him. In other words, the unclean animals in the vision symbolized the Gentiles, but Peter was being told not to consider Gentiles to be unclean. If they feared God, they were just as acceptable to God as Jews are. This point is empathized by what happens next:

⁴⁴While Peter [was] still speaking these words, **the Holy Spirit fell upon all the ones hearing the word**. ⁴⁵**And the believing ones from the circumcision were astonished**, as many as came with Peter, because **the free gift of the Holy Spirit had been poured out on the Gentiles also**. ⁴⁶For they were hearing them speaking with tongues [fig., other languages] and magnifying God. Then Peter answered, ⁴⁷**"Surely no one is able to forbid the water, can he, [for] these not to be baptized who received the Holy Spirit just as we also [did]?"** ⁴⁸And he commanded them to be baptized in the name of the Lord. Then they urgently asked him to stay several days (Acts 10:44-48).

The Jews are astonished that the Holy Spirit falls upon the Gentiles just as happened to them. But it took this dramatic event to overcome their prejudice. These Gentiles are then baptized in water, thus becoming a part of the fledging Church.

When Peter retells this story to the Jewish believers in Jerusalem to explain why he baptized Gentiles, he interprets it as follows:

¹⁷Since then **God gave the same free gift to them as also to us,** having believed on [or, having trusted in] the Lord Jesus Christ, now who was I [to be] able to forbid God?" ¹⁸So having heard these [things],

they were silent, and they began glorifying God, saying, **"In that case, God also gave to the Gentiles repentance to life!"** (Acts 11:17f).

Thus the whole story is about the Gospel being not just for Jews but also for Gentiles. That's it. It is not about clean versus unclean meats. And there is no record of Peter or any other Christian eating unclean meats in the New Testament.

Again, if this longstanding and ingrained regulation had been abrogated, you would think the New Testament would have been crystal clear about it, replete with examples of the early believers eating pig meat. But we have nothing of the sort.

There are a few other New Testament passages that could be relevant to this discussion. The first is Romans chapter 14:

[1]Now be receiving the one being weak in the faith, not for disputes over opinions. [2]**One believes [it is permissible] to eat all [things], but the one being weak eats [only] vegetables**. [3]Stop letting the one eating despise [or, look down on] the one not eating; and stop letting the one not eating judge the one eating, for God [has] accepted him. [4]Who are you, the one judging another's household bondservant? To his own master he stands or falls; but he will be made to stand, for God is able to make him stand. [5]One indeed judges [or, considers] a day [to be] above [another] day, but another judges every day [to be alike]; be letting each be fully convinced in his own mind.

[6]The one honoring [or, observing] the day, to [the] Lord he honors [it]; and the one not honoring the day, to [the] Lord he does not honor [it]. And **the one eating, to [the] Lord he eats, for he gives thanks to God; and the one not eating, to [the] Lord he does not eat, and he gives thanks to God**. [7]For none of us lives to himself, and none dies to himself. [8]For both if we live, to the Lord we live, and if we die, to the Lord we die. So both if we live and if we die, we are the Lord's. [9]Because for this [reason] Christ also died and rose and lives, so that He should exercise lordship over both dead [people] and living [people]....

[14]I know and have been persuaded in [the] Lord Jesus that **nothing [is] unclean by means of itself**, except to the one considering anything to be unclean, to that one [it is] unclean. [15]But if on account of food your brother is grieved, you are no longer walking about [fig., conducting

yourself] according to love; stop ruining with your food that one on behalf of whom Christ died.

[16]So stop letting your good be slandered [or, be spoken of as evil]. **[17]For the kingdom of God is not eating and drinking, but righteousness and peace and joy in [the] Holy Spirit.** [cp. 1Cor 8:8; Heb 13:9] [18]For the one serving as a bondservant to Christ in these [things] [is] acceptable to God and approved by people. [19]So, consequently, let us be pursuing the [things] of peace and the [things] of building up [or, edifying] one another.

[20]Stop tearing down the work of God for the sake of food. **All [things] indeed [are] clean, but** [they are] evil to the person eating with a cause of tripping [fig., eating something that causes someone else to sin]. **[21][It is] good not to eat meat nor to drink wine nor [to do anything] by which your brother is caused to stumble** [fig., to sin] or is made to fall or becomes weak. [22]You have faith? Be having [it] to yourself before God. Fortunate [or, Blessed] is the one not judging [or, condemning] himself in what he approves [of]. [23]But the one doubting, if he eats, has been condemned, because [it is] not of faith. Now all which [is] not of faith is sin (Rom 14:1-8,14-23).

I have quoted most of this chapter as it is very important. Paul starts out by saying some Christians think it is permissible to eat all things, while others will only eat vegetables. Thus the contrast here is not between clean versus unclean meats but between an omnivorous diet versus a vegetarian one. Some Christian back then ate meat while others were vegetarians, just like today. And just like today, the meat-eaters would look down on the vegetarians, and the vegetarians would look down on the meat-eaters. But both are wrong. Both the meat-eater and the person not eating meat are honoring God if they give thanks to God for their food. That's the point of the first half of the chapter. We are not to think we are better than someone else due to our dietary choices.

But starting in verse 14, Paul seems to be addressing clean versus unclean meats when he says, "nothing [is] unclean by means of itself." But the Epistle of Romans was most likely sent to Gentile Christians, who would have understood the words clean and unclean differently from Jewish Christians. By "unclean" here is meant foods or drinks that some Christians think are wrong to eat, but others do not. This is clear from verse 21, where Paul mentions meat and wine.

It would seem some Roman Christians thought that in addition to it being wrong to eat meat, they also thought it was wrong to drink alcohol. But other Roman Christians believed it was okay to eat meat and to drink alcohol. Again, this is just like today—some Christians drink alcohol in a moderate manner, while others are teetotalers. Paul is saying both practices are okay and that the alcohol drinker should not judge the teetotaler, and vice-a-versa.

But if the person who thinks it is wrong to eat meat or to drink alcoholic eats dinner with someone who thinks otherwise, and meat and alcohol are served, that "weak" brother might be tempted to eat the meat or to drink the alcohol but with still thinking it is wrong to do so. As a result, he could end up guilt-ridden afterwards, and that will be a cause of stumbling to him. If such is the case, the meat-eating, alcohol drinking Christian should forego doing so at that meal so as not be a cause of stumbling to the weaker brother.

Then the most important verse of the passage is verse 17, "For the kingdom of God is not eating and drinking, but righteousness and peace and joy in [the] Holy Spirit." In no way does eating meat, drinking wine, or consuming any other food or beverage bring a person closer to or farther away from God.

Now this general principle does apply to the eating of unclean meats in the sense that not eating unclean meats is in no way salvific. And eating unclean meats will not cause you to lose your salvation. Salvation comes by repenting of your sins and trusting in the death of Jesus Christ on the cross for the forgiveness of your sins, as Paul makes clear in chapters 3-6 in this letter.

But once you become a Christian and begin to grow in the faith, the Lord will lead you away from habits that are not beneficial to you and to ones that are beneficial. This is clear in the next two passages to be looked at, both from 1Corinthians. This first is 1Corinthians Chapter 8:

[1]Now concerning the **meats sacrificed to idols**, we know that we all have knowledge: such knowledge puffs up [fig., causes conceit], but love builds up [fig., edifies]. [2]And if anyone thinks to know anything, he has not yet known anything just as it is necessary [for him] to know. [3]But if anyone loves God, this one has been known by Him. [4]So **concerning the eating of the meats sacrificed to idols**, we know that

an idol [is] nothing in the world, and that [there is] no other God except for one.

⁵For even if they are called "gods," whether in heaven or on earth (just as there are gods many and lords many), ⁶<u>but</u> to us [there is] one God, the Father, of whom [are] all [things], and we [exist] for Him; and one Lord Jesus Christ, through whom [are] all [things], and we [exist] through Him.

⁷<u>But</u> this knowledge [is] not in all [people], but some with consciousness [or, awareness] of the idol until now, **eat [it] as meat sacrificed to an idol**, and their conscience, being weak, is defiled. ⁸But **food does not present [or, commend] us to God, for neither if we eat do we excel [or, are we better off]; nor if we do not eat do we fall short [or, are we inferior].** [cp. Rom 14:17; Heb 13:9] ⁹But be watching out [or, be aware] lest this right [or, privilege] of yours* becomes a cause of tripping to the ones being weak.

¹⁰**For if anyone sees you, the one having knowledge, in an idol's temple reclining [to eat], will not his conscience, being weak, be emboldened to be eating the meats sacrificed to idols? ¹¹And the brother being weak will perish because of your knowledge**, for the sake of whom Christ died. ¹²But sinning in this manner in regard to the brothers [and sisters], and beating [fig., wounding] their conscience, being weak, in regard to Christ you* sin.

¹³For this very reason, **if food causes my brother to stumble [fig., to sin], I shall never at all eat meats [sacrificed to idols] into the age [fig., forever], so that I do not cause my brother to stumble** (Rom 8:1-13).

Here Paul elaborates on one point from Romans. You should not do something in front of another Christian who thinks it is wrong to do so, if it will cause that person to do the same but without also being fully convinced it is okay to do so. Such will cause the person to "perish." By this is not meant to lose his salvation but that he will be guilt-ridden.

But it must be noted that this discussion is about meats sacrificed to idols, not about abut clean versus unclean meats. Paul then returns to this subject in chapter ten.

¹⁴For this very reason, my beloved, **be fleeing from idol worship**. ¹⁵I am speaking as to prudent [persons]; <u>you*</u> judge what I am saying.

[16]The cup of the blessing which we bless, it is [the] fellowship of [or, a sharing in] the blood of Christ, is it not? The loaf of bread which we break, it is [the] fellowship of the body of Christ, is it not? [17]Because we, the many, are one loaf of bread, one body, for we all partake of the one loaf of bread. [18]Be watching Israel according to [the] flesh. The ones eating the sacrifices are participants in the altar, are they not?

[19]So what am I saying? **That an idol is anything or that meat sacrificed to an idol is anything?** [20]But [I am saying that] **what the Gentiles sacrifice, they sacrifice to demons and not to God**. And I do not want you* to become participants of the demons. [21]You* are not able to be drinking [the] cup of [the] Lord and [the] cup of demons; you* are not able to be partaking of [the] table of [the] Lord and of [the] table of demons. [22]Or do we provoke the Lord to jealousy? We are not stronger than He, are we?

[23]**All [things] are lawful for me, <u>but</u> all [things] are not advantageous [or, beneficial]. All [things] are lawful for me, <u>but</u> all [things] do not build up [fig., edify].** [24]**Let no one be seeking his own [concern], <u>but</u> each the [concern] of the other.** [25]**Whatever is sold in the meat-market, eat, examining nothing, for the sake of the conscience.** [26]*"For the earth [is] the LORD's and the fullness of it."* [Psalm 24:1; 50:12; 89:11]

[27]But if someone of the unbelieving invite you*, and you* want to go, **eat all the [food] set before you*, examining nothing, for the sake of the conscience. [28]But if someone says to you*, "This is meat sacrificed to an idol,"** stop eating [it], for the sake of that one having made [it] known and his conscience, *"for the earth [is] the LORD's and the fullness of it."*

[29]Now I say conscience, not of yourself, <u>but</u> the [conscience] of the other. For why [is it] that my liberty is judged by another's conscience? [30]If I partake with thankfulness, why am I being defamed concerning what I give thanks for?

[31]**So whether you* eat or drink, or whatever you* do, be doing all [things] for the glory of God.** [32]Continue becoming without offence both to Jews and to Greeks, and to the Assembly [or, Church] of God, [33]just as I also try to please all [people] in all [things], **not seeking my own profit, <u>but</u> the [profit] of the many, so that they shall be saved.** (1Cor 10:14-33).

Creationist Diet

The background to this passage is that Corinth was a pagan city. As such, most of the meats sold in the marketplace had been sacrificed to idols. Some Christians thought it was okay to eat these meats, while others did not. In response, Paul makes it clear that idol worship is wrong, as it is the worship of demons. But that does not mean meats sacrificed to idols have been defiled. As such, a Christian could partake or not partake. Neither doing so nor not doing so would bring a person closer to God.

However, there were pagans in Corinth who, knowing the negative attitude of Christians towards idols, thought the Christians were being hypocritical by eating meats sacrificed to idols. Thus Paul is saying, if you know a meat has been sacrificed to an idol, do not purchase or eat it, as that will bring a disrepute to Christ. But if you do not know if it has been, then don't ask. Just eat it, as it is not sinful to do so.

However, some things that are lawful are not beneficial. And the eating of meats sacrificed to idols is one such thing. It is not wrong to do so, but by doing so, you are supporting the worship of idols, and you could potentially bring dispute to Christ. Therefore, it would be best not to do so. But whatever you do, let it be to the glory of God and to the spiritual benefit of others.

However, the situation in regards to unclean meat is considerably different from this one. In the case of unclean meats, God has expressly declared that they should not be eaten. As such, it is not a gray issue like eating meats sacrificed to idols, but a black and white issue. Those who believe the Bible should not partake of them.

But there are a couple of points of applicability from this passage to our subject. First, even if you are not convinced that you should not eat unclean meats, at the very least, if you are eating with someone who considers eating unclean meats to be wrong, then do not serve him pork or other unclean meats or eat them in front of him.

Second, we will see shortly that the eating of unclean meats is not beneficial health-wise. Hence, even if it were not spiritually damaging to eat unclean meats, there are health reasons not to do so.

The next passage is from 1 Timothy:

[1]Now the Spirit explicitly says that in latter times some will fall away [or, apostatize] from the faith, paying attention to deceitful spirits and teachings of demons, [2]in hypocrisy [or, insincerity] of liars, having

been seared in their own conscience, ³forbidding to be marrying, **[commanding] to be keeping distant from foods which God created for receiving with thanksgiving** by the [ones who are] faithful and have acknowledged the truth. ⁴Because **every[thing] created by God [is] good, and nothing [is to be] rejected, [if] being received with thanksgiving**. ⁵For it is sanctified through [the] word of God and prayer (1Tim 4:1-4).

Now some will read verse four and say "God created pigs, so pig meat must be good." But since the context is food, the "every[thing] created by God is good" would mean "everything created by God for food is good." This is clear from the verse three where it is said "foods which God created for receiving with thanksgiving." God did not create pigs and other unclean animals to be received as food. This point was made clear in Leviticus 11, where unclean animals are called an "abomination" and are to be "abhorred." With such designations, such animals could hardly have been created by God for food.

But Paul's statement here would apply to the vegetarian who claims Christian should not eat even clean meats. Such animals God clearly did create for food. As such, Christians can eat clean meats with thanksgiving, knowing they are eating God-given foods.

On a side note, I remember a Christian sister who used this passage to justify eating *Twinkies*. But God did not create such a processed junk food; human beings did, in a lab, using artificial ingredients that human beings created, not God. Thus *Twinkies* would not be God-given foods.

The last passage is one verse from Hebrews.

⁹Stop being carried away by varied and strange teachings, for **[it is] good [for] the heart to continue being established by grace, not by foods**, in which the ones having been walking about [in] [fig., having been occupied with] were not benefited (Hebrews 13:9).

The author's point here is clear; we are saved by grace, not by what we eat or don't eat. Such an attitude has already been seen. Do not think that your dietary choices in any way will save you. Again, salvation comes by grace through faith in Jesus Christ and His atoning death on the cross. However, your dietary choices will make a huge difference in your health. And that will affect how much you are able to serve the LORD and others. It is thus beneficial to be careful about what you eat.

The Apostolic Fathers:

Volume Seven of my *Analytical-Literal Translation of the Bible* contains the Apostolic Fathers (APF). These are the writings of the Church leaders of the late first through mid-second centuries. Most were direct disciples of the apostles, and some of their writings were seriously considered for inclusion in the NT. It is explained why this was so and why these writings were eventually rejected in Volume Three of my aforementioned *Why These Books* set.

These books are not inspired, but they do give us window into the mindset of Christians shortly after the time of the apostles. And two of these books address the issue of clean versus unclean meats.

The first is the Epistle of Barnabas. This book is purported to have been written by the Barnabas who is mentioned throughout the Book of Acts (e.g., 4:36; 9:26) and in three of Paul's epistles (1Cor 9:6; Gal 2:1,9,13; Col 4:10), but there are serious doubts as to its authenticity. It was probably written 95-135 AD, too late for that Barnabas to have written it. But this book was held in high regard in the early Church, in a secondary place to the canonical New Testament books.

The object of this letter is similar to the Book of Hebrews in the New Testament in that it finds fulfillment of Jewish regulations and rituals in Christ and the Christian faith. But it is far inferior to Hebrews and goes beyond it in being hostile toward Jewish traditions. It also contains some exaggerated allegories and strange statements.

This can be seen in the following passage about the distinction between clean and unclean meats:

[1]Now that **Moses said, "You will not eat swine [or, pig]**, nor eagle, nor hawk, nor raven, nor any all [fig., any] fish which does not have a scale with itself," **he received three dogmas [or, decrees] in the understanding**. [Lev 11:7,9f,13-16] [2]Even further, He says to them in Deuteronomy, "And I will establish My regulations towards this people." [Deut 4:1-8] So therefore **there is not a command of God not to be eating, but Moses spoke in spirit**. [3]Therefore, towards this he said the piglet {some mss, of the piglet; some mss, to the piglet}, **he means by no means will you {some mss, you will not} be joined to**

such people who are like swine. This is whenever they live in self-indulgence, they forget the Lord; but whenever they lack, they acknowledge the Lord. As also the swine, whenever it gnaws, it does not know its lord [or, master]; but whenever it is hungry, it cries out, and having received is quiet again....

⁶But also, "**You will not eat the hare [or, rabbit]**. "Towards why [or, For what reason]? He means by no **means shall you become a corrupter of boys**, nor will you be made like to such; **for according to year [or, year by year] the hare gains the [or, another] anus of hares, for as many years as it lives so many anuses it has**....

⁹Having received concerning indeed the meats, **Moses spoke three dogmas in this way in spirit [or, a spiritual sense], but they accepted [them] according to the desire of the flesh, as concerning eating** (Barnabas 10:1-3,6,9).

It can be seen this is all rather fanciful and very strange. It also says that Moses did not really mean that Jews could not eat unclean meats. The author thus denies the literal teachings of the OT. But Jews clearly understood the injunctions against the eating of unclean meats in a literal manner, as seen in the Book of Isaiah (65:4; 66:3,17) and in the Maccabean books, as was disused previously. Also, the NT never allegorizes the OT to the point of denying its literal meanings. This is probably why most translations of Barnabas add the word "merely" or "only" to the last line of verse 9 ("as only concerning eating"), making it sound as if Barnabas is not denying the literal meaning, but no such word appears in the Greek text.

This extreme negative attitude towards the Old Testament, along with the fanciful allegories, is part of the reason this book was ultimately rejected for inclusion in the New Testament.

The second book is the Epistle to Diognetus. The author of this epistle is unknown, but the recipient might have been the teacher of Roman Emperor Marcus Aurelius. If so, it was written during his reign (161-180 AD). If not, then it was written anytime from 100 to 313 AD.

This epistle is an eloquent document. It presents a scathing attack on idol worship, exposing how foolish it is; it exposes the foolishness of Jewish superstitions, using biting sarcasm, and it defends Christians as being good citizens of the emperor, who are not deserving of the persecution they are receiving. There is also a powerful presentation of the Gospel. For our purposes, part of what it considers to be Jewish superstitions is the avoidance of eating unclench meats.

[1]**But surely indeed their scrupulosity concerning the meats**, and their religion [or, superstition] concerning the Sabbaths, and their pretentious pride about circumcision, and their subterfuge about the fasting and the new moons, [which are] **utterly ridiculous and not at all worthy of a word**, I do not think you to be needing to learn [anything] from me. [2]**For to be accepting [some] of the [things] having been created by God for use of people**, which on the one hand as having been created good; on the other hand, **to be refusing [others] as useless and unnecessary [or, excessive], how [is that] not unlawful [or, superfluous]?** (Diognetus 4:1-2).

Thus the writer considers it unlawful (or, superfluous) to avoid eating meats that God created for the use of people. The writer possibly has in mind 1Timothy 4:1-4 that was discussed previously. But as we saw there, Paul is referring to the meats God gave to us for food, which would be clean meats, not unclean meats.

But more likely, the author of this book has in mind the unbiblical additions of Jews towards the food laws, such as not eating milk and meat at the same meal. Such an idea is an exaggerated expansion of Deuteronomy 14:21b, "You will not boil a lamb in its mother's milk."

This interpretation is likely given that he next says, "And to be speaking falsely of God, as forbidding to be doing anything good on the day of the Sabbaths, how [is that] not impious?" (4:3). Here the writer is thinking of Matthew 12:9-14, where Jesus declares, "Accordingly, it is lawful on the Sabbaths to be doing good" (12:12b).

Thus what the writer is criticizing is not the food laws per se, but the unbiblical attitudes and traditions that had grown up around them.

It is also possible that both of these writers are criticizing the food laws as a means of separating Christians from Jews. It was well-known even to Gentiles that Jews did not eat unclean meats, especially pig meat. That was seen in the Maccabean books. Thus for Christians to eat pig meat, it would show the Gentiles that Christians were not Jews. But interestingly, Christians by and large continued to avoid most other unclean meats. And that remains the case to this day, as we will see in a moment.

254

Conclusion:

God intends for human beings to eat clean meats, as these are the meats He gave to us for food. Conversely, He does not intend for people to eat unclean meats, as they are not God-given foods. And His intentions are always for our benefit. Therefore, even if it were now lawful to eat unclean meats, it would still not be beneficial. We will see shortly why this is so. But first, it would be good to take a closer look at which meats are clean and which are unclean.

List of Clean Versus Unclean Animals

Leviticus 11 was already quoted, with its descriptions and examples of clean versus unclean animals. But for clarity sake, the following chart lists which animals fit into which category.

Clean four-footed animals:

Antelope, Buffalo, Caribou, Cow (beef), Calf (veal), Deer (venison), Elk, Gazelle, Giraffe, Goat, Hart, Ibex, Moose, Ox, Roebuck, Reindeer, Sheep (lamb, mutton).

Unclean four-footed animals:

Armadillo, Donkey, Badger, Bear, Beaver, Boar, Camel, Cat, Cheetah, Coyote, Coney (guinea pig), Dog, Donkey, Elephant, Fox, Gorilla, Grizzly Bear, Groundhog, Hamster, Hare, Hippopotamus, Horse, Hyena, Jackal, Kangaroo, Leopard, Lion, Llama (alpaca, vicuña), Mole, Monkey, Mouse, Mule, Muskrat, Onager, Opossum, Panther, Peccary, Pig (pork, ham, bacon, sausage), Possum, Porcupine, Rabbit, Raccoon, Rat, Rhinoceros, Skunk, Slug, Snail (escargot), Squirrel, Tiger, Wallaby, Weasel, Wolf, Wolverine, Worm, Zebra.

Unclean Reptiles and Amphibians:

Alligator, Blindworm, Caiman, Crocodile, Frogs, Lizard, Newts, Salamanders, Snakes, Toads, Turtles.

Clean birds:

Creationist Diet

Chicken, Coot, Dove, Duck, Goose, Grouse, Guinea Fowl, Partridge, Peafowl, Pheasant, Pigeon, Prairie Chicken, Ptarmigan, Quail, Sagehen, Sparrow (plus any other songbirds), Teal, Turkey.

Unclean birds:

Albatross, Bat (really a mammal, but still unclean), Bittern, Buzzard, Condor, Coot, Cormorant, Crane, Crow, Cuckoo, Eagle, Falcon, Flamingo, Grebe, Grosbeak, Gull, Hawk, Heron, Ibis, Kite, Lapwing, Loon, Magpie, Nighthawk, Osprey, Ostrich, Owl, Parrot, Pelican, Penguin, Plover, Rail, Raven, Red-tail Hawk, Roadrunner, Sandpiper, Seagull, Stork, Sparrow Hawk, Swallow, Swan, Swift, Sea Gull, Stork, Vulture, Water Hen, Woodpecker.

Clean fish (any fish with scales and fins):

Albacore (Crevalle, Horse Mackerel, Jack), Alewives (Branch, River Herring), Anchovy, Barracuda, Bass, Black Drum, Black Pomfret (Monchong), Bluc Runner (Hardtail), Bluebacks (Glut Herrings), Bluebill Sunfish, Bluefish, Bluegill, Bonito, Bowfin, Buffalofish, Carp, Chubs (Bloater, Longjaw, Blackfin), Cod, Common Sucker (Fresh Water Mullet, White Sucker), Crappie (Black or White Crappies), Drum, Flounder (Dab, Gray, Lemon Sole, Summer), Flying Fish, Goldfish, Grouper (Black, Nassau, Red, or Yellowfish Grouper, Gag), Grunt (White / Yellow Grunts), Gulf Pike (Robalo, Snook, Sergeant), Haddock, Hake, Halibut, Hardhead, Hardtail (Blue Runner), Herring (Alewife, Branch, Glut, Lake, River, Sea Herrings), Kingfish, Long Nose Sucker (Northern or Red Striped Sucker), Mackerel (except snake mackerel), Mahi Mahi (Dorado, Dolphinfish, not dolphin), Menhaden, Minnow, Mullet, Muskellunge (Jacks), Orange Roughy, Perch (Bream), Pig Fish, Pike (Pickerel, Jack), Pollack (Pollock, Boston Bluefish), Pompano, Porgy (Scup), Red Drum (Redfish), Red Horse Sucker (Redfin), Red Snapper, Redfish, Robalo (Gulf Pike), Rockfish, Salmon (Chum, Coho, King, Pink or Red), Sardine (Pilchard), Scup (Porgy), Sea Bass, Sergeant Fish (Gulf Pike), Shad, Sheepshead, Silver Hake (Whiting), Jacksmelt (Silversides), Smelt, Snapper, Snook (Gulf Pike), Sole, Spanish Mackerel, Spot, Sturgeon, Steelhead, Striped Bass, Sucker (Red Horse Sucker, Redfin), Sunfish, Tarpon, Trout (Gray Sea, Lake, Sand Sea, White Sea, Spotted Sea Trouts, Weakfish), Tuna,

Turbot (all except European variety), Walleye, Whitefish, Whiting (Silver Hake), Winter Flounder, Yellow Tail, Yellow Perch.

Bass: Alaska Blackfish, Bigmouth Bass, Black Bass, Blackfish Bowfish, Crappie, Croaker, Drum, Grouper (Jewfish), Mudminnow, Sea Bass, Silver Bass, Sunfish, Tautog, White Sea Bass, Wrasse, Graysby, Stripped Bass, Redeye Bass, Northern Smallmouth Bass, White Perch, Yellow Perch.

Cod: Atlantic Cod, Cod, Haddock, Hake, Pacific Cod, Pollack, Whiting (Walleye Pollack).

Flounder: Brill, Dab, Dover Sole, Flounder, Hogchoker Sole, Halibut Turbot

Herring: Anchovy, Menhaden, Pilchards, Sardines, Shad.

Mackerel: Atlantic Horse Mackerel, Barracuda, Black Skipjack, Bonito, Chub, Cobia, Horse Mackerel, Kingfish, King Mackerel (Cavalla), Ladyfish, Mackerel, Skipjack.

Perch: Atlantic Perch, Black Perch, Breems, Lake Perch, Mahi Mahi, Ocean Perch/ Redfish/Red Drum, Pike Perch, Rockfish, Sun Perch, Surfperch, Walleyed Pike, Jacks, Pompano, Scads, Darter (Israel).

Pikes: Muskellunge, Northern Pike, Pickerel, Pike.

Pipefish: Orange Roughy

Salmon: Atlantic Salmon, Chinook Salmon, Chum/Dog Salmon, Jack Salmon, King Salmon, Pacific Salmon, Pink/Humpback Salmon, Red/Sockeye Salmon, Silver/Coho Salmon, Tripletail.

Snapper: Black Snapper, Blackfin Snapper, Bluefish, Caribbean Red Snapper, Cuberg Snapper, Gray Snapper, Grunt, Lane Snapper, Porgy (Sheepshead), Red Snapper, Silk Snapper, White Snapper, Yellowtail Snapper, Glasseye Snapper, Dog Snapper.

Creationist Diet

Sucker: Buffalo fish, Carp, Carpsucker, Hog Sucker, Minnow, Redhorse, Humpback Sucker, Smallmouth Buffalo, Bigmouth Buffalo, White Sucker, Tahoe Sucker, Webug Sucker, Spotted Sucker, Striped Jumprock (Israel).

Trout: Brook/Speckled/Square Tail, Brown trout, Char, Cisco, Cutthroat Trout, Dolly Varden/Malma Trout, Grayling, Lake Trout (Mackinaw, Salmon, Great Lakes), Mullet (Gray Mullet, Striped Mullet), Rainbow Trout, Silversides/Smelts, Tarpon, Tilapia/ Cichlids, Weakfish/ Sea Trout, Whitefish, Spotted Sea Trout.

Tuna: Albacore Tuna, Bigeye Tuna, Blackfin Tuna, Bullet Tuna, Longtail Tuna, Yellowfin Tuna, Dogtooth Tuna.

Unclean fish (do not have scales and fins):
Abalone, Billfish, Bullhead, Catfish, Clam, Crab, Crayfish, Cutlass Fish, Cuttlefish, Dolphin, Eel, European Turbot, Fire Fish, Gar, Goosefish, Jellyfish, Lamprey, Leather Jack, Limpet, Lobster, Lomosucker, Marlin, Mussels, Ocean Pout, Octopus, Oil Fish, Otter, Oysters, Paddlefish, Porcupine Fish, Porpoise, Prawn, Puffer, Rock Prickle Back, Sailfish, Sand Skate, Scallops, Sculpin, Shark, Snake Mackerel, Scallop, Seal, Shark, Shrimp, Squid (calamari), Stickleback, Stingray, Sturgeon, Swordfish, Toadfish, Triggerfish, Trunkfish, Walrus, Whale, Wolfish.

Clean insects:
Cricket, Locust, Grasshopper.

Unclean insects:
All others.
(Adapted from Bible Study Guide, Israel, Meinz, p.224, Russell, p.77).

Dr. David Meinz, author of the book *Eating by the Book*, notes, "dolphins, porpoises, and whales are mammals, not fish, and therefore are not clean." Also, "Jewish tradition counts these [sharks, sturgeon, swordfish] as unclean because of their unusual kind of 'scales'" (p.234).

258

Abiding by Distinctions

It was said previously that by and large Christians today (and most westerners for that matter) abide by the distinctions between clean and unclean animals in our diets. Notice that unclean animals include dogs and cats. Most of us would never even consider eating dog or cat meat. Such a thought would be repugnant to us, as we consider dogs and cats to be pets not food.

We would also not consider eating gorillas, monkeys, dolphins, and other relatively intelligent animals. In addition, we would not eat horses, eagles (especially the bald eagle here in the USA), swans, tigers, and other animals that we have great respect for or consider attractive. And most of us would recoil from the idea of eating "dirty" animals like bats, buzzards, rats, and vultures, or "creepy" animals like octopuses, snakes, spiders, and squid. Therefore, we are mostly following the food laws.

However, there are a few animals in these unclean lists that are becoming fashionable to eat, such as ostrich, while rabbits and squirrels are popular game animals. But the two classes of unclean meats that are most commonly eaten are pig meat and shellfish. As such, a deeper look at these two is in order.

Health Differences of Clean vs. Unclean Meats

Before looking at pig meat and shellfish, some general comments about the health effects of clean versus unclean meats would be helpful.

General Comments:

Is there a difference health-wise between clean and unclean meats? Generally speaking, animals listed as clean in the Bible are herbivores, whereas most of the unclean animals are carnivores or scavengers. An herbivorous animal would have fewer toxins in its body than a carnivorous one, as toxins get concentrated as you go up the food chain. And it would only stand to reason that animals eating garbage or dead animals would have more toxins in their flesh than ones eating greens.

Almost all of the creatures on the unclean list are scavengers. In many cases they don't hunt for their food; **they**

eat the dead and decaying matter of our environment. A catfish does that at the bottom of a pond; lobster and shrimp do it in the ocean. A pig will eat anything. Vultures, almost by definition, are known for their scavenger habits.

Could it be that God, in His wisdom, created certain animals whose sole purpose is to clean up after the others? Their entire "calling" may be to act exclusively as the sanitation workers of our ecology. God may be simply telling us that **it's better for us believers not to consume the meat of these trash collectors** (Meinz, p.225).

And in fact, Dr. Rex Russell reports about an old study of:
... the toxic effects of animal flesh on a controlled growth culture. In these tests, **the less a meat suppressed the growth of the culture the less toxic it was considered**. So the higher a percentage of culture growth, the better the meat (Russell, p.76).

Dr. Russell then gives a list of clean and unclean meats on page 77 of his book. Along with the list is the percentage of culture growth of the meats. All clean meats allowed 80% or higher culture growth, while all of the unclean meats restricted culture growth to 65% or less. Unfortunately, this study was done way back in 1954, and I haven't been able to find any more recent studies done on this subject. But this old study does give some indication that there is a significant difference between clean and unclean meats in their toxicity.

Shellfish:

In regards to all shellfish being unclean, Russell writes:
It has long been recognized that the meat of shellfish— shrimp, crabs, lobsters, etc.—is especially dangerous. Many illnesses, including instant paralysis, devastate some people every day as a result of eating shellfish (p.78).

Moreover, shellfish, along with fish like catfish, are bottom-dwellers. This means they dwell mostly in deep waters, where toxic sludge accumulates. Those toxins then get into the shrimp and other shellfish.

260

Most of the shrimp we import is "farmed"—grown in huge industrial tanks or shallow, man-made ponds that can stretch for acres. In some cases 150 shrimp can occupy a single square meter (roughly the size of a 60-inch flat-screen television) where they're fed commercial pellets, sometimes containing antibiotics to ward off disease. If ponds aren't carefully managed, **a sludge of fecal matter, chemicals, and excess food can build up and decay**. Wastewater can be periodically discharged into nearby waterways. "Bacteria and algae can begin to grow and disease can set in, **prompting farmers to use drugs and other chemicals that can remain on the shrimp and seep into the surrounding environment**," says Urvashi Rangan, Ph.D., executive director of the Consumer Reports Food Safety and Sustainability Center. Those shrimp-farming practices raise a variety of concerns—**not just about how safe shrimp are to eat but also about the environmental damage that can be caused by farming them that way** (Consumer Reports; Shrimp).

Why are lobsters cooked alive and do they feel pain?

Lobsters and other shellfish have harmful bacteria naturally present in their flesh. Once the lobster is dead, these bacteria can rapidly multiply and release toxins that may not be destroyed by cooking. **You therefore minimise the chance of food poisoning by cooking the lobster alive**...

It has been argued that lobsters do not possess a true brain and so can't feel pain. It is fair to say that they are not self-aware in the same way that we are, but they do react to tissue damage both physically and hormonally, so **they are obviously capable of detecting pain on some level** (Science Focus).

Shellfish poisoning is a risk for anyone who enjoys travelling and especially to areas of the developing world. Many species of fish such as oysters, clams and mussels contain potent toxins – known as marine toxins, which can cause food poisoning.

These marine toxins are caused by bacteria and viruses which invade shellfish, and other types of fish via consumption of contaminated algae or marine organisms in the surrounding water....

There is more than one type of food (or fish) poisoning caused by these molluscs which include:

- Paralytic poisoning
- Neurotoxic poisoning
- Diarrhoeic poisoning
- Amnesic poisoning

These are all caused by shellfish feeding on contaminated algae or plankton (dinoflagellates) which contain a variety of toxins such as saxitoxin or brevetoxins (Medic8).

Softshell clams exposed to 'red tide' events can develop a mutation that allows them to accumulate more Paralytic Shellfish Toxins (PSTs), making them more dangerous to humans.

Exposure to toxins that cause paralytic shellfish poisoning can result in a mutation that makes some clams much more resistant to the toxin, which can result in a greater danger to humans, according to a study published this week in the journal Nature. Paralytic shellfish toxins (PSTs) are produced by algae that appear in certain coastal areas in the United States in an event known as an algal bloom, commonly called a "red tide." **People who eat clams exposed to the PSTs can suffer the paralytic effects of the toxins, and there is no cure for the poisoning** (UW Today).

In the last decades, relevant efforts have been made to reduce the cancer incidence in the European Union. The prevention programmes against cancer have obtained satisfactory results except for **colorectal cancer (CRC)**. Identification of risk factors is primordial to plan preventive strategies for CRC. **We hypothesize that shellfish**

262

consumption is increasing CRC incidence. DSP toxins, present in some seafood products, seem to behave like tumour agents. There are no relevant studies on real health-risk of consuming DSP toxins, just some experimental and ecological evidence. Preventive interventions for reducing CRC risk must be approached through the collaboration of governmental, health and environmental sectors as a single regulatory agency. **Sometimes, shellfish accumulates diarrhetic shellfish poisoning (DSP) toxins** (i.e. okadaic acid and its derivatives) **which provoke a gastrointestinal illness** (DSP syndrome). **Furthermore, DSP toxins are tumour promoters that could increase CRC risk**. The current regulation about level of DSP toxins in shellfish meat is only centred on reduction of the gastrointestinal symptoms. Unfortunately, **legal levels of DSP toxins in shellfish are enough to increase CRC risk**. A review of legislation on DSP toxins is urgent (Manerio).

All of this make eating shellfish sound rather scary. But it will be acknowledged that some of these problems would apply to regular fish as well. But as we saw in the previous chapter, there are possible solutions to these problems. But to clear on one point, if you eat lobster, you are eating an animal that was slowly boiled to death, which sounds inhumane whether lobsters can feel pain or not.

Moreover, there is not near the evidence of health benefits for shellfish as there is for regular fish. Add in the Bible's clear directives against eating shellfish, and it would be best to expend our energies fixing the problems with harvesting fish and leave shellfish alone.

Pig Meat:

As for pig meat, it is well-known today that it can carry trichinosis. The trichinae parasitic worm can be killed by thorough cooking, but in ancient times, such was not known. Thus God was protecting the Jews from such food-borne diseases by forbidding unclean meats. And even today, pigs will eat just about anything, which means their meats can easily be contaminated with toxins, as can the meats of any scavenger.

The digestive system of a pig is completely different from that of a cow. It is similar to ours, in that the stomach is very acidic. **Pigs are gluttonous, never knowing when to stop eating.** Their stomach acids become diluted because of the volume of food, allowing all kinds of vermin to pass through this protective barrier. **Parasites, bacteria, viruses, and toxins can pass into the pig's flesh because of overeating.** These toxins and infectious agents can be passed on to humans when they eat a pig's flesh….

In the *Biblical Archeological Review,* **Jane Cahill examined the toilets of a Jewish household in Jerusalem, finding no parasites nor infectious agents,** but only pollen from the many fruits, vegetables and herbs they had eaten. **A similar study about Egyptians revealed eggs from Schistosoma, Trichinella, wire worm and tapeworms, all found in pork**. All of these organisms cause significant chronic diseases (Russell, p. 78).

There is also the environmental damage of large-scale hog farms. Such was mentioned in Chapter Six but was not commented upon then. But it is worth looking at in more detail now. All of the problems with factory farms mentioned in that chapter also apply to large-scale hog farming.

Since the mid-20th century, small, extensive farms have given way to massive, commercial pig production facilities. In 2009, more than 1.3 billion pigs were raised and slaughtered globally. Between 1980 and 2000, though world pork production nearly doubled, there was a decrease in the total number of farms. Large industrial farm animal production facilities, or factory farms, that often confine thousands of pigs indoors, are becoming more widespread throughout the world, particularly in developing countries. Factory farms are now responsible for more than half of all global pork production….

A significant implication of the shift toward factory farms has been the "movement of large numbers of animals from pastures and open-air lots into confined spaces with no grass or vegetation for grazing." Factory farms may have particularly severe implications for animal welfare, including **the intensive confinement of farm animals in enclosures** that prevent them from moving comfortably or expressing most basic natural behaviors. Around the world, millions of breeding sows (female pigs) in industrial systems are confined in 0.6-0.7 m (2.0-2.3 ft) by 2.0-2.1 m (6.6-6.9 ft) gestation crates for nearly their entire lives. **These crates are about the size of the animals' bodies**, denying the sows the ability to exercise, turn around for months on end, or perform other integral, instinctual, and natural behaviors, including rooting, foraging, nest-building, and grazing. In addition to causing tremendous animal suffering, factory farms degrade the environment and negatively impact public health and rural communities...

Much of the environmental damage caused by industrial pig production facilities is due to the volume and content of animal waste, and the consequent challenges of storage and disposal. **Pigs produce four times more waste than human beings** and "one animal facility with a large population of animals can easily equal a small city in terms of waste production." **While traditional farming systems combine animal agriculture with crop agriculture, thereby balancing the number of animals with the crops' ability to absorb the animals' manure, at industrial farm animal production facilities, the amount of manure typically exceeds the ability of the surrounding land to absorb it**. Waste from pig factory farms is often stored in lagoons or pits, which have been known to leak or break, contaminating nearby water sources with excess nitrogen and phosphorous, pathogens, and other pollutants that are found in the manure. The minimally treated (or even untreated) waste is also often sprayed on nearby fields, potentially contaminating water, soil, and air (Humane Society).

The collapse of a dike on a rain-soaked industrial swine farm in Onslow County sent 25 million gallons of hog waste surging across roads and crops and into the headwaters of the New River.

The state's worst spill of agricultural waste began Wednesday afternoon, just as state legislators were debating whether to put new restrictions on the state's booming corporate swine industry. The proposal was rejected in favor of a study.

Adding further irony, the 1 ½-year-old farm involved in the accident was the first to be sanctioned under new regulations designed to protect the state's waters from livestock waste. Pork industry officials have maintained that farms built under the new guidelines are environmentally safe.

On Thursday, state investigators linked the accident to a fish kill in at least one tributary of the New River and were **bracing for bigger problems today as the waste plume moves downstream.**

The full impact of the spill may not be known for days or weeks. **Widespread fish kills, for example, often occur hours or days after a spill of sewage or animal waste**, when the oxygen level in the water has been depleted.

The risks to humans were believed to be minor (Learn NC).

Animal agriculture in the United States for the most part has industrialized, with negative consequences for air and water quality and antibiotic use. **We consider health and environmental impacts of current US swine production** and give an overview of current federal, state, and local strategies being used to address them.... **the vast majority of animals now raised for food in the United States live within concentrated animal feeding operations (CAFOs)....**

In Iowa, the largest producer state, 70% of farms had hogs as part of their farming operations in the 1960s, compared with approximately 12% in 2000. Until the late 1980s, a typical hog farm raised fewer than 1000 animals from farrow (birth) to finish (ready for slaughter), and feed was from crops largely grown on-farm. Now **it is common to have 4000 sows within a single breeding facility**, each sow producing litter after litter. After early weaning, "feeder" piglets by the thousands are moved to "finisher" barns, where **in 6 months as many as 12,000 pigs grow from about 50 to 250 pounds before being slaughtered**. Industrialization also means that

266

food animals have been largely brought indoors, and grain and other feed-stuffs must be imported by the ton to serve them....

Manure waste must be disposed of, also by the ton. Manure from confined animal operations is 3 times the nation's volume of human waste. Because it is uneconomical to transport for any distance, manure typically is stored in pits under buildings, or in lagoons adjacent to buildings, and later is applied to nearby fields. However, the largest CAFO facilities typically lack sufficient acreage to absorb manure nutrients. According to a survey by the US Department of Agriculture (USDA), "**Large operations tend to view manure as a waste rather than a resource** and dispose of it on land closest to the facility....

... **manure can contain arsenic and other heavy metal compounds, as well as antibiotics, that are routinely added to animal feeds**. Manure and manure-related contaminants **readily move off-site in water and air**....

Current farming practices are responsible for 70% of the pollution in the nation's rivers and streams....

CAFOs have public health impacts. **CAFO workers suffer documented ill effects from manure-related gases, odors, and degradants; dust; bacteria; and endotoxins**. CAFOs, including swine CAFOs, produce water and air emissions that may affect the health of neighbors, surrounding communities, and the environment. **CAFOs also make routine use of antibiotics and other feed additives to offset the greater risk of infection from the concentration and accelerated production of animals. This contributes to the global crisis of antibiotic resistance** (Osterberg).

It would be good to point out a couple of statements mentioned in the last quote that were discussed previously. First, with old-fashioned farms, manure is a resource that naturally fertilizes the land the animals graze on. But in a factory farm, manure is a waste product that can cause environmental damage.

Second, proactive antibiotic use is needed in a factory farm to offset the greater risk of widespread infection of packed in animals in factory farms. But such is not needed in old-fashioned farms.

That said; as with factory cattle farms, factory hog farms carry many potential problems. When accidents happen, these problems become particularly acute, but even without an accident, the problems are real and ongoing.

However, there are ways to raise hogs that are not environmentally damaging and inhumane to the hogs.

If you choose to eat pig meat then you can make a statement on what you do and don't support with where you put your dollar. **Buying free-range, pastured and if possible organic pig meat say "I care about the environment" and "I care about the animals welfare."** It will mean the farms have the ability to use an outdoor, rotation system, that allows regeneration of the land and evenly spreads the waste of the pigs. **When stocking densities are kept low and outdoors, the amount of waste is able to go onto the land without a problem**, and without the high amounts of toxic bacteria created in an over populated factory shed.

When choosing to eat the meat from a pig, you should choose to buy from a farm where the pigs:

- have freedom to move in generous space, with low stocking densities
- live outside in nature
- are able to graze, fed no antibiotic/additives
- have the ability to root with their snout
- have protection from extreme weather
- are provided farrowing huts for the sows
- Get to keep their tails and teeth intact! (Compassionate Road).

Thus like old-fashioned farms for beef, it is possible to find pig meat from farms that do not carry the problems of factory farms. And similar to grass-fed beef, there is a difference between the meat from grass-fed pigs versus factory farm pigs, but it is not as significant or clear-cut:

> **... a 2012 review that tried to make an overall comparison between free-range and factory-farmed pork had a difficult time, because the studies found widely different results. Some found no significant difference at all**; others found the free-range pork to be **anywhere from 18% to 291% higher in Omega-3s**, with a difference in O6:O3 ratio anywhere from 7% to 42%. **Whenever there was a difference, it was a difference in favor of the free-range animals.**
>
> This variation in results is frustrating but not surprising. First of all, not all pigs are the same; it's unreasonable to expect totally uniform results. The type of plants on the pasture can also have an effect. Then you have to consider that all these studies raised the pigs in different ways. It would really be more surprising if the research all agreed!
>
> **The results for micronutrient content are less impressive.** For Vitamin E, the 2012 review found that free-range pork provides 1.7-5% of the RDA, compared to 0.8-2.5% for CAFO pork. For iron, the difference was even smaller: 3.6% for free-range vs. 1.1% for CAFO. This could potentially make a difference if pork is your only source of Vitamin E or iron, but **it's not extremely significant in the context of an otherwise balanced diet** (Paleo Leap).

Thus if you are going to eat pork, then you should try to find pork from an old-fashioned farm. And in fact, Pittsburgh's East End Food Co-op that I mentioned about previously sells such pork from small local farms. But like grass-fed beef, it is rather expensive. It fact, it costs as much as the steak at the Co-op. And given that the benefits are not as significant or clear-cut and given the Bible's directives against eating pig meat, then one's money would be better spent on grass fed beef, for which there are significant and clear cut benefits.

Moreover, pork is only one form in which pig meat is eaten. It is more commonly eaten via processed meats like ham, sausage, and bacon, and that is a double-whammy against pig meat, as we will see shortly. But first, we need to revisit another important issue.

269

Mercury in Fish

The potential problems of mercury and other contaminations in fish was mentioned in the previous chapter. Many claim fish should not be eaten for such reasons. However, the levels of mercury in fish vary greatly from one species to another. Below is a list of the respective mercury levels in a wide variety of fish.

Least mercury: Less than 0.09 parts per million:
Enjoy these fish:
Anchovies, Butterfish, Catfish, Clam, Crab (Domestic), Crawfish/Crayfish, Croaker (Atlantic), Flounder, Haddock (Atlantic), Hake, Herring, Mackerel (N. Atlantic, Chub), Mullet, Oyster, Perch (Ocean), Plaice, Pollock, Salmon (Canned), Salmon (Fresh), Sardines, Scallops, Shad (American), Shrimp, Sole (Pacific), Squid (Calamari), Tilapia, Trout (Freshwater), Whitefish, Whiting.

Moderate mercury: From 0.09 to 0.29 parts per million
Eat six servings or less per month:
Bass (Striped, Black), Carp, Cod (Alaskan), Croaker (White Pacific), Halibut (Atlantic), Halibut (Pacific), Jacksmelt (Silverside), Lobster, Mahi Mahi, Monkfish, Perch (Freshwater), Sablefish, Skate, Snapper, Tuna (Canned chunk light), Tuna (Skipjack), Weakfish (Sea Trout)

High mercury: From 0.3 to 0.49 parts per million
Eat three servings or less per month:
Bluefish, Grouper, Mackerel (Spanish, Gulf), Sea Bass (Chilean), Tuna (Canned Albacore), Tuna (Yellowfin)

Highest mercury: More than .5 parts per million.
Avoid eating:
Mackerel (King), Marlin, Orange Roughy, Shark, Swordfish, Tilefish, Tuna (Bigeye, Ahi). (Disabled World).

If you compare the lists of clean and unclean fish with this list, you will see that for the most part, clean fish are in the first two levels with lower mercury contamination, while unclean fish are in the latter two with higher contamination. Thus by obeying God, you will avoid most varieties of the most contaminated fish. It should also be noted that there are other contaminants in seafood besides just mercury. Thus shrimp might be low in mercury, but it is often high in other contaminates, as we have already seen.

The best approach would be to avoid all of the fish listed on the Biblically unclean list **or** on the latter two mercury lists, while eating those fish on the Biblically clean list **and** on the first two mercury lists. The latter would be:

Biblical Clean and Low in Mercury:

Anchovies, Bass (Striped, Black, and probably others), Carp, Cod (Alaskan), Croaker (White Pacific), Flounder, Haddock (Atlantic), Halibut (Atlantic), Halibut (Pacific), Hake, Herring, Mackerel (N. Atlantic, Chub), Jacksmelt (Silverside), Mahi Mahi, Mullet, Perch (Ocean), Perch (Freshwater), Plaice (Right-eyed Flounder), Pollock, Salmon (Canned), Salmon (Fresh), Sardines, Shad (American), Sole (Pacific), Snapper, Tilapia, Trout (Freshwater), Tuna (Canned chunk light), Tuna (Skipjack), Weakfish (Sea Trout), Whitefish, Whiting.

If you consume only these fish, you will attain the benefits while avoiding the drawbacks of fish.

Blood and Fat

In the next verse after God's decree about giving "Every moving thing that lives" for food, God says, "However, flesh with blood of life you* will not eat" (Gen 9:4). Therefore, while God intends for us to eat meat, it is wrong to eat it with the blood still in it. This commandment is repeated throughout the Old Testament:

[26]'**All blood you* will not eat** in all your* habitations, both from birds and from animals. [27]**Every soul which shall eat blood, that soul will perish from his people**'" (Lev 7:26f).

[10]'And a person, a person [fig., Any person] of the sons [and daughters] of Israel, or of the strangers abiding among you, **who shall eat any blood, I will even set My face against that soul, the one**

271

eating blood, and will destroy it from its people. [11]For the life of all flesh is its blood, and I have given it to you* on the altar to be making atonement for your* souls; for its blood will make atonement for the soul. [cp. Heb 9:22] [12]Because of this, I said to the sons [and daughters] of Israel, '**No soul of you* will eat blood, and the stranger, one abiding among you* will not eat blood**' (Lev 17:10-12).

[15]**"But you will kill in [or, according to] all your desire, and will eat meat according to the blessing of the LORD your God**, which He gave to you in every city; the unclean among you and the clean will eat it the same, as a gazelle or a deer. [16]**However, you* will not eat the blood; you* will pour it out on the ground as water** (Deut 12:15).

[23]**Take diligent heed [that] you do not eat blood, for the blood [is] the life of it;** the life will not be consumed with the meat. [24]You* will not eat [it]; **you* will pour it out on the ground as water** (Deut 12:23f).

[23]**Only you* will not eat the blood; you will pour it out upon the ground as water** (Deut 15:23).

[32]And the people turned to the spoil; and the people took flocks, and herds, and children of cows [fig., calves], and slaughtered [them] on the ground, and **the people were eating with the blood!** [cp. Gen 9:4; Lev 3:17; 17:10-14] [33]And it was reported to Saul, saying, "**The people have sinned against the LORD, having eaten with the blood!**" And Saul said, "In Getthaim roll a great stone to me here." [34]And Saul said, "Disperse among the people, and tell them to bring here each [one] his calf, and each [one] his sheep; and let them slaughter [it] on this [stone] and **by no means sin against the LORD in eating with the blood**." And all the people were bringing each [one] the [animal] in his hand, and they were slaughtering [them] there. [35]And Saul built an altar there to the LORD. This [was the] first altar Saul built to the LORD (1Sam 14:32-35).

Note that it is assumed people will eat meat, "according to all your desire." In fact, doing so is a blessing of the LORD. But note how strongly the command against eating blood is asserted and how often it is repeated in the Torah. And at the time of Saul, a great sin was committed when people ignored this law.

Notice also the prescribed manner of eliminating the blood, "pour it on the ground as water." This is important as some vegetarians try to use this command against eating blood as a backdoor way of claiming the Bible forbids the eating of meat. It is said that it is impossible to remove every drop of blood, so meat should not be eaten at all.

But again, these passages assume meat will be eaten, even calling it a blessing of God. Simply pouring out the blood until it no longer pours like water will suffice for removing the blood.

In this case, there is no doubt this command is applicable to Christians, as it is repeated in the New Testament:

[28]For it seemed good to the Holy Spirit and to us to lay no more burden on you*, except [for] these necessary things: [29]**to be keeping distant** from meats sacrificed to idols and **from blood** and from [anything] strangled **and from fornication.** From which keeping yourselves, you* will do well (Acts 15:20).

Notice that consuming blood is as much as of a sin as fornication.

Dr. Russell comments on this restriction, "Blood is the body's transport system, carrying in it all waste products for disposal" (p.34). And in fact, in the culture tests mentioned previously, the blood of all animals, clean and unclean, significantly inhibited culture growth. Blood was thus considered to be very toxic.

In the Mosaic Law, God combines the restriction about blood with another one. It is in the context of the animal sacrifices in the temple:

[1]'Now if his gift to the LORD [is] a sacrifice of a peace-offering, if he should bring it **from the herd**, both male and female, he will bring it unblemished before the LORD. [2]And he will lay his hands on the head of the gift and will slaughter it by the doors of the tabernacle of witness. And the sons of Aaron, **the priests, will pour the blood on the altar of burnt-offerings round about**. [3]And they will bring from the sacrifice of the peace-offering a burnt-sacrifice to the LORD, **the fat covering the belly, and all the fat on the belly. [4]And the two kidneys and the fat upon them; the [fat] upon the thighs**, and the lobe above the liver together with the kidneys he will take away. [5]And **the sons of Aaron,**

the priests, will offer them on the altar on the burnt-offering, on the wood on the fire upon the altar; [it is] a burnt-offering, a sweet smell, a fragrant aroma to the LORD (Lev 3:1-5).

Notice that the blood and fat of cattle are to be offered to the LORD. The same is said of the blood and fat of sheep and of goats in the next two paragraphs (Lev 3:6-16). Then is the following command:

¹⁷[It is] a statute into the ages [fig., forever] into [or, throughout] your* generations, in all your habitations; all fat and all blood you* will not eat [or, you* will eat no fat and no blood]'" (Lev 3:17).

Thus just as blood is not to be eaten, so also the fat should not be eaten. This command is repeated a few chapters later:

²²And the LORD spoke to Moses, saying, ²³"Speak to the sons [and daughters] of Israel, saying, 'All fat of oxen and sheep and goats you* will not eat. ²⁴And [the] fat of animals that died [of themselves] and eaten by wild beasts, will be employed for any work; but it will not be consumed for food. ²⁵Everyone eating fat from animals, which he will bring [as] a burnt-offering to the LORD, that soul will perish from his people.
²⁶'All blood you* will not eat in all your* habitations, both from birds and from animals. ²⁷Every soul which shall eat blood, that soul will perish from his people'" (Lev 7:22-27).

Notice that the command against eating fat is worded just as strongly as the command against eating blood. To be clear, the fat being referred to here is not the marbling within the muscle, it is the cover fat, the fat outside of the muscle that can easily be cut away. The command is to cut it off and either offer it to the LORD or to discard it. But under no circumstances should it be eaten.

Dr. Meinz comments on these restrictions:
> It goes without saying we should never eat blood today. The idea is disgusting. It almost suggests some type of satanic involvement. If it was discovered that someone at your church was drinking blood, a special meeting of the pastor and

church leadership most likely would be called. This kind of action would be addressed quickly and decisively. We seem to know in our very beings that eating blood is unacceptable.

As we've just seen in Leviticus 3:17, in God's sight, *eating animal fat* **is just as unacceptable. And that prohibition is for all the generations.** Consuming blood would cause real indignation in your church, and yet eating animal fat is practiced by many church members today without any thought whatsoever. **It may be that animal fat was never designed for human consumption. We may be better off just not eating it** (pp. 200-201, italics in original).

It would thus be prudent for Christians today when eating meat to be sure the blood is drained from the meat before cooking and any outer or cover fat is trimmed from it. Note also, the skin of chicken and turkey would also qualify as a "fat" that should not be eaten, as it also can be easily removed. But is there any evidence that removing the outer fat of meat or the skin of poultry is beneficial? Consider the following study:

Temporal trend and migrant studies have indicated that the etiology of **colorectal cancer** is predominantly environmental and, hence, modifiable. **Animal fat intake has been frequently, but inconsistently, associated with the risk of this disease.** We conducted a population-based case-control study in Hawaii (United States) among ethnic groups at different risks of the disease to evaluate the role of dietary lipids and foods of animal origin on the risk of colorectal cancer....

Odds ratios (OR), adjusted for caloric intake and other dietary and non-dietary risk factors, were estimated using conditional logistic regression. **Intakes of total fat, saturated fat (S) and polyunsaturated fat (P) were not related to the risk of colorectal cancer.** However, an inverse association was found for the P/S ratio, with ORs of 0.6 in both genders (95 percent confidence interval [CI] = 0.4-1.0 for males; CI = 0.3-0.9 for females) for the highest compared with the lowest quartile (P < 0.05 for trend). **Intakes of red meat and processed meat were associated with the risk of cancer in the right colon and rectum, respectively, in men only. Fat-**

275

trimmed red meat and fish intakes were not related to risk. Chicken eaten without skin was associated inversely with risk in both genders. The strongest association was found for eggs...

These data suggest that the ratio of polyunsaturated to saturated fat may be a better indicator of colorectal cancer risk than the absolute amount of specific fats in the diet. They also suggest that eggs and, possibly, **untrimmed red meat and processed meat increase, and chicken eaten without skin decreases, colorectal cancer risk** (Marchand).

Note that red meat and processed meat were associated with an increased risk of colorectal cancer, but not trimmed red meat. Therefore, it is the cover fat and not the meat itself that increases risk. This is another important point that is not usually accounted for in studies. Note also that chicken without skin was associated with a reduced risk, so it is important to remove the skin from poultry. This means science is finally catching up with what God decreed millennia ago.

Meat is a good source of dietary proteins in many countries and provides high biological value. Apart from being important sources of proteins, vitamins and minerals, it also provides fat including saturated fatty acids (SFA), unsaturated fatty acids (USFA), cholesterol, triacylglycerol and phospholipids. Thus, consumers often associate meat with a negative image as a high fat and cancer-promoting food (Valsta et al. 2005). Some of these **negative nutrients can be minimized by selection of lean meat cuts, removal of adipose fat, dietary manipulation to alter fatty acid composition and proper portion control** to decrease fat consumption and caloric intake. As **meat is by itself rich in nutrients such as fatty acids, minerals, dietary fiber, antioxidants and bioactive peptides**, their incorporation into other products would alter the nutritional and biofunctional value of the product positively (Swapna).

Note that "adipose fat" is what was just called the cover or outer fat. Note also the emphasize on how nutritious meat is. Moreover, "dietary manipulation to alter fatty acid composition" would refer to grass-fed beef being better in the type of fat it contains as compared to grain-fed beef. But "proper portion control" is needed.

Miscellaneous Meats

So far, this discussion on meats has been primarily on whole meats, such as steaks, roasts, and whole chicken pieces. But meat is often eaten in more treated forms.

Processed Meats:

The first miscellaneous meats are processed meats.

> Processed meat is meat that has been preserved by curing, salting, smoking, drying or canning. Food products categorized as processed meat include: Sausages, hot dogs, salami, bacon, ham (Authority. Why Processed).

Processed meats are altered to such a degree that they bear little resemblance to whole meats. In addition, the processing used is often such that it would not have been possible in Biblical times. Thus sausage and the like is not mentioned in the Bible.

In the processing, the cover fat of the meat is usually ground into the product, so eating processed meats would break the command against eating the fat of meat. That is also why processed meats are usually much higher in fat content than their whole meat counterparts.

In addition, processed meats also often contain artificial ingredients or other food stuffs that would not be God-given, such as nitrates. "One thing is clear, processed meat contains harmful chemical compounds that may increase the risk of chronic disease" (Authority. Why Processed). They also contain a significant amount of salt.

Processed meats are also often made with pig meat. And they are made by grinding together an assortment of "leftovers" in the meat processing plants.

All of this is why it was said previously that sausage and other pig-based processed meats are a double-whammy, as they break both the unclean food law and the don't eat fat law, along with having these other problems with them.

Consequently, it is no surprise processed meats are associated with an increased risk of cancer, as seen in a preceding quote. And such studies could easily be multiplied, as an association between processed meats and various health problems is commonly found in studies.

For instance, a meta-analysis was done of 20 studies. They "included 1,218,380 individuals and 23,889 CHD [coronary heart disease], 2,280 stroke, and 10,797 diabetes cases." The results were:

Red meat intake was not associated with CHD (n=4 studies, RR per 100g serving/day=1.00, 95%CI=0.81–1.23,p-for-heterogeneity=0.36) **or diabetes** (n=5, RR=1.16, 95%CI=0.92–1.46,p=0.25). **Conversely, processed meat intake was associated with 42% higher risk of CHD** (n=5, RR per 50g serving/day=1.42, 95%CI=1.07–1.89,p=0.04) **and 19% higher risk of diabetes** (n=7, RR=1.19, 95%CI=1.11–1.27,p<0.001). Associations were intermediate for total meat intake. Red and processed meat consumption were not associated with stroke, but only 3 studies evaluated these relationships.

Conclusions:

Consumption of processed meats, but not red meats, is associated with higher incidence of CHD and diabetes. These results highlight the need for better understanding of potential mechanisms of effects, and for particular focus on processed meats for dietary and policy recommendations (Renata).

A study of ovarian cancer found:

Although there was no association between total or red meat intake and ovarian cancer risk, women with the highest intake of processed meat had a significantly increased risk of ovarian cancer in the 2 case-control studies (combined OR: 1.18; 95% CI: 1.15, 1.21) and the meta-analysis [7 studies; pooled relative risk (RR): 1.20; 95% CI: 1.07, 1.34]. In contrast, **a frequent intake of poultry was associated with borderline significant reductions in risk in the 2 case-control studies** (combined OR: 0.83; 95% CI: 0.67, 1.03) and the meta-analysis including 7 additional studies (pooled RR: 0.90; 95% CI: 0.79, 1.01). **High fish intake was associated with a significantly reduced risk** in the 2 case-control studies (combined OR: 0.76; 95% CI: 0.62, 0.94) and a smaller borderline significant reduction in the meta-analysis (6 additional studies; pooled RR: 0.84; 95% CI: 0.68, 1.03).

Our results suggest that **low consumption of processed meat and higher consumption of poultry and fish may reduce the risk of ovarian cancer** (Kolahdooz).

Thus processed meats are associated with an increased risk of cancer, heart disease, and even diabetes. But whole red meats are not, while chicken and especially fish intake can reduce the risk. This all fits with what we have seen previously. And it should be noted that these studies do not take into account if the red meat was from a factory or old-fashioned farm. If the latter, it might also decrease risk.

Putting all of this together, if a processed meat is made with factory farm meat, and/ or pig meat, and/or the cover fat is ground into the product, and/or it contains artificial ingredients, then it would not be a God-given food. Just one of these factors would disqualify it.

All of this makes the common practice of serving ham at Christmas and Easter gatherings very dubious. It makes no sense to celebrate the birth and the resurrection of our Lord and Savior Jesus Christ with an unhealthy food that Jesus Himself would never have eaten.

But what about all-natural processed meats that are made from clean, old-fashioned meats, like all-beef hot dogs, chicken sausage, or turkey kielbasa? Would they be God-given?

Well first you might still have the problem of cover fat or skin being ground into the product. The amount of fat in the product could be a clue in this regard. Second, they would still be processed in a way that was not possible in Bible times. Third, they probably still contain a large amount of added salt.

These three factors together would mean they would be borderline God-given foods at best, and if they are consumed, it should only be in very limited amounts. But what the health-effects of such would be is hard to say, as such have not been studied separately from other forms of processed meats. Though given their nutritional profiles, it would be logical to assume they would not have near the adverse health effects of commercial processed meats.

Ground Meats:

The next miscellaneous meats would be ground meats. If they are God-given would depend on how they are made. The reason for this caveat is that when beef is ground into ground meat, sometimes the cover fat is ground in with the muscle. If it is, then such meat would not be God-given. But if it is not, then it could be. The way to know the difference is to check the fat content. If the meat is labeled as "extra lean" then the cover fat was probably not ground in, while "regular" ground meat probably contains cover fat.

As for ground turkey, if the skin is ground into the meat, then it would not be God-given, but if it is not, it could be. Again, check the fat content for a clue if it is or not.

I say "could be" as the difference between factory farm and old-fashioned meats would also apply. If you are purchasing meats from a local farm, you can ask if the cover fat or skin is ground into the meat. But even without a label or asking, it is possible to tell the difference simply by cooking the meat. Fatty ground meat has far more drippings that lean ground meat. At the very least, pour off those fat drippings before consuming the cooked meat.

Another potential problem with factory farm ground meat that would render it non-God-given is the presence of non-food items in the meat. Consider the following disturbing report:

> **Ring in the new decade with yet another disturbing story about commercial hamburger**. A New York Times expose, published on December 30, 2009, revealed that Beef Products, Inc (BPI), a South Dakota meat processor, has been **injecting ammonia into "fatty slaughterhouse trimmings" to kill bacteria and render it safe for human consumption**.
>
> The USDA has approved this novel process. Indeed, studies conducted by BPI showed the product to be so effective that the government agency exempted BPI products from routine testing. In another bow to the company, **the USDA agreed with BPI that the word "ammonia" need not appear on**

ingredient labels. Instead, it can be described as a generic "processing agent."

Why does this matter to you? **If you eat commercial hamburger, the chances are very good that you've eaten ammoniated beef** (eat Wild. Notes).

Dried Meats:

Drying meat is a form of processing, but it differs from other treated meats in that only salt is added in the processing, and it was commonly practiced by all people in ancient times, even though it is not specifically mentioned in the Bible. It is still popular among hunters today. It is thus a natural way of preserving meat without refrigeration.

In physical terms, drying is the lowering of the water activity in meat and meat products. Water activity is the measure of free unbound water available for microbial growth. **Microorganisms need certain amounts of free water for growth, and their growth is halted below defined minimum levels of moisture**. Minimum levels vary from species to species of microorganisms....

Meat drying is a simple but efficient food preservation activity. Dried meat can be stored under ambient temperatures for many months. Due to the low water content, microbial spoilage of the muscle proteins can be safely prevented. However, deterioration of adhering fatty tissue through rancidity cannot be stopped. It is therefore **advisable to use lean meat only. Beef and buffalo meat as well as goat and certain game meats (deer, antelopes) are best suited**. The same applies to meat of livestock used in some regions for meat production, such as camels or yaks. The suitability of mutton is ranked slightly lower. **Pork, even from very lean muscle parts, is less suitable**, as it contains higher amounts of intermuscular and mostly invisible intramuscular (within the muscle cells) fat, which is prone to oxidation and hence turns quickly rancid (FAO. Meat Drying).

Thus to dry meat, the cover fat must be removed, and only lean meats used. And unclean meats like pork cannot be used. This all means

281

drying meat would be a process consistent with Creationist Diet principles. Therefore, dried meat could be a God-given form of meat.

However, the same standard of old-fashioned meats being used rather than factory farm meat would still apply. You also have to look out for the addition of artificial ingredients. And there is usually a significant amount of salt added. But then, it is salt's preservation qualities that led Jesus to declare, "salt is good" (Luke 13:34).

Starting with the next chapter, we will consider animal foods other than meats. But first, an interesting tidbit I heard while working on the final draft of this book.

"The Oldest in the World"

CBN News had a report on the world's oldest living person. Violet Moss Brown turned 117 years old in 2017, having been born in 1900. She attributes her long life to her Christian faith. She stated, "I've done nearly everything in the church. I spent all my time in the church, from a child right up."

When asked what she eats, she replied, "Anything at all. What makes my belly full. **I don't eat pork**, I don't eat chicken, but I eat many other things. **Greens, mutton, beef, fish, that's what I eat.**"

Note that mutton is meat from a sheep that is over a year old, usually about three years old, while lamb comes from a sheep less than a year old (Spruce). It would thus seem that this world's oldest living person is following a Creationist Diet, lots of variety, with eating various clean meats while avoiding unclean meats, plus lots of veggies.

Bibliography:

Authority Nutrition. Why Processed is Bad for You. https://authoritynutrition.com/why-processed-meat-is-bad/

Bible Study Guide. Clean and Unclean Foods in the Bible. http://www.biblestudy.org/cleanfood.html

CBN News on WPCB Pittsburgh, April 21, 2017.

Compassionate Road. The damage Pig Farming is doing to the Environment and how you can avoid playing a part. http://thecompassionateroad.com/the-damage-pig-farming-is-doing-to-the-environment-and-how-you-can-avoid-playing-a-part/

Consumer Reports. How safe is your shrimp?

http://www.consumerreports.org/cro/magazine/2015/06/shrimp-safety/index.htm

Disabled World. Mercury Levels in Fish: Chart & Information. https://www.disabled-world.com/calculators-charts/fish-mercury.php

Eat Wild; Notes & News. http://www.eatwild.com/news.html

Humane Society. The Environmental, Public Health, and Social Impacts of Pig Factory Farming. http://www.hsi.org/assets/pdfs/hsi-fa-white-papers/an_hsi_factsheet_the.pdf

Knowledge Nuts. The Difference Between Pigs, Hogs, And Wild Boars. http://knowledgenuts.com/2014/08/06/the-difference-between-pigs-hogs-and-wild-boars/

Kolahdooz F1, et. al., *American Journal of Clinical Nutrition*. 2010 Jun;91(6):1752-63. doi: 10.3945/ajcn.2009.28415. Epub 2010 Apr 14. Meat, fish, and ovarian cancer risk: Results from 2 Australian case-control studies, a systematic review, and meta-analysis. https://www.ncbi.nlm.nih.gov/pubmed/20392889

Israel of God Research Committee. Clean. http://www.theisraelofgodrc.com/Clean_Animals.html

Learn NC. The impact of hog farms. http://www.learnnc.org/lp/editions/nchist-recent/6172

Manerio E1, Rodas VL, Costas E, Hernandez JM. *Medical Hypotheses*. 2008;70(2):409-12. Epub 2007 Jul 2. Shellfish consumption: a major risk factor for colorectal cancer. https://www.ncbi.nlm.nih.gov/pubmed/17606330

Marchand, Le L. Wilkens LR. Hankin JH. Kolonel LN. Lyu LC. *Cancer Causes & Control*. 8(4):637-48, 1997 Jul). A case-control study of diet and colorectal cancer in a multiethnic population in Hawaii (United States): lipids and foods of animal origin. https://www.ncbi.nlm.nih.gov/pubmed/9242481

FAO. Meat Drying. http://www.fao.org/docrep/010/ai407e/AI407E18.htm

Medic8. Shellfish toxins. http://www.medic8.com/healthguide/food-poisoning/shellfish-toxins.html

Meinz, David L. *Eating by the Book*. Virginia Beach, VA: Gilbert Press, 1999.

Osterberg, David, MS and David Wallinga, MD. *American Journal of Public Health*. 2004 October; 94(10): 1703–1708. PMCID: PMC1448520. Addressing Externalities From Swine Production to Reduce Public Health and Environmental Impacts.
https://www.ncbi.nlm.nih.gov/pmc/articles/PMC1448520/

Paleo Leap. Not Just the Cows. Pastured Pork and Poultry.
http://paleoleap.com/just-cows-pastured-pork-poultry/

Renata Micha, RD, PhD, et. al. *Circulation*. 2010 Jun 1; 121(21): 2271–2283. Red and processed meat consumption and risk of incident coronary heart disease, stroke, and diabetes: A systematic review and meta-analysis.
https://www.ncbi.nlm.nih.gov/pmc/articles/PMC2885952/

Ruminates. What is a Ruminant Animal?
http://aitc.ca/bc/uploads/ruminants.pdf

Russell, Rex MD. *What the Bible Says about Healthy Living*. Grand Rapids, MI: Baker Book House, 1999.

Science Focus. Why are lobsters cooked alive and do they feel pain?
http://www.sciencefocus.com/qa/why-are-lobsters-cooked-alive-and-do-they-feel-pain

Spruce, The. Lamb vs Mutton. https://www.thespruce.com/the-difference-between-lamb-and-mutton-2356034

Swapna C., et. al., *Journal of Food Science Technology*. 2012 Dec; 49(6): 653–664. Characteristics and consumer acceptance of healthier meat and meat product formulations—a review.
https://www.ncbi.nlm.nih.gov/pmc/articles/PMC3550835/

UW Today. Paralytic shellfish toxins cause mutation that allows clams to accumulate 100 times more toxin.
http://www.washington.edu/news/2005/04/08/paralytic-shellfish-toxins-cause-mutation-that-allows-clams-to-accumulate-100-times-more-toxin/

Chapter Nine:
Additional Animal Foods

The Noahic decree gave "every moving thing that lives" to humans to eat. As discussed previously, this decree would include various kinds of meats, with some restrictions. But besides meats, there are various other kinds of animal foods. Would these other animal foods be included in the Noahic decree? When did such foods enter the human diet? And do they have a place in a Creationist Diet? These questions will be discussed in this and the following chapters.

But before we proceed, the distinction between factory farms and old-fashioned farms would also apply to other animal foods besides meats, as there are significant differences between the two. Keep that in mind as we proceed.

Eggs

Eggs are living things, but they are not "moving things." However, they do come from living and moving things, so most likely they would have been included in the Noahic Decree. Eggs are mentioned twice in regards to food in the Old Testament and once in the New Testament.

The earliest reference is in the somewhat humorous statement in the Book of Job, "Can flavorless food be eaten without salt? Or is there any taste in the white of an egg?" (6:6; NKJV).

Debates abound as to the dating of the book of Job, as I discuss in Volume One of my three volume set, *Why Are These Books in the Bible and Not Others?* But whatever the date of the actual writing, the time period covered is most likely about the same as that of Abraham's. I explain why in that book. But here, Abraham lived a couple of centuries after the Flood. Thus very early in human history, eggs were being consumed. In fact, the tone of Job's statement is such that he assumes the three friends he is talking too have eaten eggs and thus understand what he is referring to.

Abraham's time would be after the Tower of Babel incident. As mentioned at the beginning of this book, Biblical decrees about food mentioned before the Tower of Babel would be most important, as they would be given to all people. After the Tower of Babel, people would have "scattered over the face of the earth." As such, different people groups would begin to develop unique eating habits, so what one group might become adapted to eating another might not become adapted to. This might have been the case with Job and his friends.

Moreover, if these "new" foods are not included in the Adamic or Noahic food decrees, then they could not be considered to be God-given foods. The exception to this general rule would be if God's statements about a food later would be such as to indicate the new food is being "given" to humans for food. This verse in Job does no such thing for eggs. In fact, if anything, it tells us that least part of an egg is actually "tasteless."

The second Old Testament verse is best read in context:

[4]No one calls for justice, Nor does *any* plead for truth. They trust in empty words and speak lies; [5]They conceive evil and bring forth iniquity. They hatch **vipers' eggs** and weave the spider's web; **He who eats of their eggs dies**, And from that which is crushed a viper breaks out. [6]Their webs will not become garments, Nor will they cover themselves with their works; Their works are works of iniquity, And the act of violence is in their hands (Isaiah 59:4-6; NKJV).

The comment about anyone who eats vipers' eggs dies is not a very flattering thing to say about eggs, so this verse would seem to be discouraging egg consumption. But one point needs to be noted, vipers "creep on the ground." As such, they would be unclean animals (Lev 20:25). Therefore, what this verse is teaching is that humans should not eat the eggs of unclean animals. And this observation would fit with Job 14:4, "Who can bring a clean thing out of an unclean? No one!" (NKJV).

Eggs are mentioned once in the New Testament, by Jesus Himself. This important verse was quoted previously, but it bears repeating:

[11]"Now which father [among] you*, [if] his son will ask [for] a loaf of bread, he will not give to him a stone, will he? Or also [if he asks for] a fish, he will not give to him a serpent instead of a fish, will he? [12]Or also if he asks [for] an **egg**, he will not give to him a scorpion, will he? [13]If you* then being evil know [how] to be giving **good gifts** to your*

286

children, how much more will the Father of heaven [fig., your* heavenly Father] give [the] Holy Spirit to the ones asking Him?" (Luke 11:11-13).

In this verse, Jesus puts eggs alongside of fish and bread, and He declares all three to be "good gifts." This is thus strong evidence that eggs are indeed a God-given food and can have a place in a Creationist Diet. But this is the only verse that supports egg eating, so eggs would have a smaller place in Creationist Diet than foods mentioned much more frequently.

As far as the scientific evidence about eggs goes, most readers are probably aware that eggs have received a "bad rap" in recent decades due to their high cholesterol content. However, some recent studies show that eating up to three eggs (about 600 mg of cholesterol) a day does not significantly increase cholesterol levels (Authority Nutrition. Eggs). Furthermore:

> **The recommended daily allowance [of 300 mg] has sometimes come into question**. The reason for this is because **dietary cholesterol is only responsible for about 15 percent of total blood cholesterol. The rest is manufactured by the body**. Other factors that contribute to blood cholesterol levels include smoking, obesity, physical activity and the **consumption of saturated fat**" (Livestrong. How).

> **Cholesterol levels in the human body tend to be affected less by cholesterol in our diets than they are by the saturated fats** and trans fats we eat, according to Tara Linitz, a registered dietitian at Massachusetts General Hospital who also has a master's degree in exercise science" (Boston Globe.).

> The 2015 Dietary Guidelines Advisory Committee (DGAC) has already garnered headlines because its members are advocating revisions to a decades-old warning about cholesterol consumption. An overview of the committee's Dec. 15, 2014 meeting says, '**Cholesterol is not considered a nutrient of concern for overconsumption.**'" …

As for cholesterol, the changes being considered there are backed by **many studies that have questioned the relationship between dietary cholesterol and heart disease**. Experts now believe that saturated fats in foods like red meat and cheese have a bigger impact on blood cholesterol levels than the cholesterol in foods like eggs" (Fiscal Times).

Moreover, I remember back at Penn State a professor teaching that the body will decrease its production of cholesterol when dietary cholesterol is increased. At that time, the professor was not sure how much the body could down-regulate its production. But "Your liver can produce about 1,000 mg of cholesterol a day. A little more is added by the small intestines" (HowStuffWorks). So there is a limit to how much the body can reduce its production, but it is far more than the generally recommended 300 mg.

This is important due to the connection between cholesterol and testosterone that was discussed in Chapter Four. There it was seen that too low of a cholesterol intake could lower testosterone levels, which has adverse health effects, especially for men.

However, some studies find an association between egg consumption and degenerative diseases. This was seen in the previous chapter in the study on colorectal cancer. "The strongest association was found for eggs" (Marchand). But the amount was no indicated.

Similar results were found in a study on prostate cancer:

We examined the association between intakes of total red meat, processed and unprocessed red meat, poultry, fish, and eggs and prostate cancer recurrence. We conducted a prospective study of 971 men treated with radical prostatectomy for prostate cancer between 2003 and 2010. Men completed a food frequency questionnaire at diagnosis. We used logistic regression to study the association between diet and high-grade or advanced-stage disease. We used Cox models to study the risk of progression [N = 94 events, mainly prostate-specific antigen (PSA) recurrence]. **Total red meat intake was marginally associated with risk of high-grade disease** [Gleason ≥ 4+3; adjusted OR top vs. bottom quartile: 1.66; 95% confidence interval (CI), 0.93-2.97; Ptrend = 0.05], **as was very**

high intake of eggs (OR top decile vs. bottom quartile: 1.98; 95% CI, 1.08-3.63, Ptrend = 0.08). **Well-done red meat was associated with advanced disease** (≥pT3; OR top vs. bottom quartile: 1.74, 95% CI, 1.05-2.90; Ptrend = 0.01). **Intakes of red meat, fish, and eggs were not associated with progression. Very high poultry intake was inversely associated with progression** (HR top decile vs. bottom quartile: 0.19; 95% CI, 0.06-0.63; Ptrend = 0.02). **Substituting 30 g/d of poultry or fish for total or unprocessed red meat was associated with significantly lower risk of recurrence.** Lower intakes of red meat and well-done red meat and higher intakes of poultry and fish are associated with lower risk of high grade and advanced prostate cancer and reduced recurrence risk, independent of stage and grade (Wilson).

Note that total red meat intake was only marginally associated with risk, and it took a high intake of eggs to increase the risk, though "high" is not defined. But in other studies, an increase risk of prostate cancer is found even with low intakes. See Chapter Fourteen for details.

But here; a meta-analysis was done in regard to egg consumption and heart disease and stroke:

The possible relationship between dietary cholesterol and cardiac outcomes has been scrutinized for decades. However, recent reviews of the literature have **suggested that dietary cholesterol is not a nutrient of concern**. Thus, we conducted a meta-analysis of egg intake (a significant contributor to dietary cholesterol) and risk of coronary heart disease (CHD) and stroke. A comprehensive literature search was conducted through August 2015 to identify prospective cohort studies that reported risk estimates for egg consumption in association with CHD or stroke. Random-effects meta-analysis was used to generate summary relative risk estimates (SRREs) for high vs low intake and stratified intake dose-response analyses.,,,

Based on the results of this meta-analysis, consumption of up to one egg daily may contribute to a decreased risk of total stroke, and daily egg intake does not appear to be associated with risk of CHD. • Overall, summary associations indicate that intake of up to 1 egg daily may be associated with reduced risk of total stroke. • Overall, summary associations show no clear association between egg intake and increased or decreased risk of CHD. • **Eggs are a relatively low-cost and nutrient-dense whole food that provides a valuable source of protein, essential fatty acids, antioxidants, choline, vitamins, and minerals** (Alexander).

Thus eating up to one egg per day (seven/ week) is not associated with an increased risk of heart disease and can actually decrease the risk of stroke. This fits with what was said previously that eggs have a place in a Creationist Diet, but in lesser amounts than other God-given foods.

Note also the last line of the preceding study. Eggs are a very nutritious food. And this is even more so if old-fashioned eggs are consumed rather than factory farm eggs.

Most of the eggs currently sold in supermarkets are nutritionally inferior to eggs produced by hens raised on pasture. That's the conclusion we have reached following completion of the 2007 Mother Earth News egg testing project. Our testing has found that, compared to official U.S. Department of Agriculture (USDA) nutrient data for commercial eggs, **eggs from hens raised on pasture may contain**:

- 1/3 less cholesterol
- 1/4 less saturated fat
- 2/3 more vitamin A
- 2 times more omega-3 fatty acids
- 3 times more vitamin E
- 7 times more beta carotene

These amazing results come from 14 flocks around the country that **range freely on pasture** or are housed in moveable pens that are rotated frequently to maximize **access to fresh pasture** and protect the birds from predators (Mother).

Pastured eggs are also higher in vitamin D:

Eggs from hens raised outdoors on pasture have from three to six times more vitamin D than eggs from hens raised in confinement. Pastured hens are exposed to direct sunlight, which their bodies convert to vitamin D and then pass on to the eggs (Eat Wild. Notes).

Thus the negative health effects of eggs can be minimized and the beneficial aspects maximized by choosing old-fashioned eggs. Such are better for the chickens as well, as they have room to roam outside rather than being confined in cages inside.

Honey

Honey is not a "moving thing that lives." But it is made by bees, which are moving things that live. As such, it would fall under the Noahic Decree. Moreover, honey has a prominent place in the Bible. This is mainly because of the phrase "milk and honey," as in God saying the Promised Land would be "flowing milk and honey." This phrase occurs twenty times in the Bible. Honey is mentioned 37 additional times.

The first reference to the Promised Land flowing milk and honey is in Exodus 3:8. But why is the Promised Land so described?

> This poetic description of Israel's land emphasizes the fertility of the soil and bounty that awaited God's chosen people. The reference to **"milk" suggests that many livestock could find pasture there; the mention of "honey" suggests the vast farmland available—the bees had plenty of plants to draw nectar from**....
>
> God's description of the Promised Land as "a land flowing with milk and honey" is **a beautifully graphic way of highlighting the agricultural richness of the land**. God brought His people out of slavery in Egypt to a prosperous land of freedom and blessing and the knowledge of the Lord (GotQuestions?org).

Thus the emphasis of the phrase is on the abundance to be found in the Promised Land. Lots of land for cattle, and lots of land for growing

291

plants. Therefore, God was telling the Israelites there would be an abundance of both animal and plant foods in the Promised Land. And one of these animal foods would be honey.

The first reference to honey in the Bible is Genesis 43:11. The time period here is after Joseph had risen to prominence in Egypt, so we are talking a couple of centuries later than the time of Abraham. Thus honey seems to have entered the human diet later than eggs.

But note how honey is described in this verse:
[11]Then Israel, their father, said to them, "If thus it be, do this; take from the [Heb., +best] **fruits of the land** in your* vessels, and carry down to the man gifts of resin and **honey**, incense and oil of myrrh, and pistachio nut[s] and tree nuts [Heb., almonds] (Gen 43:11).

Following the Hebrew text, notice honey is said to be a part of "the best fruits of the land" along with pistachio nuts and almonds. Similar is Moses' description of the Promised Land:

[7]"For the LORD your God is bringing you into **a good and extensive land**, where [there are] brooks of waters, and bottomless fountains going [or, flowing] through the plains and through the mountains; [8]**a land of** wheat and barley, grapevines, fig trees, pomegranate trees; a land of olive oil and **honey**; [9]a land on which you will not eat your bread with poverty, and **you will not want anything upon it**; a land whose stones [are] iron, and out of its mountains you will dig copper. [10]And **you will eat and be filled**, and will bless the LORD your God on the good land, which He has given to you" (Deut 8:7-10).

Notice that Moses emphasizes how abundant the Promised Land is. This confirms the aforementioned definition of "flowing milk and honey" as indicating abundance. And honey is again grouped together with very healthy foods: wheat, barley, grapes, figs, pomegranates, and olive oil.

Then very significant is the prophesied diet of the coming Messiah:
[14]Because of this, the Lord Himself will give to you* a sign: Look! The virgin will have [fig., conceive] in [the] womb and will give birth

to a Son, and you will call His name Emmanuel ["God with us" – Matt 1:23]. [15]Butter and **honey** He will eat, before <u>He</u> knows either to be preferring evil [or] will choose the good (Isaiah 7:14,15).

The first verse is well-known from being often repeated at Christmastime. But the next verse concerns us here. The Messiah will eat butter and honey. Therefore, if Jesus is to eat these foods, they must be good foods to eat.

Similar is the already mentioned diet of John the Baptist. It is said, "his nourishment was migratory locusts and wild honey" (Matt 3:4). Thus both the Messiah and His forerunner are said to eat honey.

Then there's an interesting reference in 1Samuel. This was when King Saul had given a decree that none of his soldiers were to eat until the enemy had been defeated. But his son Jonathan had not heard the decree and had eaten. When told of the decree, Jonathan replied:

[29]But Jonathan said, "My father has troubled the land. Look now, how **my countenance has brightened because I tasted a little of this honey**. [30]How much better if the people had eaten freely today of the spoil of their enemies which they found! For now would there not have been a much greater slaughter among the Philistines?" [31] Now they had driven back the Philistines that day from Michmash to Aijalon. So the people were very faint (1Sam. 14:29-31, NKJV).

Thus Jonathan was revived by a "little" honey, but the rest of the soldiers who had not eaten the honey remained very weary.

Then note how honey is described in Proverbs, "**Eat honey**, O son, **for [the] honeycomb [is] good**, that your throat shall be sweetened" (24:13). Therefore, honey should be eaten, as it is good.

With honey being eaten by such prominent people as Jonathan, John the Baptist, and Christ Himself, and with such glowing references to it in Scripture, even though it entered late in the human diet, it can still be said honey is a God-given food. However, since honey is a "late" food, it should not be consumed in significant amounts.

In fact, Proverbs also says about honey, "**Having found honey, eat [only] the sufficient [amount]**, lest having been filled, you vomit" (25:16). And, "**[It is] not good to be eating much honey**, but it is necessary to be honoring splendid words" (25:27). So honey is a good food, but it should only be eaten in limited amounts.

Another point to note is the only sweetener mentioned in Scripture other than honey is raisins. They are mentioned eight times, always in a good light (e.g., 1Sam 25:18; 30:12; 2Sam 6:19). Therefore, raisins are a healthy God-given food, being just dried grapes. But they are not easily used in most recipes. Thus honey would be the most easily used Biblical sweetener.

However, the form that honey is generally used today is not the form that it would have been most commonly used in Bible times. What most people know as honey today, the thick liquid that pours but very slowly (like molasses), is actually cooked or processed honey. Raw honey is a solid at room temperature. It has the consistency of butter, so it can be spread but not poured.

What is raw honey?

While there is no official U.S. federal definition of raw honey, the National Honey Board **defines raw honey as "honey as it exists in the beehive** or as obtained by extraction, settling or straining **without adding heat**." This definition does not have any legal authority, but is provided to help in the understanding of honey and honey terms (National Honey Board. FAQ).

But is there a difference between raw and cooked honey? There is a debate in this regard. This same webpage states:

Honey is produced by honey bees from the nectar of plants, not pollen. Pollen occurs only incidentally in honey. **The amount of pollen in honey is miniscule and not enough to impact the nutrient value of honey**....

A 2012 study by the National Honey Board analyzed vitamins, minerals and antioxidant levels in raw and processed honey. The study showed that **processing significantly reduced the pollen content of the honey, but did not affect the nutrient content or antioxidant activity**, leading the researchers to conclude that the micronutrient profile of honey is not associated with its pollen content and is not affected by commercial processing (National Honey Board. FAQ).

But others claim there is a significant difference:

Generally speaking, the basic difference between raw honey and "regular" honey is the way it's processed. **Raw honey has not been heated to high temperatures** in order to achieve the golden, syrupy look we're used to. Some people think that this heating, also called pasteurization, is necessary to make the honey fit for human consumption, as **it kills bacteria and filters out bits of pollen and other debris**.

But proponents of raw honey disagree that pasteurization is necessary, or even helpful….

Just like most foods that are processed or pasteurized, **liquid honey loses a lot of its beneficial nutrients when it undergoes a heating process. Raw honey is loaded with nutrients like energizing B vitamins and immune-boosting vitamin C. It contains antibacterial and antioxidant properties, helping fight off free radicals in your body and keeping your immune system strong**….

The anecdotal evidence from raw honey devotees is overwhelming. In fact, **even some vegans have decided to use it** (technically it's an animal product, so it shouldn't be included in a vegan diet)….

Almost everyone I spoke to discussed the **reported benefits of eating local honey as a way to combat allergies**, too. Holistic nutritionist Andrea Palen commented:

The idea behind eating honey as a remedy for allergies is kind of like gradually vaccinating the body against pollen allergens, a process called immunotherapy. Honey contains a variety of the same spores that give allergy sufferers so much trouble when the seasons change. Introducing these spores into the body in small amounts by eating honey might make the body more accustomed to their presence and decrease the chance of an allergic immune response (Bliss Tree).

However, as the first quote showed, the amount of pollen is miniscule in raw honey, so its absence in cooked honey is insignificant.

295

And in regards to vitamins, minerals, and antioxidants, the amounts are miniscule in both forms of honey. But there is a difference, with raw honey containing higher amounts.

As for combatting allergies, since the level of pollen is low, this is unlikely. But given that there is some pollen, a caveat is in order:

> While All Allergy discloses that **allergic reactions to honey are rare, it can happen** if the pollen an individual is allergic to is present in honey. Honey eaten right from the comb could be especially harmful to those with pollen allergies. Symptoms of an allergic reaction to honey can range from itching to anaphylactic shock. **Some people believe consuming small amounts of local honey daily will help prevent seasonal allergies. Honey should not be given to an infant under one year of age** because botulism can be contracted from the clostridium bacteria that may be present in honey (Leaf.TV).

Bottom line is there is a difference between cooked and raw honey, with raw honey being the more natural of the two. Therefore, it would be the preferred form of honey to be used on a Creationist Diet, though cooked honey would not necessarily be excluded. Note also the caveat about not giving honey to infants.

However, the most prominent sweetener in use today is white sugar, aka sucrose. It is a disaccharide, containing one molecule of glucose and one of fructose.

> **Americans eat about 20 teaspoons of sugar a day** according to a report from the 2005–10 NHANES (National Health and Nutrition Examination Survey) database. **Teens and men consume the most added sugars.** Average daily consumption for men: 335 calories, women: 230 calories, boys: 362 calories, girls: 282 calories (AHA).

> However, the American Heart Association set a recommended limit, so you don't get too many extra calories in your diet. **Men shouldn't have more than 9 teaspoons daily, while women shouldn't have more than 6 teaspoons.** This

amounts to a max of 37.5 grams of sugar or 150 calories from sugar for men, and 25 grams of sugar or 100 calories from sugar for women (SFGate).

Thus Americans on average are consuming two to three times the recommended amount of added sugar a day. But it should be noted:

Some foods have naturally occurring sugars. These sugars aren't part of the added sugar allotment though. **Fruits**, for example, have a fruit sugar called fructose, while **milk and dairy foods** have a sugar called lactose. These types of foods give you a variety of vitamins, minerals and sometimes fiber, making them a beneficial part of your diet -- unlike sugary snacks (SFGate).

Meanwhile, white sugar is a highly processed food, having all of the naturally occurring nutrients in the sugar beet removed. Thus while whole natural foods with naturally occurring sugars like fruits are part of a Creationist Diet, a highly processed, nutritionally worthless food like white sugar would not be. The type of processing it undergoes is far beyond what was possible in Bible times. And such high amounts of ingested added sugar were unheard of before the twentieth century.

Moreover, white sugar is just one of many types of processed sugars that are added to foods.

Added sugars are sugars and syrups that are added to foods or beverages during processing or preparation. They do not include naturally occurring sugars such as those found in milk (lactose) and fruits (fructose). **Added sugars (or added sweeteners) include** natural sugars (such as white sugar, brown sugar and honey) as well as other caloric sweeteners that are chemically manufactured (such as high fructose corn syrup). Some names for added sugars include agave syrup, brown sugar, corn sweetener, corn syrup, sugar molecules ending in "ose" (dextrose, fructose, glucose, lactose, maltose, sucrose), high-fructose corn syrup, fruit juice concentrate, honey, invert sugar, malt sugar, molasses, raw sugar, sugar, syrup (AHA).

Creationist Diet

Note all the different kinds of sugar that are used in processed foods. In addition to honey and sucrose, food processors might use fructose (fruit sugar), lactose (milk sugar), corn syrup, high fructose corn syrup, maltodextrin, maltose, and others.

This is important to know as ingredients lists on food packages often list several different kinds of sugar. The reason for this is to make it appear there is less sugar in the food than there really is.

For instance, say a breakfast cereal has "wheat" as the first ingredient. This would mean, by weight, there is more wheat than anything else in the food. But if the next four ingredients are sugar, high fructose corn syrup, maltodextrin, and maltose, then if these four sweeteners were added together, there is probably more sugar in the cereal than wheat. And someone following a Creationist Diet would want to avoid such an item.

Note also that honey is listed alongside of sugar in the preceding quote. But should it be? Are there any differences between white sugar and honey? There are some important differences:

The manufacturing process for sugar often eliminates many healthy components, such as protein, vitamins, minerals, organic acids, and nitrogen elements.

Honey, doesn't go through this type of process and is usually only subjected to minimal heating.

Honey contains other beneficial ingredients that have antimicrobial and antioxidant properties that aren't contained in sugar (Hive & Honey).

First, **honey is a whole food and sucrose is not**. In other words, sucrose is an isolate – technically only one chemical compound – lifted from a background of hundreds of other components within the whole plant, whereas honey is composed of an equally complex array of compounds, many of which are well-known (including macronutrients and micronutrients, enzymes, probiotics and prebiotics, etc.), others whose role is still completely a mystery.

Even **the "sugar" in honey**, which we might mistakenly equate (due to caloric and nutrient classification equivalencies) to the "sugar" from sugarcane, **is a complex mixture of the** monosacharrides (one-sugars) glucose and fructose, and at least 25 different oligosaccharides (which are sugars composed of between two to ten monosaccharides linked together), including small amounts of the disacchardide sucrose, as well as trisaccharides (three-sugars) like melezitose and erlose.

Interestingly, if you were to isolate out the fructose from honey, and consume it in isolation in American-size doses (over two ounces a day), it would likely contribute to over 70 fructose-induced adverse health effects; primarily insulin resistance, fatty liver, obesity, hypertension and elevated blood sugar. But place that fructose back into the complex nestled background of nutrient chemistries we call honey, and the fructose loses its monochemical malignancy to our health. **Food is the ultimate delivery system for nutrition. Reduce whole foods to parts, and then concentrate and consume them excessively, and you have the recipe for a health disaster that we can see all around us today** in the simultaneously overnourished/malnourished masses **who still think a 'calorie is a calorie,' and a 'carb is a carb,' without realizing that the qualitative differences are so profound that one literally heals, while the other literally kills** (Green Med).

The last paragraph is a basic tenant of the Creationist Diet. Nutrients are best consumed from whole, natural foods, while highly processed foods should be avoided. On that basis alone, honey, especially raw honey, would be preferred to white sugar.

Further comments on the carbs in honey are needed. Honey ranks lower on the "glycemic index" than sugar does. The glycemic index (GI) measures how rapidly a food causes blood sugar to rise. This is important as too quickly a rise can cause a "rebound effect" from too much insulin being released. This can then lead to low blood sugar and resulting fatigue or hunger. It is especially a problem for diabetics or those with hypoglycemia (low blood sugar). The lower the GI number, the less quickly a food causes the blood sugar to rise.

The GI ranks specific carbohydrates from zero to 100, based on how they affect your blood sugar levels after eating them. Typically, **eating foods that have a high GI (such as white bread and soda) causes a spike in blood sugar levels. When you consume these foods, you may feel a surge of get-up-and-go at first, but will have an energy crash soon afterward.** High GI foods have also been linked to an increased risk for cancer, type 2 diabetes, acne, Alzheimer's, and weight gain. **Foods that are low on the GI have been associated with feeling full, which can prevent you from overeating** (Pop Sugar).

Foods with **a high glycemic index rating -- above 70 --** generally make your blood sugar quickly go up and then rapidly drop back down in a short period of time. If a food has a **moderate score, between 55 and 69**, it will still raise your blood sugar, but probably not as much as something with a higher ranking. Ideally, all the foods in your diet should be **low GI**, with a rating **under 55**. These types of foods often keep your blood sugar stable for a while.

Pure honey has a typical ranking of 58 on the scale. But some varieties are even lower. The glycemic index of honey depends on how much fructose is in that particular batch. Honeys that contain 35 to 45 percent fructose, for example, score around **35 to 48** on the glycemic index. **White table sugar, also known as sucrose, is higher, with a glycemic index between 58 and 65** (Livestrong. Glycemic).

The above value of 35-58 is for cooked honey. Raw honey is lower at 30 (Pop Sugar). Thus raw honey is a low GI food with a small amount of naturally occurring nutrients, while white sugar is a moderate to near high GI food with zero nutrients.

Moreover, white sugar is a highly-refined substance, while honey, especially raw honey, is unrefined. As such, honey might have "something" in it we simply have not yet discovered is beneficial. Given the glowing statements about honey in Scripture, this is a distinct possibility, and the following study seems to confirm it:

This study included the following experiments: (1) **effects of dextrose solution** (250 mL of water containing 75 g of dextrose) **or honey solution** (250 mL of water containing 75 g of natural honey) **on plasma glucose level (PGL), plasma insulin, and plasma C-peptide** (eight subjects); (2) **effects of dextrose, honey, or artificial honey** (250 mL of water containing 35 g of dextrose and 40 g of fructose) **on cholesterol and triglycerides (TG)** (nine subjects); (3) **effects of honey solution, administered for 15 days, on PGL, blood lipids, C-reactive protein (CRP), and homocysteine** (eight subjects); (4) **effects of honey or artificial honey on cholesterol and TG** in six patients with hypercholesterolemia and five patients with hypertriglyceridemia; (5) **effects of honey for 15 days on blood lipid and CRP** in five patients with elevated cholesterol and CRP; (6) **effects of 70 g of dextrose or 90 g of honey on PGL in seven patients with type 2 diabetes mellitus**; and (7) **effects of 30 g of sucrose or 30 g of honey on PGL, plasma insulin, and plasma C-peptide** in five diabetic patients.

In healthy subjects, **dextrose elevated PGL at 1 (53%) and 2 (3%) hours, and decreased PGL after 3 hours (20%). Honey elevated PGL after 1 hour (14%) and decreased it after 3 hours (10%). Elevation of insulin and C-peptide was significantly higher after dextrose than after honey. Dextrose** slightly reduced cholesterol and low-density lipoprotein-cholesterol (LDL-C) after 1 hour and significantly after 2 hours, and **increased TG after 1, 2, and 3 hours. Artificial honey** slightly decreased cholesterol and LDL-C and **elevated TG. Honey reduced cholesterol, LDL-C, and TG and slightly elevated high-density lipoprotein-cholesterol (HDL-C). Honey consumed for 15 days decreased cholesterol (7%), LDL-C (1%), TG (2%), CRP (7%), homocysteine (6%), and PGL (6%), and increased HDL-C (2%).** In patients with hypertriglyceridemia, **artificial honey increased TG, while honey decreased TG.** In patients with hyperlipidemia, **artificial honey increased LDL-C, while honey decreased LDL-C. Honey decreased cholesterol (8%), LDL-C (11%), and CRP (75%) after 15 days.**

In diabetic patients, **honey compared with dextrose caused a significantly lower rise of PGL**. Elevation of PGL was greater after honey than after sucrose at 30 minutes, and was lower after honey than it was after sucrose at 60, 120, and 180 minutes. Honey caused greater elevation of insulin than sucrose did after 30, 120, and 180 minutes.

Honey reduces blood lipids, homocysteine, and CRP in normal and hyperlipidemic subjects. Honey compared with dextrose and sucrose caused lower elevation of PGL in diabetics (Al-Waili).

To sort all of this out, dextrose is the name for glucose, the sugar found in blood, when it is used as a food ingredient. The artificial honey contained a mixture of refined dextrose and fructose.

What these experiments found is honey caused less of a rise and a less of a drop of blood sugar than dextrose or artificial honey did. Honey decreased LDL ("bad") cholesterol but increased HDL ("good") cholesterol. Honey also decreased triglycerides, C-reactive protein, and homocysteine (all good things). None of these beneficial effects were found with dextrose or artificial honey.

To sum up, honey is a healthy, God-given food, so it can be included in a Creationist Diet. But since it is a later addition to the human diet, and since Scripture specifically warns against eating too much of it, honey should only be consumed in limited amounts.

One point to note, most vegan societies disallow the use of honey, but many vegans eat it anyway. It's hard to make a case that bees are so mistreated in honey production that someone who is concerned about the treatment of animals should avoid honey.

Gelatin

Yes, gelatin is an animal food. Many people don't realize this:
Gelatin is: ... foodstuff obtained from connective tissue (found in hoofs, bones, tendons, ligaments, and cartilage) of vertebrate animals by the action of boiling water or dilute acid. It is largely composed of the protein collagen. Pure gelatin is brittle, transparent, colorless, tasteless, and odorless. It dissolves in hot water and congeals when cooled. **Gelatin**

> is widely used to give food a proper consistency, in photographic emulsions, and as a coating for pills (*Concise Columbia Encyclopedia*).

Sounds appetizing, doesn't it? Just knowing what gelatin is made of is enough to turn many people off of it. Eating something that is used to process photographs just doesn't sound that appealing. Moreover, it is a highly-processed food ingredient that is taken from otherwise inedible parts of animals. As such, it would not be a God-given food.

Moreover, the main problem with gelatin is the way it is most commonly used, as an important ingredient in gelatin desert, usually called by the trade name *Jell-O*. But what is *Jell-O?*—sugar, gelatin, and various artificial colorings and flavorings.

The problem with sugar has already been discussed. As for artificial flavorings and colorings, by definition they are human-created ingredients and thus in no sense God-given foods. The same would go for artificial sweeteners like saccharin and aspartame. No such artificial ingredients would have a place in a Creationist Diet.

A note on aspartame (trade name *NutraSweet*); the producers of it claim it is made from natural food stuff. This is true, in part. Aspartame is made from two amino acids (the building blocks of protein). But these amino acids have been altered significantly through an eight-stage process. As such, it is not a natural nor God-given food.

> Although **its components**—aspartic acid, phenylalanine, and methanol—**occur naturally in foods, aspartame itself does not and must be manufactured**. NutraSweet' (aspartame) is made through fermentation and synthesis processes (How. Aspartame).

In fact, other than honey and raisins, all sweeteners, natural and artificial, would not be considered to be God-given foods or would be borderline God-given at best. A detailed discussion of other sweeteners is found in Chapter Fourteen of my *God-given Foods Eating Plan* book (see Appendix One).

But getting back to gelatin, since it is an animal food, most vegan societies disallow it, and most vegans do avoid it. And besides gelatin desert, gelatin is used as a binder in many processed foods. So strict vegans have to be careful to read labels. However, there is a vegetable based alternative, "Vegetable gelatin, or AGAR, is made from seaweed" (*Concise Columbia Encyclopedia*).

Those following a Creationist Diet should read labels also. Not only to avoid gelatin but also to avoid artificial ingredients and sweeteners like the ones just mentioned.

That covers three additional animal foods besides meats. The issues surrounding the remaining class of animal foods are so complex, they will be discussed in the next three chapters. But first; a study about soda that was released while I was working on the final draft of this book will be relevant to a couple of issues raised in this chapter. It shows that both sugar and artificial sweeteners are deleterious.

The Brain and Soda and Diet Soda

A new study has found that **people who frequently drink soda** are more likely to have poorer memory, smaller overall brain volume, and a significantly smaller hippocampus, an area of the brain important for learning and memory.

But researchers caution you should wait before you give up sugar-filled soda and reach for the diet soda. The study also found that **people who drank diet soda daily** were almost three times as likely to develop stroke and dementia….

"It looks like there is not very much of an upside to having sugary drinks, and substituting the sugar with artificial sweeteners doesn't seem to help. **Maybe good old-fashioned water is something we need to get used to**" (Psych Central).

Bibliography:

AHA. American Heart Association. Frequently Asked Questions About Sugar. http://www.heart.org/HEARTORG/HealthyLiving/HealthyEating/Heal thyDietGoals/Frequently-Asked-Questions-About-Sugar_UCM_306725_Article.jsp#.WI8QFUTQeUk

Al-Waili, NS, *Journal of Medicinal Food*. 2004 Spring;7(1):100-7. Natural honey lowers plasma glucose, C-reactive protein, homocysteine, and blood lipids in healthy, diabetic, and hyperlipidemic subjects: comparison with dextrose and sucrose.

https://www.ncbi.nlm.nih.gov/pubmed/15117561.

Alexander DD, et. al, *Journal of American College of Nutrition.* 2016 Nov-Dec;35(8):704-716. Epub 2016 Oct 6. Meta-analysis of Egg Consumption and Risk of Coronary Heart Disease and Stroke. https://www.ncbi.nlm.nih.gov/pubmed/27710205

Authority Nutrition. Eggs and Cholesterol - How Many Eggs Can You Safely Eat? https://authoritynutrition.com/how-many-eggs-should-you-eat/

Bliss Tree. The Benefits Of Raw Honey vs Conventional Honey. http://www.blisstree.com/2012/10/05/food/benefits-of-raw-honey-832/

Boston Globe. Six myths about nutrition and health. http://www.bostonglobe.com/lifestyle/2015/01/23/six-myths-about-nutrition-and-health/BRiFwWBn6l8rFZQbdaYD1O/story.html

Concise Columbia Encyclopedia is licensed from Columbia University Press. Copyright © 1995 by Columbia University Press. All rights reserved.

Eat Wild. Notes & News. http://www.eatwild.com/news.html

Fiscal Times, The. Why the Government's New Dietary Guidelines Could Set Off a Food Fight. http://www.thefiscaltimes.com/2015/02/18/More-Eggs-Less-Meat-Why-Government-s-New-Nutrition-Guidelines-Could-Set-Food-Fight

GotQuestions?org. Why was Israel called the land of milk and honey? https://www.gotquestions.org/Israel-milk-honey.html

Hive & Honey Apiary. Honey vs Sugar - Are There Really Any Differences? http://www.hiveandhoneyapiary.com/honeyvssugar.html

How Products are Made. Aspartame. http://www.madehow.com/Volume-3/Aspartame.html

HowStuffWorks. What's the difference between LDL and HDL cholesterol? http://health.howstuffworks.com/diseases-conditions/cardiovascular/cholesterol/difference-between-ldl-and-hdl-cholesterol1.htm

Hu FB, Stampfer MJ, Rimm EB, Manson JE, Ascherio A, Colditz GA, Rosner BA, Spiegelman D, Speizer FE, Sacks FM, Hennekens CH, Willett WC..*Journal of the American Medical Association.* 1999 Apr 21;281(15):1387-94. *A prospective study of egg consumption and risk of cardiovascular disease in men and women.*

Kushi LH. Mink PJ. Folsom AR. Anderson KE. Zheng W. Lazovich D. Sellers TA. *American Journal of Epidemiology.* 149(1):21-31, 1999 Jan 1). *Prospective study of diet and ovarian cancer.*

Leaf.TV. Difference Between Raw Honey & Regular Honey. https://www.leaf.tv/articles/difference-between-raw-honey-regular-honey/

Livestrong. How Many Milligrams of Cholesterol Should I Have a Day? http://www.livestrong.com/article/254182-how-many-milligrams-of-cholesterol-should-i-have-a-day/

Livestrong. Glycemic Index of Honey vs. Sugar. http://www.livestrong.com/article/270875-honey-vs-sugar-glycemic-index/

Marchand, Le L. Wilkens LR. Hankin JH. Kolonel LN. Lyu LC. *Cancer Causes & Control.* 8(4):637-48, 1997 Jul). A case-control study of diet and colorectal cancer in a multiethnic population in Hawaii (United States): lipids and foods of animal origin. https://www.ncbi.nlm.nih.gov/pubmed/9242481

Mendosa, Rick. *Glycemic Index Lists –* http://www.mendosa.com/gilists.htm

Mother Earth News. Meet Real Free-Range Eggs. http://www.motherearthnews.com/real-food/free-range-eggs-zmaz07onzgoe

National Honey Board. FAQ. https://www.honey.com/faq

Pop Sugar. Glycemic Index: Where Do Sweeteners Fall? http://www.popsugar.com/fitness/Glycemic-Index-Where-Do-Sweeteners-Fall-3031565

Psych Central. Soda Linked to Faster Brain Aging. https://psychcentral.com/news/2017/04/23/soda-linked-to-accelerated-brain-aging/119475.html

SFGate. How Much Sugar Should Someone Consume a Day? http://healthyeating.sfgate.com/much-sugar-should-someone-consume-day-9919.html

Wilson KM, et. al. *Cancer Prevention Resource* (Phila). 2016 Dec;9(12):933-941. Epub 2016 Sep 20. Meat, Fish, Poultry, and Egg Intake at Diagnosis and Risk of Prostate Cancer Progression. https://www.ncbi.nlm.nih.gov/pubmed/27651069

Chapter Ten:
Milk Products and the Bible

The last class of animal foods to be looked at is milk and other dairy products. Milk and milk products in themselves are not "moving things that live." However, they come from living and moving animals, so they would have been included in the Noahic decree. And milk is mentioned quite often in the Bible.

Milk in the Bible

The first reference to milk is in Genesis 18:8, in a passage we have looked at before:

⁶And Abraham hurried to the tent to Sarah, and he said to her, "Hurry, and knead three measures of fine wheat flour, and make loaves. ⁷And Abraham ran to the herd, and took a young calf, tender and good, and gave it to his bond-servant, and he quickly made [or, prepared] it. Then he took **butter and milk**, and the calf which he had made [or, prepared]; and he set [them] before them, and they ate, but he stood by them under the tree (Genesis 18:6-8).

Abraham lived about the same time as Job, so this gives us about the same time-period as for eggs. Again, this is later in human history than for other foods. And more importantly, it is after the scattering of people at the Tower of Babel. That will be important later

However, the "they" that ate this butter and milk are the LORD and two angels. Therefore, if God Himself in incarnate form ate dairy products, they are surely God-given.

Moreover, as with honey, milk has a prominent place in the Bible. It is, of course, included in God's statement about the Promised Land "flowing milk and honey." This phrase, as mentioned previously, occurs twenty times in Scripture. Milk is mentioned thirty additional times, and various other milk products are also mentioned.

As with honey, being included in the phrase "milk and honey" indicates the abundance to be found in the Promised Land. And other references to milk support it as being God-given.

But it must be asked, what kind of milk was generally drunk in Biblical times? Was it cow's milk as is the norm today, or the milk of some other mammal? A look at Abraham's possession might help to answer this question.

When Abraham (then called Abram) was in Egypt, his wife Sarah was taken by the Pharaoh because of her beauty. We are then told, "He treated Abram well for her sake. He had sheep, **oxen,** male donkeys, male and female servants, female donkeys, and camels" (Gen 12:16; NKJV). Note that sheep, donkeys, and camels are mentioned, but not cattle.

However, that is the Hebrew text. The Greek text of the LXX is a bit different, "And they treated Abram well on her account, and there became to him [fig., he acquired] sheep and **calves** and donkeys, male bond-servants and female bond-servant, mules and camels" (ALT). Here, sheep and donkeys are again mentioned, but instead of oxen are calves. These would have of course grown into cows.

A similar incident happened with Sarah later, only this time with Abimelech. When Abimelech discovered Sarah was Abraham wife, it is written, "Then Abimelech took **sheep, oxen**, and male and female servants, and gave them to Abraham; and he restored Sarah his wife to him" (Gen 20:14; NKJV).

But again, the LXX is worded differently, "Now Abimelech took a thousand didrachma [about 15.6 pounds or 7 kilograms of silver], **sheep and calves**, and male bond-servants and female bond-servants, and gave [them] to Abraham, and he returned to him Sarah his wife." Thus once again the Hebrew text says Abraham is given sheep, but not cattle. But in the LXX, he is given calves.

Therefore, the evidence indicates Abraham had sheep, camels, and possibly calves, so Abraham would could have been drinking or serving milk from any of these animals.

Moreover, it is reported of Abraham's nephew, "Lot also, who went with Abram, had **flocks and herds** and tents" (Gen 13:5; NKJV). The term "flocks" usually refers to sheep or goats, and "herds" to cattle. But here, we have the exact opposite situation with the LXX, "And to Lot, the one going out with Abram, was **sheep and oxen** and tents." Thus the LXX has "oxen" instead of herds, but it confirms that flocks refers to sheep, so Lot probably had sheep and possibly cattle.

As previously mentioned, Job lived at about the same time as Abraham, and there are two references to milk in the Book of Job (10:10; 21:24). And again, a description of Job's possessions will give an indication of what kind of milk this was:

Also, his possessions were **seven thousand sheep, three thousand camels, five hundred yoke of oxen, five hundred female donkeys**, and a very large household, so that this man was the greatest of all the people of the East" (Job 1:3; NKJV).

And his livestock was **seven thousand sheep, three thousand camels, five hundred yoke of oxen, [and] five hundred female-donkeys in the pastures**, also a very great household. And great works were to him. And upon the earth that man was [most] noble of the [men] from [the] sun rising [fig., east] (Job 1.3; ALT).

Here, both the Hebrew text and the LXX are the same in indicating Job had sheep, camels, and donkeys, but not cows. So the references to milk in the book of Job are most likely to be sheep or camel milk.

Another interesting reference in the time period of Genesis is when Jacob was returning to his brother after his stay with Laban. And here again there is a difference between the Hebrew text and the LXX:

So he lodged there that same night, and took what came to his hand as a present for Esau his brother: **two hundred female goats and twenty male goats, two hundred ewes and twenty rams, thirty milk camels with their colts, forty cows and ten bulls**, twenty female donkeys and ten foals (Gen 32:13-15; NKJV).

[13]And he fell asleep there that night, and he took [the] gifts which he was carrying and sent [them] out to Esau his brother: [14]**two hundred female-goats, twenty male-goats, two hundred sheep, twenty rams, [15]thirty milking camels, and their colts, forty oxen, ten bulls, twenty donkeys, and ten colts** (Gen 32:13-15; ALT).

Note that in the LXX (ALT) "colts" can refer to "the young of the horse or donkey" (Friberg).

So Jacob's livestock possibly consisted of cows. But interestingly, it is with reference to camels that milk is mentioned. Note also that Abraham was also said to have had camels.

Putting this information together, it is possible that during the time period from Abraham to Jacob, that cow's milk was being drunk, but it seems more likely it was sheep or camel's milk. The import of all of this is some people who cannot tolerate cow's milk can tolerate other kinds of milk.

Looking at other books of the Bible, there is the command, "You will not boil a lamb [Heb., young goat] in its mother's milk" (Exod 23:19a; also Exod 34:26; Deut 14:21). So it would seem lamb or goat's milk was used for cooking purposes, but with this limitation to teach the Israelites respect for feed animals.

The next relevant reference to milk is Moses' prophecy about how the Israelites would act once they were in the Promised Land:

13"He brought them up on the strength of the land; He fed them with the produce of [the] fields. They sucked **honey out of a rock and olive oil out of a solid rock.** 14**Butter [Heb., curds] of cows and milk of sheep**, with [the] fat of lambs and rams, of sons of bulls [fig., calves] and male-goats, with fat kidneys of wheat [fig., abundant wheat kernels]; and he drank wine, [the] blood of grape[s]. 15And Jacob ate and was filled, and the one having been loved kicked off; he grew fat, he became thick, he became broad; then he forsook God, the One having made him, and departed from God his Savior (Deut 32:13-16; ALT).

Note that "Jacob" is a figurative way of referring to the nation of Israel. That said; the first part of this description is to symbolically indicate how good the Israelites had it. God had truly blessed them, to the point that honey and olive oil was flowing from rocks. But rather than being thankful to God for this abundance, the Israelites gluttonously consumed this abundant food, while ignoring God. Sound like the USA today?

In any case, relevant to this discussion are two points. First, the Israelites are said to have "milk of sheep." But notice that "butter" is said to come from cows.

But the Hebrew text is again a bit different, with "flocks" instead of "sheep" and "curds" instead of "butter." Again, flocks probably refer to sheep, so there is no difference there. And like butter, curds are a dairy food. They are, "a soft, white substance formed when milk sours, used as the basis for cheese." (Oxford). So the Israelites did milk cows and use that milk for food, whether for butter or as curds for cheese making. But there is still no definite reference to cow's milk.

The first such reference is when the Philistines captured the Ark of the Covenant. After plagues broke out on the Philistines because of the Ark, they asked their "priests and the diviners and their enchanters" what they should do (1Sam 6:2). They replied:

[7]"And now take [wood] and make a new wagon, and two cows, giving birth to calves for the first time [Heb., **two milk cows which have never been yoked**], without their calves; and yoke the cows to the wagon and lead away the calves from behind them into [their] home. [8]And you* shall take the ark and put it on the wagon, and you* will give back with it the golden articles for the plague; and you will place [them] as a deposit in a sack by [the] side of it; and you* will let it go and send it away, and it will depart. [9]And you* will see if it will go the way of its boundaries along by Beth Shemesh [LXX, Baethsamys], [then] He has brought upon us this great affliction; but if not, then we will know that His hand has not touched us, but this [is] a chance [which] has happened to us" (1Sam 6:7-9).

Not surprisingly, "the cows went straight on the road to [the] way of Beth Shemesh" (1Sam 6:12a). This showed that all of the events that happened were in fact from the LORD, the God of the Israelites. I expound on this passage at length in my book *The LORD Has It Under Control* (see Appendix One).

But here, what concerns us is the reference in the Hebrew text to "milk cows." Therefore, cows were being milked not just by the Israelites, but by their enemies the Philistines. This shows that using cow's milk for food was not restricted to just the Israelites but other people in the region used it as well.

However, a reference from the New Testament shows non-Jews also used sheep or goat's milk:

Who ever serves as a soldier at his own expense? Who plants a vineyard and does not eat of the fruit of it? Or [who] **tends a flock and does not eat of the milk of the flock?**" (1Cor 9:7).

Note: The Christians in Corinth were mostly Gentiles, not Jews.

A reference to milk from the Book of Proverbs is very instructive, "You shall have enough **goats' milk for your food**, For the food of your household, And the nourishment of your maidservants" (Prov 27:27; NKJV). Here goat's milk is specifically said to be for food. This is strong evidence that milk is a God-given food, at least goat's milk.

Similar to the promise about the Promised Land, is the following prophecy about the future of Jerusalem:

[18]"And it will be in that day, the mountains will drop sweetness, and **the hills will flow [with] milk**, and all the remissions [fig., fountains] of Judah will flow [with] waters, and a fountain will go forth out of [the] house of the LORD and will water the valley of the reeds. [19]Egypt will be for a vanishing [fig., desolation], and Edom [LXX, Idumea] will be a vanishing [or, desolate] plain, because of [the] unrighteousnesses of [the] sons [and daughters] of Judah, because they shed righteous blood in their land. [20]But **Judea will be inhabited into the age** [fig., forever], and Jerusalem into generations of generations [fig., for all generations]. [21]And I will avenge their blood, and by no means will I let it go unpunished; and the LORD will dwell in Zion!" (Joel 3:1-208).

This prophecy declares the glorious future of Israel. And this glory is demonstrated by the hills flowing with milk. With the reference to the Promised Land flowing milk and honey, the preceding verse in Proverbs, and this prophecy, without a doubt, milk is a God-given food, whether it comes from cows, sheep, or goats.

Claims about Differences in Today's Milk

Despite this strong Biblical evidence that milk is a God-given food, there are some today who claim the milk we generally drink today is far different from the milk drunk in Bible times. It is further said that due to these differences, today's milk is not healthy and should not be drunk.

Homogenization:

The first difference has to do with homogenization of milk. The anti-milk crowd will start with Proverbs 30:33, "For **as the churning of milk produces butter**, And wringing the nose produces blood, So the forcing of wrath produces strife" (NKJV).

This verse is worded quite differently in the LXX, "**Be milking milk, and there will be butter**, and if you squeeze [one's] nostrils there will come out blood; so if you drag out words, there will come out judgments [fig., quarrels] and strifes" (ALT). But the import is still the same. Both say butter is made from milk. Of that there is no doubt.

However, it is said churning homogenized milk does not produce butter, so homogenized milk is not milk by Biblical standards. The first claim is true and has been known since homogenization first began to be used. This is seen in a medical journal way back in 1915:

> Milk and similar emulsions are homogenized by forcing them through extremely fine openings, under great pressure, with the result that the fat globules are broken up into fragments of such minute size that they are no longer capable of agglutinating together again. Hence **no cream will rise to the surface of perfectly homogenized milk and no butter can be made from homogenized cream**; neither can it be whipped or even separated in a mechanical separator (Baldwin).

Why is this important? Dr. Rex Russell claims in this regard:
> The **normal larger butterfat molecules in unhomogenized milk bounce through the intestine, and only small portions are absorbed** as they travel through the intestines because of the limited surface area in contact with the mucosa of the small bowel. **The smaller particles of butterfat resulting from homogenization** created a marked increase in surface area of butterfat presented to the mucosa of the small bowel. The small particles **pass quickly into the bloodstream**. The result is that **nearly all of the fat in homogenized milk enters the bloodstream, raising our triglycerides and cholesterol levels** unnecessarily, according to Jack Mathis (Russell, p.109).

Thus it is claimed that homogenization increases the deleterious effects of the saturated fat in milk. It is also sometimes claimed that homogenization increases the likelihood of being allergic to milk, of being lactose intolerant, or in other ways for people not being able to tolerate or digest milk. However, the evidence does not support any of these contentions. In fact, it is the exact opposite. Homogenized milk is easier to digest.

When you homogenize milk, you not only change the size of the fat globules, you also rearrange the fat and protein molecules—which could alter how they act in the human body. **In the 1970s, Kurt Oster proposed the hypothesis that homogenized milk might increase your risk of heart disease.**

There wasn't (and still isn't) any evidence that the widespread adoption of homogenization led to an increase in heart disease rates. Nonetheless, researchers spent the next decade or so testing various aspects of Dr. Oster's rather ornate hypothesis. Ultimately, **research failed to validate any part of this theory** and most scientists considered the matter settled—but **the notion that homogenized milk is a culprit in heart disease lives on in certain corners of the internet, among other outdated myths and rumors** (Quick).

On the **supposed influence of milk homogenization on the risk of CVD, diabetes and allergy**.

Commercial milk is homogenized for the purpose of physical stability, thereby reducing fat droplet size and including caseins and some whey proteins at the droplet interface. This seems to result in a **better digestibility than untreated milk**. Various casein peptides and milk fat globule membrane (MFGM) proteins are reported to present either harmful (e.g. atherogenic) or beneficial bioactivity (e.g. hypotensive, anticarcinogenic and others). Homogenization might enhance either of these effects, but this remains controversial.

The effect of homogenization has not been studied regarding the link between early cow's milk consumption and occurrence of type I diabetes in children prone to the disease

314

and no link appears in the general population. **Homogenization does not influence milk allergy and intolerance in allergic children and lactose-intolerant or milk-hypersensitive adults**. The impact of homogenization, as well as heating and other treatments such as cheese making processes, on the health properties of milk and dairy products remains to be fully elucidated (Michalski).

No difference in symptoms during challenges with homogenized and unhomogenized cow's milk in subjects with subjective hypersensitivity to homogenized milk.

It has been hypothesized that certain consumers tolerate untreated cow's milk, but react to processed (i.e. homogenized and pasteurized) cow's milk although they do not suffer from IgE-mediated cow's milk allergy or lactose intolerance. The aim of the study was to compare the tolerance of unhomogenized and homogenized cow's milk in lactose tolerant adults who had repeatedly experienced better tolerance of unhomogenized than homogenized milk. Forty-four subjects were challenged with homogenized and unhomogenized cow's milk for five days in a randomized, double-blind, cross-over study. **No differences in the symptoms during the challenges were found. Roughly half the subjects tolerated the homogenized milk better and the other half tolerated the unhomogenized milk better**. The results of this study show no difference in the tolerance of homogenized and unhomogenized milk in adults with self-reported symptoms suggestive of hypersensitivity to homogenized milk (Paajanen).

According to its detractors, homogenized milk contributes to heart disease, diabetes and other chronic disorders, as well as allergies, largely **by boosting the absorbability of an enzyme in milk called xanthine oxidase (XOD)**. They claim that the resulting higher blood levels of XOD increase disease-promoting inflammatory processes.

While it's true that elevated activity of XOD (along with other enzymes) produced in the body can increase inflammation, the adverse effects of XOD in milk remain

315

theoretical. In any case, the point is moot, because **XOD is not absorbed from any food**.

The notion that homogenization, and milk's XOD in particular, is a health hazard was originally **disproven by researchers from the University of California at Davis in a paper published in the** *American Journal of Clinical Nutrition* **back in 1983**. Subsequent research has also debunked it.

In addition, studies have shown that **homogenization actually improves the digestibility of milk and that it does not increase the risk of milk allergy or intolerance in children or adults** (Berkeley).

Thus the claims about deleterious effects from the homogenization of milk are all bogus, although you will still see these claims circulating on the Internet.

Pasteurization:

Similar claims circulate on the Internet about supposed deleterious effects from another processing method, namely that of pasteurization. The reason milk is pasteurized is to kill food borne pathogens. But it is claimed that pasteurization also destroys much of the nutrient content and other beneficial elements of milk.

The alternative to pasteurized milk is called raw milk. Raw milk is milk that has not been heat-treated. Advocates of raw milk claim that it is better tolerated than pasteurized milk, meaning that it can be drunk by those who are lactose intolerant or allergic to milk. They also make many other claims about health benefits of raw milk over pasteurized milk, complete with numerous testimonies on their websites, such as the afore-referenced Real Milk site.

For instance, in a chart in his book, Dr. Russell claims that pasteurizing milk causes the loss of: 50% of the vitamin C, 66% of vitamins A and D, 50% of the calcium and magnesium, and 90% of the enzymes. This loss of enzymes is said to be important as, "Calcium and magnesium require the enzymes present in raw milk for best absorption" (108).

There are also many other claims about supposed detrimental health effects from pasteurized milk.

If you're drinking conventional milk, you must stop! Why? Because it's dangerous for your health. Pasteurization is the process used to heat milk to a specific temperature for a set time. The goal is to kill potentially bad bacteria that may have found its way into the milk supply. **The problem with pasteurization is that it kills all the beneficial bacteria we call probiotics as well as damaging the vitamins, minerals and denaturing the proteins leading to some of our health issues** (Dr. Axe).

Many nutrients and immune-enhancing components are destroyed by exposure to high heat and the temperatures used during pasteurization. **Vitamin A is degraded, proteins and enzymes are denatured, and immunoglobulins are destroyed** (Real Milk).

Are any of these claims true? It is true that like any other heating method, pasteurization does cause some loss of nutrients. But the amounts of loss are greatly exaggerated by pasteurization detractors.

Scientific research has demonstrated that **pasteurization does not significantly alter the nutritional qualities of milk. The important nutrients in milk are not affected by heat**. Pasteurized milk is an excellent source of calcium, protein, riboflavin, vitamin A, and phosphorus. It is a good source of thiamine and vitamin B12. Pasteurized milk is also fortified with vitamin D, making it a good source of this essential vitamin that many Canadians are deficient in (BC Dairy).

An extensive review of various claims of raw milk advocates was done by the New Zealand government titled, "An Assessment of the Effects of Pasteurisation on Claimed Nutrition and Health Benefits of Raw Milk." It reviewed dozens of studies that have been done on this subject and these claims.

The report found that there were slight changes in the proteins in milk (casein and whey), but these changes "have no significant effect on their digestibility and nutritional properties" (p.3).

Creationist Diet

It looked at the effect of pasteurization on vitamins A, B1, B2, B6, B12, C, E, and folate. There was "no significant effect of pasteurization was found in the concentration of B1 or B6 in milk, yet concentrations of B2, folate and vitamin C were significantly lower."

But in regards to folate and vitamin C, since milk is not a good source of these nutrients anyhow, the loss of them was insignificant. In other words, even if the previous claim that "50% of the vitamin C" is loss, since a cup of whole milk contains less than four milligrams (mg) while the recommended intake is 60 mg, reducing this to 2 mg is irrelevant. The same goes for folate.

As for vitamin A, E and B12, there was too much variation in milk to come to a conclusion, but the differences were considered to probably be insignificant. And interestingly, the level of vitamin A was higher in pasteurized milk than in raw milk—the exact opposite of a claim in an earlier quote. Only vitamin B2 was left as being significantly lower in pasteurized versus raw milk (p.4).

As for minerals, "**heat treatment appears to have no significant effect on the amount or bioavailability of calcium**. A number of studies demonstrated that there is no impact of pasteurisation on milk mineral content and mineral bioavailability" (p.5). As such, the previous claims that pasteurization destroys "50% of the calcium and magnesium" and that it damages vitamins and minerals are false.

As for claims about beneficial enzymes in milk and that those with lactose intolerance can digest milk, it first must be said that lactose intolerance is due to a lack of the enzyme lactase that digests milk. All humans produce this enzyme in infancy, but the ability to do so is lost in many people by the time they reach adulthood. This lost ability is more common in some races than in others.

An estimated 65% of human adults (and most adult mammals) downregulate [decrease] the production of intestinal lactase after weaning. Lactase is necessary for the digestion of lactose, the main carbohydrate in milk, and without it, milk consumption can lead to bloating, flatulence, cramps and nausea. **Continued production of lactase throughout adult life (lactase persistence, LP) is a genetically determined trait** and is found at moderate to high frequencies in Europeans and some African, Middle Eastern and Southern Asian populations (ProCon).

This situation is exactly what we would expect given the previous Biblical information about when milk entered the human diet. It was after the Tower of Babel incidence. It was because of that incident that the human population separated into different areas of the world, and that separation led to the development of the races.

The genetics behind this are rather complicated and beyond the scope of this book. But it will be said that each people group would develop unique characteristics due to environmental and other factors. One of those factors is that in some of these people groups, people began to drink milk while others did not. Those that did retain the ability to produce lactase into adulthood, while those that did not do not.

How this relates to this discussion is that raw milk advocates claim that raw milk contains lactase and other enzymes that enable lactose intolerant individuals to consume raw milk. However, the New Zealand study found:

> **Lactase does not occur naturally in raw milk**. Lactase-producing strains of bacteria potentially can be present in small amount in raw milk, but that their growth and hence lactase production, is inhibited at the refrigeration temperature used to store raw milk. **The number of these bacteria and their activity are too limited to have any physiological effect for consumers**. The destruction of these bacteria by heat treatment has no consequent net health effects (Claeys et al. 2012 and references therein)....
>
> Currently there is only one case-control study that has evaluated lactose intolerance and raw milk consumption. **The authors did not find any significant association as the lactose intolerant participants reported symptoms after the consumption of both, raw milk and pasteurised milk and the severity of these symptoms were not significantly different** (Korpela et al. 2005, MacDonald et al., 2011) (p.6).

The next claim the New Zealand researchers looked at was the claim that raw milk contains beneficial bacteria and enzymes that are

319

destroyed by heating. But the researchers found the growth of beneficial bacteria is inhibited by refrigeration, while not refrigerating the milk would lead to the growth of harmful bacteria.

Another benefit attributed to the bacteria occurring naturally in milk is that they are probiotics. **Probiotic bacteria** (specific strains belonging to Lactobacillus, Bifidobacterium and Enterococcus species), **are described as health-promoting micro-organisms**.

However, the levels found in raw milk are far too tiny to have any beneficial effects. "It has been shown, that the ingested amount required to have an effect, needs to be 1000 to 10,000 times higher than the amount actually present in raw milk" (p.7).

The next claim of raw milk advocates is that raw milk contains enzymes that prevent the growth of pathogens in milk. This is to evade the need for pasteurization. But the New Zealand researchers found:

Overall **there is little evidence that "good" bacteria or other components of raw milk reduce pathogen numbers**. This is supported by the observation that live bacterial pathogens are routinely found in bulk tanks of raw milk on farms. (Jayarao et al., 2001, Olivier et al., 2005, van Kessel et al, 2011, Hill et al., 2012). **Pasteurisation does not significantly reduce the biological activity of naturally occurring antimicrobial components of milk** (p. 8).

The next claim of raw milk advocates is that raw milk contains enzymes that aid in the digestion of milk. It is for this reason that they claim it is better tolerated than pasteurized milk. But the researchers found:

Heat treatment may inactivate some milk enzymes like proteases and lipoprotein lipase (LPL). There is no evidence of physiological role of these enzymes in human protein digestion. Protease and lipase that help the process of digestion are proteins secreted by organs in the human gastrointestinal tract. Although raw milk contains various protease and lipoprotein lipase, there is no described role of milk proteases in human protein digestion or LPR in lipids digestion. **Milk enzymes, like other proteins, are denatured in the acid gastric environment and digested by human proteases secreted in the gastrointestinal tract**. Therefore, inactivation of proteases and LPR by pasteurisation has no impact on the nutritional value of milk (Olivecrona et al., 2003; FDA, 2011) (p.9).

We saw this in Chapter Three. There it was claimed the enzymes in raw produce aided in digestion. But just like with those enzymes, the enzymes in raw milk are destroyed by the stomach acid and thus do not reach the small intestine where digestion and absorption of nutrients occur and where the pancreas secretes digestive enzymes into.

Another claim of raw milk advocates is raw milk contains beneficial immunoglobulins that are destroyed by pasteurization. However, most of these immunoglobulins are heat stable and thus are not destroyed by pasteurization, and the amounts in raw milk are too tiny to have any significance anyways (p.10).

The last issue the New Zealand researchers studied is rather complicated. The claim is that children who drink raw milk develop less allergies than those who drink pasteurized milk. The reason it is said is that the naturally occurring bacteria in raw milk strengthen the immune system of children against allergies. This would be similar to the way allergy shots strengthen the immune system in adults against allergies. The evidence for this claim is epidemiological studies that have found fewer allergies amount children raised on a farm who drink raw milk versus children raised in urban areas who drink pasteurized milk.

However, there are many other differences between the lives of farm kids versus city kids than just the type of milk that is drunk. As such, it is not possible to draw any conclusions from such observations. As the researchers state:

> it is not always clear if the observed reduction in risk of developing asthma and other allergies is completely independent of **other factors such as the exposure to a farm environment or to animals** (Claeys et al., 2012) (p.11).

Bottom line of all of this is none of the claims of raw milk advocates hold up under investigation. To put it another way, there is no significant difference between the health benefits of raw versus pasteurized milk.

But is raw milk as dangerous as advocates of pasteurization make it out to be? We turn to that question next.

Dangers of Raw Milk:

It does seem more natural to consume raw milk rather than pasteurized milk. And it would seem more consistent with the main principles of the Creationist Diet to consume raw milk. However, it has already been discussed that humans learned how to cook food very early in human history on a Creationist timescale, and pasteurization is simply a form of heating or cooking food. Therefore, it would not be out of line with a Creationist Diet. Meanwhile, the reason for heating milk is the same as for heating meat—to reduce the risk of food poisoning.

According to the United States Center for Disease Control and Prevention (CDC):

> **Raw milk can carry harmful bacteria and other germs that can make you very sick or kill you.** While it is possible to get foodborne illnesses from many different foods, raw milk is one of the riskiest of all.
>
> Getting sick from raw milk can mean many days of diarrhea, stomach cramping, and vomiting. Less commonly, it can mean kidney failure, paralysis, chronic disorders, and even death....
>
> **A wide variety of germs that are sometimes found in raw milk**, can make people sick, including bacteria (e.g., Brucella, Campylobacter, Listeria, Mycobacterium bovis (a cause of tuberculosis), Salmonella, Shiga toxin-producing Escherichia coli [e.g., E. coli O157], Shigella, Yersinia), parasites (e.g., Giardia), and viruses (e.g., norovirus). Each ill person's symptoms can differ, depending on the type of germ, the amount of contamination, and the person's immune defenses (CDC).

This is not just theory. There have been many outbreaks of illnesses due to the consumption of raw milk.

From 1998 through 2011, 148 outbreaks due to consumption of raw milk or raw milk products were reported to CDC. These resulted in 2,384 illnesses, 284 hospitalizations, and 2 deaths. Most of these illnesses were caused by Escherichia coli, Campylobacter, Salmonella, or Listeria. It is important to note that a substantial proportion of the raw milk-associated disease burden falls on children; among the 104 outbreaks from 1998-2011 with information on the patients' ages available, 82% involved at least one person younger than 20 years old (CDC).

It is because of these dangers that raw milk is banned for sale in most states in the USA.

However, raw milk advocates do not accept this evaluation. They claim that the risks of raw milk are overblown by the CDC. They further claim that other foods pose a greater risk of food poisoning. In responding to headlines proclaiming raw milk causes more illnesses than pastured milk, one raw milk website states:

While two of these headlines are technically accurate – raw milk is responsible for more illnesses than pasteurized milk when the number of people who consume each is taken into account – the concern they convey about the risk of drinking unpasteurized milk is dramatically overstated....

Foodborne illness is a concern for many types of food. According to the most recent review of foodborne disease outbreaks in the U.S. in 2008 by the Center for Science in the Public Interest (CSPI), seafood, produce and poultry were associated with the most outbreaks. Produce is responsible for the greatest number of illnesses each year (2,062), with nearly twice as many illnesses as poultry (1,112). Dairy products are at the bottom of the list. They cause the fewest outbreaks and illnesses of all the major food categories – beef, eggs, poultry, produce and seafood....

According to these data, it's true that you have a higher chance of getting sick from drinking raw milk than pasteurized milk. But **the risk is 9.4 times higher, not 150 times higher as the CDC claimed**.

Perhaps this is a good time to review the difference between absolute and relative risk. When you hear that you have a roughly 9 times greater (relative) risk of getting sick from drinking raw milk than pasteurized milk, that might sound scary. And indeed it would be, if we were talking about the absolute risk moving from 5% to 45%.

But when the absolute risk is extremely small, as it is here, a relative 9-fold increase is rather insignificant. If you have a 0.00011 percent chance of getting sick from drinking pasteurized milk, and a 9.4 times greater risk of getting sick from drinking unpasteurized milk, **we're still talking about a miniscule risk of 0.00106%** (one one-thousandth of a percent)....

That said, hospitalizations from raw milk are extremely rare. During the 2000 − 2007 period, there were 12 hospitalizations for illnesses associated with raw fluid milk. That's an average of **1.5 per year**. With approximately 9.4 million people drinking raw milk, that means **you have about a 1 in 6 million chance of being hospitalized from drinking raw milk** (Kresser).

All of the points raised in this article are valid. Although people have gotten sick from raw milk, far more people have gotten sick from other types of foods. Simply put, you are always taking a risk when you eat a food raw, be it a plant or an animal food. This is especially true with today's large scale food operations and long transport systems. Just one mistake in the whole chain from farm to table can cause a food borne pathogen to be present in any food.

It is also true that the number of people who have gotten seriously sick from raw milk is tiny in proportion to the number of people who consume raw milk.

Between a belief in the benefits of raw milk and a disbelief in the dangers, raw milk advocates ignore the law and buy and drink raw milk. As NPR reports:

Raw milk — milk that comes straight from the cow or goat without being pasteurized — has been effectively banned in many states because the Food and Drug Administration says it presents a health threat. But **people who believe it's an important part of a diet with more local and natural foods are finding ways to get it, and they say it's worth the risk** (NPR).

And those who drink raw milk think the laws against it are silly, and they go to great extremes to attain raw milk:

> **But because it's illegal to sell raw milk in Maryland, Duncan's milk is practically contraband.** The milk isn't pasteurized, and it's hard to get. Reitzig drives more than two hours to farms in Pennsylvania for it, and pays $5 to $7 a gallon.
>
> In other states where sales are banned, people buy shares of cows or goats raised on dairy farms, and then collect the milk from their animals at pre-established drop-off points.
>
> "**Well, I just think it's so silly. I can go out and get a six pack of beer anywhere and a carton of cigarettes,**" Reitzig says of the ban. If you're going to eat, you have to take risks, she says. **Any food can be contaminated.**
>
> "**Legally, I can feed my children fast food three meals a day. But then to get this incredible, nutrient-dense, fresh local food, the farmer in my state is criminalized for selling that to me,**" she says.
>
> Her family started drinking raw milk about six years ago, after her second child was born. And she says the family has not had to make many trips to the doctor's office since; **allergies have cleared up, and milk intolerances have gone away.** (NPR).

Conclusion on Raw Milk:

The evidence indicates that both the claimed benefits and the claimed dangers of raw milk have been overblown. In other words, raw milk is not near as beneficial as raw milk advocates claim, nor is it near as dangerous as the USA government claims.

But given the risks (even if overblown) and the lack of evidence for benefits, I cannot in good faith recommend people drink raw milk. However, given my conservative, limited government political beliefs, I think people should be able to make this decision for themselves, without the government dictating the decision. Just be sure to investigate the issue thoroughly before consuming raw milk and especially before giving it to children. And the next chapter will raise another concern that should be considered before consuming raw milk.

But here; this whole debate is summed up well on the website for the United States Food and Drug Administration (FDA):

Raw Milk & Pasteurization: Debunking Milk Myths

While pasteurization has helped provide safe, nutrient-rich milk and cheese for over 120 years, some people continue to believe that pasteurization harms milk and that raw milk is a safe healthier alternative. **Here are some common myths and proven facts about milk and pasteurization**:

- Pasteurizing milk DOES NOT cause lactose intolerance and allergic reactions. Both raw milk and pasteurized milk can cause allergic reactions in people sensitive to milk proteins.
- Raw milk DOES NOT kill dangerous pathogens by itself.
- Pasteurization DOES NOT reduce milk's nutritional value.
- Pasteurization DOES NOT mean that it is safe to leave milk out of the refrigerator for extended time, particularly after it has been opened.
- Pasteurization DOES kill harmful bacteria.
- Pasteurization DOES save lives (FDA).

Unnatural to Drink Milk?

Another question is whether adults should even be drinking milk in the first place. Although the preceding and other references to milk in the Bible show that adults in Biblical times drank some kind of milk, the anti-milk crowd will point out other references in Scripture that seem to indicate milk drinking is only for infants. The first such reference is in Isaiah 28:9:

⁹To whom did we report evil [deeds]? And to whom did we report a message? [To] **the ones having been weaned from the milk**, the ones having been withdrawn from [the] breast."

Thus Isaiah seems to be saying that normally people are "weaned" off of milk. Then in the New Testament, Paul writes to the Corinthians, ²"I gave you* **milk to drink and not solid food**, for you* were not yet able [to receive it]. Indeed, neither are you* now yet able" (1Cor 3:2). Thus adults should be eating solid food, not drinking milk.

Similar, is the following passage from Hebrews:
¹²For indeed, [though] you* ought to be teachers by this time, you* again have need [for someone] to be teaching you* what [are] the rudimentary elements [or, basic teachings] of the beginning of the oracles of God, and you* have become [ones] **having need of milk and not of solid nourishment** (Heb 5:12).

Peter also indicates it is "babes" who should be drinking milk, "as newborn babies long for the rational [or, spiritual] pure milk, so that you* shall grow by it" (1Peter 2:2).

However, in all of these references, the "milk" being drunk and weaned from would be human breast milk. As such, these passages are just making the observation that only infants suckle at the breast, but then solid food is gradually introduced as they are weaned from breast milk, as specifically stated in the first passage. These passages are not addressing the consumption of cow's or other forms of milk.

Other Dairy Foods

That covers liquid milk. But what does the Bible have to say about other kinds of dairy products?

Curds:

Curds have already been referred to. This item is mentioned five times in the NKJV, more than any other dairy product besides milk. IN addition to Deuteronomy 32:14, mentioned previously, curds are mentioned in 2Samuel 17:29; Isaiah 7:15,22 (twice).

The most important reference is Isaiah 7:15, which has been quoted previously in reference to honey, "Curds and honey He shall eat, that He may know to refuse the evil and choose the good" (NKJV). Again, this is a prophecy about the coming Messiah. So along with honey, Jesus also ate curds. Add this to the Biblical evidence that dairy foods in general are God-given foods.

But as for curds, today, the most common way curds are consumed is via cottage cheese. Hence why there is "small curd" and "large curd" cottage cheese.

Cheese:

Cheese is mentioned twice in the Bible (2Sam 17:29; Job 10:10). The first reference is the most important:

[27]And it happened when David came to Mahanaim, [that] Uesbi son of Nahash from Rabbah of [the] sons of Ammon, and Machir son of Amiel from Lodabar, and Barzillai the Gileadite from Rogellim, [28]brought ten beds (and double-sided), and ten caldrons and earthenware, and wheat and barley and wheat flour and peeled barley, and bean[s] and lentil[s], [29]and honey and **butter** and sheep and **cheese of cows**. And they brought [them] to David and to the people with him to eat; **for they said, "The people [are] hungering and growing faint and thirsting in the wilderness** (2Sam 17:27-29).

This is an interesting list of foods, all of which have already been discussed. The important point is that all of these foods are considered to be good for people who are "hungering and growing faint." And note that here cheese of cows (NKJV: "of the herd") are mentioned. Thus along with curds, the Israelites also made cheese from cow's milk.

Butter:

Butter is mentioned three times in the NKJV, but at least one more time in the LXX (the preceding passage from 2Samuel, where the NKJV has "curds" instead).

The first additional reference is the Biblical quote that opened this chapter, Genesis 18:8, and the last is Proverbs 30:33 quoted previously.

328

The other reference is Psalm 55:21. But it simply tells us butter is "smooth," so it doesn't add anything to this discussion. But the others are strong evidence that butter is a God-given food.

But isn't butter an unhealthy food due to its high saturated fat content? That could be true, except for the alternative being unnatural margarine.

The biggest knock against margarine used to be that it contained hydrogenated oils, which is to say, trans fats. But, "the FDA has now banned trans fat from processed food, and after the deadline of June 2018, we will no longer find any trans fat in any food sold in the United States" (Florida).

But even without the trans fats, margarine is still an artificial food that often contains artificial colorings, flavorings, and other artificial ingredients. As such, it would not fit within the paraments of a Creationist Diet. Therefore, butter would be a better choice. And it can be included in a healthy diet, if used in limited amounts.

Here's the lowdown on the difference between the two: Butter contains 5 grams of saturated fat per tablespoon, and 33 mg of cholesterol. All animal products, including butter, contain cholesterol, and there's no getting around that.

Tub margarine, on the other hand, contains about 1.5 grams of saturated fat and no cholesterol. Margarine is made from vegetable oil, which is not an animal product, and therefore does not contain cholesterol.

Considering that most of us should consume no more than about 15 grams of saturated fat per day, the 5 grams contained in a tablespoon of butter is a big sacrifice to make.

But what if you just really prefer the taste of butter? **Is it okay to use a little bit? Well, sure it is**. It's all about controlling your total intake of saturated fat, and not going over your daily limit. If you want to use a little butter, **just be cautious about other sources of saturated fat in your diet,** so you don't end up going overboard.

An even better choice would be to use olive oil whenever you can, rather than either butter or margarine (Florida).

Creationist Diet

The last paragraph is very true. Although butter is a God-given food, olive oil is even more so, being mentioned far more often in the Bible than butter. And as we saw previously, olive oil is a very healthy food.

Cream:

Cream is mentioned three times in the NKJV (Judges 5:25; Job 20:17; Job 29:6). But none of these references add anything to this discussion.

Yogurt:

Yogurt is not mentioned in the Bible, but "curds" are. And the Hebrew word rendered curds can mean "a type of curdled milk, similar to yoghurt" (Holladay). It occurs ten times in Scripture, though it is sometimes rendered as "butter" (Gen 18:8; Deut 32:14; Judg 5:25; 2Sam 17:29; Job 20:17; 29:6; Prov 3-:33; Isa 7:15; 7:22, 2x).

A couple of these passages have been quoted before, and they strongly indicated the mentioned foods are God-given foods. Therefore, if these curds are in fact a form of yogurt, then yogurt would be a Biblical food; but even if not, it is still a God-given food as it just fermented milk. That a form of yogurt would be used in Bible times is not surprising, as fermented milk products tend to keep a little longer without refrigeration than milk. It is also not surprising that there are known health benefits of eating yogurt:

> And just what are the health benefits of yogurt?
>
> First off, **let us not forget that yogurt comes from milk**. So yogurt eaters will get a dose of **animal protein** (about 9 grams per 6-ounce serving), plus several other nutrients found in dairy foods, like **calcium, vitamin B-2, vitamin B-12, potassium, and magnesium**.
>
> But one of the words we're hearing more and more of regarding yogurt is "probiotics." **Probiotics are "friendly bacteria" that are naturally present in the digestive system. Live strains of these "good bacteria" are also found in many yogurt products**. While more research needs to be done, there's some evidence that **some strains of probiotics can help boost the immune system and promote a healthy digestive tract** (WebMD. Yogurt).

Eating yogurt is one of the most common ways to consume the healthy bacteria beneficial to the gut known as probiotics. **Probiotics are effective in regulating the digestive system and decreasing gas, diarrhea, constipation and bloating**.

Some research has suggested that **probiotics can boost the immune system, help with weight management and reduce the risk of cancer**. Consuming yogurt and other probiotic foods may even **enhance absorption of vitamins and minerals**.

The two most common bacteria used to ferment milk into yogurt are Lactobacillus bulgaricus and Streptococcus thermophiles, but many yogurts contain additional bacteria strains.

To help consumers identify yogurts with live and active cultures, **the National Yogurt Association has implemented the LAC (Life & Active Cultures) seal**, found on the product container. In most cases, the number of live bacteria declines the longer the product sits on the shelf....

People who experience discomfort, bloating or gas after consuming liquid milk or ice cream can often tolerate yogurt without symptoms. **The lactose content in yogurt is very low, and the bacteria help the digestion process**.

Try a small amount of yogurt (1/4 cup) first to see how your body reacts. **Because many people who are lactose intolerant are calcium deficient, yogurt can be a very important component of their diet** (MNT).

Yoghurt is fermented milk, and fermented foods contain probiotics. So, logic would dictate that all yoghurts are probiotic-rich, but unfortunately that's not the case. **If yoghurt has been heated or pasteurised, probiotics are destroyed and may not be added back in. Look for the words "live active cultures," or check ingredient lists for names of specific probiotics** (lactobacillus acidophilus, L bulgaricus, etc.) to ensure you're getting these beneficial bacteria, which aid digestion and support the immune system (Sydney).

Check the label to be sure the yogurt you are eating contains live, active cultures. Also be sure it is plain yogurt. Add your own fruit and honey if you need to sweeten it, but do not purchase fruit-flavored yogurt as it contains a large amount of added sugar. And be sure it does not contain artificial ingredients. Frozen yogurt would not fit any of these standards, as it generally does not contain live cultures, and it generally contains added sugar and often artificial ingredients.

Thus plain, natural yogurt would be God-given, while all others would not be God-given.

Ice Cream:

Ice cream is the final dairy food to be discussed. Not surprisingly, it is not mentioned in the Bible. Needless to say, without freezing technology, it would not have been possible to make ice cream in Biblical times. And given that it is not particularly healthy, containing a large amount of added sugar and often artificial ingredients, it would not be a God-given food.

Conclusion

There is strong Biblical evidence that milk and milk products are God-given foods. As such, they would be included in a Creationist Diet. In fact, given how often milk and milk products are mentioned in Scripture and the contexts in which they are mentioned, it is disingenuous for some to claim their diet plan is based on the Bible and to not include dairy products. But given that milk and milk products entered the human diet relatively late, they should be consumed in lesser amounts than the previously discussed foods.

Looking back at the past two chapters, the two animal foods besides meats that stand out are milk and honey. Since these foods are both mentioned in reference to the Promised Land, a version of the Creationist Diet that includes these foods will be called the "Promised Land Diet."

But there are some other factors worth considering in regards to the consumption of milk and other dairy products. These will be addressed in the next chapter.

Bibliography:

Baldwin, Herbert B. Some Observations on Milk and Cream. *The American Journal of Public Health.* Read before the Laboratory Section, American Public Health Association, Rochester, N. Y., September 9, 1915.
https://www.ncbi.nlm.nih.gov/pmc/articles/PMC1286925/pdf/amjphea lth00096-0072.pdf

Berkeley Wellness. Homogenized Milk Myths Busted.
http://www.berkeleywellness.com/healthy-eating/food/article/homogenized-milk-myths-busted

BC Dairy. Does Pasteurization Destroy Nutrients in Milk?
bcdairy.ca/milk/articles/does-pasteurization-destroy-nutrients-in-milk

CDC. Raw Milk Questions and Answers.
https://www.cdc.gov/foodsafety/rawmilk/raw-milk-questions-and-answers.html

Dr. Axe. The Truth About Pasteurization.
https://draxe.com/pasteurization-homogenization-raw-milk/

FDA. The Dangers of Raw Milk: Unpasteurized Milk Can Pose a Serious Health Risk.
www.fda.gov/Food/ResourcesForYou/Consumers/ucm079516.htm

Florida Today. Nutrition for Today: Is butter better?
http://www.floridatoday.com/story/life/wellness/2017/01/31/nutrition-today-butter-better/97220720/

Friberg, Timothy and Barbara. *Analytical Lexicon to the Greek New Testament.* Copyright © 1994. As found on *BibleWorks™ for Windows™.*

Kresser, Chris. Raw Milk Reality: Is Raw Milk Dangerous?
https://chriskresser.com/raw-milk-reality-is-raw-milk-dangerous/

Michalski, MC, *British Journal of Nutrition.* 2007 Apr;97(4):598-610. On the supposed influence of milk homogenization on the risk of CVD, diabetes and allergy.
https://www.ncbi.nlm.nih.gov/pubmed/17349070

MNT (Medical New Today). Is yogurt good for you?
http://www.medicalnewstoday.com/articles/295714.php

New Zealand. An Assessment of the Effects of Pasteurisation on Claimed Nutrition and Health Benefits of Raw Milk.

http://www.foodsafety.govt.nz/elibrary/industry/2014-13-Assessment-of-effects-of-Pasteurisation-on-Claimed-Nutrition-and-Health-Benefits-of-Raw-Milk.pdf

Oxford Dictionary. As found on Microsoft *Word 365*™.

NPR. Drinking Raw Milk Is Worth The Risk, Advocates Say.
http://www.npr.org/templates/story/story.php?storyId=128547897

Paajanen, L. et. al. *Journal of Dairy Research.* 2003 May;70(2):175-9. No difference in symptoms during challenges with homogenized and unhomogenized cow's milk in subjects with subjective hypersensitivity to homogenized milk.
https://www.ncbi.nlm.nih.gov/pubmed/12800871

Parsonnet, Mia, M.D. *What's in Our Food?* New York: Madison Books, 1996.

ProCon. Lactose Intolerance by Ethnicity and Region.
http://milk.procon.org/view.resource.php?resourceID=000661

Quick and Dirty Tips. Is Homogenized Milk Bad For You?
http://www.quickanddirtytips.com/health-fitness/healthy-eating/is-homogenized-milk-bad-for-you

Real Milk. Pasteurization Does Harm Real Milk.
http://www.realmilk.com/health/pasteurization-does-harm-real-milk/

Robbins, John. *Spotlight on Soy.*
http://www.earthsave.org/news/spotsoy.htm

Russell, Rex MD. *What the Bible Says about Healthy Living.* Grand Rapids, MI: Baker Book House, 1999.

Sydney Morning Herald. Ten nutrition mistakes even really healthy people make.
http://www.smh.com.au/lifestyle/health-and-wellbeing/nutrition/ten-nutrition-mistakes-even-really-healthy-people-make-20170314-guy7y9.html

WebMD. The Benefits of Yogurt.
http://www.webmd.com/food-recipes/features/benefits-yogurt#1

Webster's Talking Dictionary/ Thesaurus. Copyright 1996 by Exceller Software Corp. Based on Random House *Webster's College Dictionary.* Copyright 1995 by Random House, Inc.

Chapter Eleven: Arguments Against Dairy Consumption

Milk and other dairy products have traditionally been considered to be very healthy foods. This is evidenced by the recommendations of the United States Department of Agriculture [USDA], as seen in the "Basic Four Food Groups" of the past, the more recent "Food Pyramid," and the current "MyPlate." In all of these, it is recommended that everyone consume 2-3 servings of dairy foods. But this viewpoint and recommendation has been coming under fire from many quarters in recent years.

There are many websites with articles discussing the supposed problems with milk consumption. There are even entire websites dedicated to the anti-milk crusade. In this chapter, some of reasons for the anti-milk position be will summarized and evaluated.

Lactose Intolerance

The anti-milk crowd claims it is not "natural" for adults to drink milk. The first evidence given for this idea is the widespread rate of lactose intolerance. This issue was already mentioned in the previous chapter. But to reiterate, lactose intolerance refers to the inability to digest lactose, the sugar in milk. This inability is due to the lack of the production of lactase—the enzyme needed to digest lactose, the sugar naturally found in milk.

All humans produce this enzyme in infancy, but the majority of people lose this ability in childhood. "Symptoms of intolerance, when they occur, may variously consist of bloating, abdominal rumbling, cramps, nausea, flatulence, and diarrhea" (Parsonnet, p.122).

It is said that if milk were an "early" food, people would have adapted to digesting lactose by continuing to produce lactase throughout their lives. And more importantly, the consumption of milk would be more widespread. But throughout history, and even today around the world, the vast majority of adult humans have not consumed milk products as part of their normal diet.

Creationist Diet

Lactose tolerance, and the consumption of milk and other dairy products, has historically been limited to isolated people groups. Specifically, northern Europeans are the only ones with significant numbers of people who are lactose tolerant. Only 10% of northern Europeans are lactose intolerant. However, the next lowest percentage is 75% for Mediterranean Europeans. The world as a whole is 70% lactose intolerant (Parsonnet, p.122).

As was said previously, this situation is probably due to milk entering the human diet after the Tower of Babel incident. Some of the scattered people groups began drinking milk while others did not. Those that did retained the ability to digest lactose, and for them, milk would be a natural food. But this does not mean it is "unnatural" for those who did not consume milk. Even those with lactose intolerance can consume certain dairy foods, like yogurt and cheese. And such foods, especially yogurt, can be a healthy and yes natural part of one's diet.

However, one interesting point is that the rate of lactose intolerance among Jews is 80% (Parsonnet, p.122). This is somewhat surprising since, as indicated in the previous chapter, milk and other dairy products are mentioned dozens of times in the Bible. But if dairy consumption was so common in Biblical times, why are so many Jews still lactose intolerant? It could be because the Jews were drinking milk from animals other than cows, as we saw in the previous chapter. However, further details on lactose intolerance might give another answer.

Important to know is not all dairy foods cause problems for the lactose intolerant:

Skim milk, low fat milk, whole milk, and buttermilk (in that order) are most likely to cause difficulties. Yogurt, **although high in lactose, contains an enzyme in its culture that aids in lactose digestion**, so that symptoms are less common and less severe. (This is not true of frozen yogurt as freezing destroys this enzyme.) **The various other dairy products are rarely a problem**. One would have to eat 10 ounces of processed cheese, or a stick of butter, or a cup of sour cream to consume the lactose found in 8 ounces of milk (Parsonnet, p.122).

Thus again, those who are lactose intolerant can consume some dairy foods. Moreover, an article in the *Journal of the American Dietetic Association* reported, "Scientific findings indicate that the prevalence of lactose intolerance is grossly overestimated." So the preceding figures for the prevalence of lactose intolerance, including the 80% figure among Jews, might be too high. This article further reports:

> Scientific findings also indicate that people with laboratory-confirmed low levels of the enzyme lactase **can consume 1 serving of milk with a meal or 2 servings of milk per day in divided doses at breakfast and dinner without experiencing symptoms** (McBean and Miller).

Thus it is possible though milk was consumed among ancient Jews, it was not consumed in large amounts or they ate dairy in forms that are not problematic. This is probable in that the second most popular dairy food in the Bible is "curds." Curds are made from casein, the protein in milk. They do not contain lactose, so curds do not require lactase to digest. Also as noted previously, this term could refer to a yogurt-like food, which is usually not a problem for those with lactose intolerance.

Cheese, butter, and cream are the other Biblical dairy foods. As indicated, cheese does not contain much lactose, neither does butter nor cream. The reason for this is these foods are made primarily or solely from the fat in milk, not the sugar.

Therefore, the reason so many Jews today do not retain the ability to produce lactase in adulthood is their early ancestors were consuming only small amounts of milk, along with dairy products that don't require lactase to digest. So what we see today is what would be expected given the Biblical evidence, a partial adaptation to lactose digestion among Jews, whether it be 20% or somewhat higher.

But other than in the Mediterranean area (where the Jews originated), and in Europe, most of the rest of the world's population have not historically consumed milk and milk products. That is why the rates of lactose intolerance among Africans, Asians, and others is 90% or greater. This intolerance is confirmed by an article in the *Journal of the National Medical Association*:

... research has shown that lactase nonpersistence, the loss of enzymes that digest the milk sugar lactose, occurs in a majority of African-, Asian-, Hispanic-, and Native-American individuals. Whites are less likely to develop lactase nonpersistence and less likely to have symptoms when it does occur (Bertron, et al).

Such high rates of lactose intolerance, especially among non-whites, are taken by many to be a "sign" milk consumption is not natural for human adults. But again, as is the case with the Jews, it is also possible other populations only used milk in small quantities and/ or used dairy products in the past that don't need lactase to digest. These would include curds, cheese, and yogurt. And those with lactose intolerance could consume such dairy foods today, along with limited amounts of milk.

Cow's Milk Allergy and Casein Intolerance

Lactose intolerance is not the only difficulty some people have with consuming milk. There are also those who cannot digest the casein (protein) in milk (casein intolerance) and those who are allergic to cow's milk. In regard to the former, an article in the journal *Clinical and Experimental Allergy* reported:

> **Cow's milk protein intolerance** is caused by an inability to digest casein (milk protein) which is 300 times higher in cow's milk than human milk. It can cause diarrhoea and colic in very young babies. Later in life, it shows itself mainly as respiratory problems such as asthma (Iacono).

In regard to the latter, the potential to be allergic to milk is taken by some to indicate that milk consumption is not "natural." But milk is by no means the only food that people are commonly allergic to.

> Eight foods account for the majority of all reactions: milk, eggs, peanuts, tree nuts, soy, wheat, fish and shellfish. Even trace amounts of a food allergen can cause a reaction (FARE).

338

To be consistent, to say milk is an unnatural food due to it being allergenic, one would have to say all of these foods are unnatural as well. Moreover, the percentage of people who are casein intolerant or allergic to milk is actually quite low:

> **Between 5% and 15% of infants show symptoms suggesting adverse reactions to cow's milk protein** (CMP), while estimates of the prevalence of **cow's milk protein allergy (CMPA) vary from 2% to 7.5%.** Differences in diagnostic criteria and study design contribute to the wide range of prevalence estimates and underline the importance of an accurate diagnosis, which will reduce the number of **infants on inappropriate elimination diets...**
> **CMPA persists in only a minority of children** (Vandenplas).

> Even though milk allergies in infants and very young toddlers are the most common food allergy, they still occur in **only about 2.5 percent of the population** in the US and other Western groups (Science Blogs).

Thus from 7-22.5% of infants have one or the other condition. The lower end is less than one-tenth of infants, while the higher end is still less than one-quarter of infants, and even then, most of those infants will "outgrow" the allergy.

The second quote it taken from a blog titled "Milk allergy is the most common form of food allergy found in humans, but you don't have one and neither does your baby." The point is that many people think they or their child is allergic to milk, but most often, that is not the case.

After going through the possible reasons for this misconception, this blogger concludes:

> So, to summarize, **human babies rarely have milk allergies**. One in fifty babies, roughly, might have one. People over diagnose this condition, so you probably know far more babies said to have a milk allergy than actually have one. In order for a baby to demonstrate an allergy to cows milk it must drink cows milk. **Milk allergy is not lactose intolerance**, and

is an utterly different thing, with a different biology and mostly different symptoms. And finally (not mentioned above) **a human baby's allergy to cow's milk is likely to go away by itself**, probably while the baby is a toddler (Science Blogs).

The point is, new parents are so concerned about their children that they find problems where there are none. Note also the emphasis on the difference between milk allergy and lactose (or casein) intolerance. An allergy concerns the immune system, while an intolerance concerns the digestive system—they are two completely different conditions.

It is also worth noting:

> Breast feeding is the gold standard for milk feeding in infant nutrition and is recommended exclusively for the first 4 months of life at least. **The incidence of CMPA is lower in exclusively breast-fed infants compared to formula-fed or mixed-fed infants.** Indeed, only about **0.5%** of exclusively breast-fed infants show reproducible clinical reactions to CMP and most of these are mild to moderate…
>
> **Breast feeding should be promoted for the primary prevention of allergy** (Vandenplas).

It is thus possible that the prevalence of cow's milk allergy is due to the widespread practice of babies being bottle-fed rather than breast-fed. The latter is of course the most natural way for infants to be fed and would help to prevent a cow's milk allergy from developing.

But there is the following caveat:

> There is evidence that food proteins from milk, egg, peanut and wheat are excreted in breast milk and may cause adverse reactions during exclusive breast feeding in sensitised infants. Due to the many benefits of breast feeding to the infant and the mother, clinicians should advise mothers to continue breast feeding but avoid the causal foods in their own diet (Vandenplas).

Leukemia Caused by Milk?

The preceding are not the only problems the anti-milk crowd claims there is with milk. Robert M. Kradjian, MD says he studied over 500 indexed medical journal articles on milk consumption. In his article, *The Milk Letter: A Message to My Patients*, he summarizes what he found:

> The main focus of the published reports seems to be on intestinal colic, intestinal irritation, intestinal bleeding, anemia, allergic reactions in infants and children as well as infections such as salmonella. **More ominous is the fear of viral infection with bovine leukemia virus** or an AIDS-like virus as well as concern for childhood diabetes. Contamination of milk by blood and white (pus) cells as well as a variety of chemicals and insecticides was also discussed. Among children the problems were allergy, ear and tonsillar infections, bedwetting, asthma, intestinal bleeding, colic and childhood diabetes. In adults the problems seemed centered more around heart disease and arthritis, allergy, sinusitis, and **the more serious questions of leukemia**, lymphoma and cancer.

It would take an entire book in itself to go through each of these claims. But it will be worthwhile to investigate an important one—the claim of leukemia being caused by drinking milk. It is true that dairy cows can be infected by bovine leukemia virus (BLV), and this can get into the milk.

A 2007 U.S. Department of Agriculture survey of bulk milk tanks found that **100 percent of dairy operations with large herds of 500 or more cows tested positive for BLV antibodies**. This may not be surprising since milk from one infected cow is mixed in with others. **Even dairy operations with small herds of fewer than 100 cows tested positive for BLV 83 percent of the time** (Berkeley).

Then a 2015 study found:
The frequency of BLV DNA in mammary epithelium from women with breast cancer (59%) was significantly

higher than in normal controls (29%) (multiply- adjusted odds ratio = 3.07, confidence interval = 1.66–5.69, p = .0004, attributable risk = 37%). In women with premalignant breast changes the frequency of BLV DNA was intermediate (38%) between that of women with breast cancer and normal controls (p for trend < .001) (Buehring).

What this study is saying is the bovine leukemia virus has been found in human breast tissue, and more often in those with breast cancer than those without it. The anti-milk crowd has jumped on this as "proof" that milk causes breast cancer. However, it is important to know that pasteurization inactivates BLV.

The survival of bovine leukemia virus (BLV)-infected lymphocytes in milk was studied to determine whether treatments similar to those on a dairy farm would inactivate BLV. **Bovine leukemia virus was found in milk stored for 72 hours at 1.1 C (34 F)**; milk constituents, such as protein, total solids, minerals, fat, and somatic cell concentration did not affect the presence of BLV. Infectivity also was found in the cream layer of milk. **Pasteurization at 63 C for 30 minutes did inactivate BLV-infected lymphocytes** (Rubino).

Thus what we have here is not an argument against drinking milk *per se* but an argument against drinking raw milk that can be added to the concerns raised in the previous chapter. But since most people today drink pasteurized milk, how did the virus get into the women? And is the virus in fact the cause of their breast cancer? The researchers theorized on these questions:

How humans become infected with BLV is not known. Transmission from cattle to humans is plausible, as BLV is widespread in both beef herds and dairy herds. Although **pasteurization renders the virus non-infectious and presumably thorough cooking of beef also does, many people have drunk raw milk and/or eaten raw or undercooked beef at some point in their life.** Breast cancer incidence is markedly higher in countries with high milk consumption [49–52]. Numerous prospective studies on dairy consumption in various defined populations [53], however, including one study that carefully evaluated unpasteurized milk consumption [54], **found no significant relationship between cow's milk consumption and breast cancer incidence.**

Human to human transmission is also plausible. Milk-borne transmission of BLV from cow to calf occurs naturally and HTLV, the human virus closely related to BLV, is transmitted primarily **from nursing mother to child** in endemic areas. Epidemiologic studies on human breast milk consumption, **however, have not found a significant increase in breast cancer among women who were ever breast-fed as infants compared with those who were never breast fed.**

One potential challenge confronting the elucidation of BLV's route of transmission to humans is the long agricultural association of humans with cattle, which began over 2,000 years ago, while **milk pasteurization in western countries was not standard practice until around 1925. This would have allowed ample time for BLV to enter the human population and become established, yet still be reentering the human population under certain circumstances. The current reservoir for transmission to humans could, therefore, be cattle, humans, or both** (Buehring).

"The association between BLV infection and breast cancer was surprising to many previous reviewers of the study, but it's important to note that **our results do not prove that the virus causes cancer,**" said study lead author Gertrude Buehring, a professor of virology in the Division of Infectious Diseases and Vaccinology at UC Berkeley's School of Public Health. "However, this is the most important first step. We still need to confirm that the infection with the virus happened before, not after, breast cancer developed, and if so, how." ...

Buehring emphasized that **this study does not identify how the virus infected the breast tissue samples in their study. The virus could have come through the consumption of unpasteurized milk or undercooked meat, or it could have been transmitted by other humans** (Berkeley).

343

There is thus no evidence that drinking milk, even milk tainted with BLV, causes cancer. There is also no evidence that the women got the virus from drinking milk. More likely, it survives in the human population from the days before pasteurization, being transmitted from mother to child or other human to human contact. But the important point is, pasteurization solves the problem. This is why the CDC is so adamant in its recommendation against drinking raw milk.

But despite the fact that pasteurized milk is perfectly safe to drink in this regard, that does not satisfy the anti-milk crowd. One anti-milk crusader exclaims, "What happens if they incorrectly pasteurize the milk? What happens to those drinking raw milk? I shudder at the thought" (Cohen. Leukemia).

But it could just as easily be asked in exasperation, "What happens if the farmer doesn't follow correct procedures and my lettuce gets contaminated with listeria?" Or, "What happens if the cannery doesn't follow correct protocols and my canned corn get contaminated with botulism?" Or "What happens if the rancher doesn't follow correct procedures and my beef gets contaminated with salmonella?" Or "What happens if the cook at the restaurant doesn't wash his hands after going to the bathroom and contaminates my food?"

The point is, as mentioned previously, just one mistake in the whole chain from farm to table could leave any food contaminated with a pathogen. You are thus taking a chance every time you eat any food that you did not grow and prepare yourself. You can live in paranoia, or you can trust that 99.99% of the time the prescribed procedures are followed and work, and your food is safe to eat. And that is the case with pasteurized milk.

Comparison to Other Mammals

Another major argument used by milk opponents is that no other mammal consumes the milk of another species and no other mammal consumes milk past the age of weaning.

These points are true, but whether they are relevant or not is another matter. The reason animals in the wild do not consume milk past weaning is simple—they simply are not capable of doing so. It takes God-given human intelligence to domesticate animals and attain their

344

milk for consumption. In fact, this would be part of the dominion God granted to human beings over animals (Gen 1:26). Even anti-milk Dr. Kradjian admits as such, "Of course, it is not possible for animals living in a natural state to continue with the drinking of milk after weaning" (*Milk Letter*).

However, domesticated animals will consume milk when humans give it to them, so there is not a "natural" aversion to milk in adult animals. Anyone who owns a cat knowns this. I remember well when I owned a cat as a kid, opening up an empty carton of ice cream, laying it on the floor, and "Buttons" having a really good time licking it clean.

Ethical/ Environmental Considerations

The ethical and environmental considerations for milk consumption would be similar to those for meat consumption. People's picture of dairy cows today is often the idyllic scene of "Betsy the Cow" being kept on a family farm, almost as a member of the family. But this picture is far from the situation in factory dairy farms:

> An older article on the website for the Vegan Society of the UK reported:
> **The dairy industry has undergone considerable change during the past 50 years. Machines replaced hand milking at the beginning of the [nineteen] fifties and cows were taken to the milking parlour more frequently.** Cows are currently milked two or three times a day. However, fully robotic milking parlours will probably eventually be programmed to milk the cow four or even five times a day. Frequent milking stimulates feed intake, thus increasing milk yield (*The Dairy Cow*).

A newer article on PETA's website states similarly:
> Cows produce milk for the same reason that humans do: to nourish their young. In order to force them to continue producing milk, factory farm operators typically impregnate them using artificial insemination every year. Calves are generally torn away from their mothers within a day of birth, which causes them both extreme distress. Mother cows can be

345

heard calling for their calves for days. Male calves are destined to end up in cramped veal crates or barren feedlots where they will be fattened for beef, and females are sentenced to the same sad fate as their mothers.

After their calves have been taken away from them, mother cows are hooked up, two or more times a day, to milking machines. Their reproductive systems are exploited through genetic selection, despite the negative effects on their health. **Artificial insemination, milking regimens, and sometimes drugs are used to force them to produce even more milk—the average cow today produces more than four times as much milk as cows did in 1950....**

A cow's natural lifespan is about 20 years, but cows used by the dairy industry are typically killed after about five years because their bodies wear out from constantly being pregnant or lactating. A dairy-industry study found that by the time they are killed, **nearly 50 percent of cows are lame because of standing on concrete flooring and filth in intensive confinement**. Cows' bodies are often turned into soup, food for dogs and cats, or ground beef because they are too "spent" to be used for anything else (PETA).

Another animal rights advocacy groups states:

Over 90% of U.S. dairy cows are confined in primarily indoor operations, with more than 60% tethered by the neck inside barren stalls, unable to perform the most basic behaviors essential to their well-being...

Of the 9 million dairy cows in the U.S., 3 million are **slaughtered each year at only a fraction of their natural lifespan**. Their worn out bodies become ground beef and restaurant hamburgers (Free from Harm).

Those concerned with the treatment of animals need to realize the impact factory farming has on dairy cows.

Environmentally, vegan advocate John Robbins reports, "The 1,600 dairy farms in California's Central Valley generate more waste than 21 million people" (*Factory Farm Alarm*). Multiply this by the millions of dairy cows throughout the USA and around the world, and the impact on the environment from the manure dairy cows produce is immense.

According to a July 2011 study conducted by the USDA's Agricultural Research Service, a 10,000 cow confinement dairy in Idaho **produces staggering amounts of greenhouse gases**. Every day, 37,075 pounds of pollution spew into the air. This breaks down into 33,092 pounds of methane, 3,575 pounds of ammonia, and 409 pounds of nitrous oxide. Most of the emissions come from the bare dirt lots where the cows spend their time between milkings. The 25-acre manure holding pond is the next biggest source (Eat Wild. News).

While milk carton imagery pictures bucolic, small farms, more than 50 percent of U.S. milk is now produced by just 3 percent of the country's dairies — those with more than 1,000 cows, according to the U.S. Department of Agriculture (USDA). The very largest U.S. dairies now have 15,000 or more cows.

With this increased concentration of milking cows comes a corresponding concentration of manure production. And what happens to this manure is at the heart of the pollution issues surrounding the dairy industry....

According to the EPA, **a 2,000-cow dairy generates more than 240,000 pounds of manure daily or nearly 90 million pounds a year**. The USDA estimates that the manure from 200 milking cows produces as much nitrogen as sewage from a community of 5,000 to 10,000 people.

This year and last, **Wisconsin has fined several dairy operations for manure spills and manure runoff**. According to an analysis by the Milwaukee Journal Sentinel, in 2013 a record number of manure spills — more than 1 million gallons worth — were recorded in Wisconsin. The newspaper reported that from 2007 to 2013, the state experienced an average of 15 manure spills annually from dairy farms....

Wisconsin is hardly alone in grappling with this problem. Similar pollution issues — primarily from spills related to manure storage — have been cropping up across the country (Yale).

Thus not only is the treatment of dairy cows in factory farms inhumane, but the large scale farming method is terrible for the environment. All of this is true. But where some animal rights advocates and environmentally concerned people are disingenuous is when they try to claim the situation is the same on old-fashioned farms. The only comparison is that eventually all farm animals die. But otherwise, the situation is far different, and the lives of dairy cows much better and longer, and the farming process not detrimental to the environment.

Raise dairy cows outside on pasture—the time-honored way—and the world benefits. This is the conclusion of a just-released study conducted by the USDA Agricultural Research Service (ARS).

Compared with dairy cows raised in factory farms, letting Bossie graze in the fresh air **lowered the amount of ammonia released into the atmosphere by about 30 percent. It also cut emissions of other greenhouse gasses**, including methane, nitrous oxide and carbon dioxide. Furthermore, **the carbon footprint of the pasture-based dairy was 6 percent smaller** than that of a high-production dairy herd kept indoors. **The milk of grass-fed cows is much healthier for you as well** (Eat Wild. News).

Two years and Bossy is hamburger

The typical dairy cow raised in a confinement dairy is injected with hormones to increase her milk production. Then after only two years on the job, she's slaughtered and turned into hamburger because she's either sick, lame, fails to breed, or is a less than stellar producer. The average cull rate in the dairy industry is 30 percent. That means that each year, almost a third of our dairy cows are slaughtered and replaced with new heifers.

A cow that's treated well, spared the hormones, and raised on pasture can be expected to produce milk for ten years or more. The cull rate in a grass-based dairy can be as

348

low as 7 percent. The money that a farmer saves by not having to replace a third of the herd every year helps offset the fact that a cow free of artificial hormones produces less milk. **Bossy gets the respect that she deserves and consumers get hormone-free, nutrient-rich milk** (Eat Wild. Pasture Based).

One day this winter, I visited one of the dwindling number of smaller U.S. dairies —Double J Jerseys, **a 200-cow dairy operation in Oregon's Willamette Valley**. As I arrived cows munched clover in the barnyard, near the Bansens' front door. Jon Bansen, a third-generation dairy farmer who produces milk for the Organic Valley co-op, said that **the ratio of cows to pasture on smaller farms leads to a sustainable nitrogen balance**. The steady rise of large-scale dairy operations, he said, has been "fueled by cheap fuel and cheap feed," adding, "More is not always better" (Yale).

Long-lived cows reduce global warming

Bossy has a short lifespan when she is raised in a confinement dairy, which is the way most cows are raised today. She provides a very high volume of milk, partly due to hormone injections and a high-grain diet, but she lasts for only 2-3 years. Then infertility, disease, physical problems, or inflammation end her milking career, and she is sold at auction for hamburger.

Cows raised on grass are healthier and more fertile, making them good milk producers for up to twelve years. These long-lived and more contented cows may reduce greenhouse gas production (methane) between 10 and 11 percent according to a British Study (Eat Wild. News).

As a bonus, as with grass-fed beef versus grain-fed beef, milk from grass-fed cows is much more nutritious than milk from grain-fed cows. On the page on Eat Wild's website where they list old-fashioned dairy farms, it is stated:

100-Percent Grass-Fed Dairies

Milk from 100-percent grass-fed animals is much healthier than ordinary milk. **It has a higher concentration of vitamins and antioxidants, fewer "bad" fats, and more "healthy" fats such as omega-3 fatty acids and CLA (conjugated linoleic acid)**.

The following dairies raise their animals on forage alone. Typically, the forage includes grass and a legume such as clover or alfalfa. The animals are given hay or grass silage when there is not enough high-quality pasture…

All of the dairy farmers listed on Eatwild produce delicious, superior milk that is free of antibiotics and added hormones. We have made a separate list of these 100-percent grass-fed dairies because they are very rare, and because of the premium products they sell. **You can expect to pay more for these products because the farmers are sacrificing volume for quality** (Eat Wild. Pastured Products Directory).

As last line indicates, as with pasture-raised meat, pasture-raised dairy is more expensive. But again, a tenant of the Creationist Diet is that later foods should be consumed in lesser amounts than earlier foods. Thus a reduced intake of dairy but switching to pasture-raised dairy where possible would be the best approach.

Bovine Growth Hormone

One last issue in regards to dairy is worth exploring. Recombinant bovine growth hormone (rBGH) is a very hot topic in the anti-milk crusade. There is usually at least one article about it on every anti-milk website. An older article on the AFPA Fitness website explains the problem:

It may be the newest carcinogen, but the FDA and Monsanto, the chemical giant that makes **rBGH (recombinant bovine growth hormone, used on cows to increase milk yield)**, apparently don't want the public to know. Rumors and insinuations of research cover-up and possible government-industry collusion abound...

350

The problem with rBGH is a hormone, common to cows and humans, called **IGF-1 (insulin-like growth factor)**. IGF-1, normally found in the human body (in the blood and saliva), **causes cells to divide and grow to proliferate and it is this factor that directly increases milk production in cows**. But when additional amounts of **IGF-1 enter the human body in the presence of milk protein (casein), the body is unable to destroy it, stomach enzymes are unable to digest it, and it is absorbed by the colon**, which is known to have cell receptor sites for IGF (*Tainted Milk Mustache*).

Cows may be dosed with recombinant bovine growth hormone (rBGH), which contributes to an increased incidence of mastitis, a painful inflammation of the udder. (In the U.S., rBGH is still used, but it has been banned in Canada and the European Union because of concerns about human health and animal welfare.) According to the U.S. Department of Agriculture, **16.5 percent of cows used for their milk suffer from mastitis, which is one of the leading causes of death in adult cows in the dairy industry** (PETA).

It was because of this hormone and perceived cover-up that Robert Cohen wrote the book *MILK—The Deadly Poison* and founded the Dairy Education Board (www.notmilk.com).

Cohen summarizes his fears:
By continuing to drink milk, one delivers the most powerful growth hormone in nature to his or her body (**IGF-I**). **That hormone has been called the key factor in the growth of breast, prostate, and lung cancer**. At the very best, or worst, this powerful growth hormone instructs all cells to grow. **This might be the reason that Americans are so overweight**. At the very worst, this hormone does not discriminate. **When it finds an existing cancer, usually controlled by our immune systems, the message it delivers is: GROW!** (Dairy Industry. Capitalization in original).

And it isn't just rBGH, there are also many other hormones that can find their way into milk. Cohen writes:

> **Every sip of milk contains 59 different bioactive hormones** according to endocrinologist Clark Grosvenor who published a list of those hormones in the *Journal of Endocrine Reviews*, Vol. 14, No. 6, 1992. That same list can be found on the NOTMILK homepage or on page 238 of *MILK—The Deadly Poison"* (*New America*).

Whether these hormones are truly a cause for concern or not is a matter of great debate. The main debate is whether rBGH and other hormones survive stomach acids. The FDA and the dairy industries say they do not, while writers such as the preceding claim they do. An article on the website for the American Cancer Society (ACA) explains up the situation well.

> **Recombinant bovine growth hormone (rBGH) is a synthetic (man-made) hormone that is marketed to dairy farmers to increase milk production in cows.** It has been used in the United States since it was approved by the Food and Drug Administration (FDA) in 1993, but **its use is not permitted in the European Union, Canada, and some other countries.** This document summarizes what is known about the product and its potential effects on health....
>
> Concerns about possible health effects on humans from milk produced using rBGH have focused on 2 main issues.
>
> First, **does drinking milk from rBGH-treated cows increase blood levels of growth hormone or IGF-1 in consumers?** If it does, would this be expected to have any health effects in people, including increasing the risk of cancer? Several scientific reviews have looked at these issues and are the main focus of this document.
>
> Second, **cows treated with rBGH tend to develop more udder infections (mastitis). These cows are given more antibiotics than cows not given rBGH. Does this increased use of antibiotics lead to more antibiotic-resistant bacteria,**

and is this a health concern for people? This remains a concern, but it has not been fully examined in humans....

Bovine growth hormone levels are not significantly higher in milk from rBGH-treated cows. On top of this, **BGH is not active in humans,** so even if it were absorbed from drinking milk, it wouldn't be expected to cause health effects....

At this time, **it is not clear that drinking milk, produced with or without rBGH treatment, increases blood IGF-1 levels into a range that might be of concern regarding cancer risk or other health effects.**...

One study estimated that the additional amount of IGF-1 that might be absorbed by humans drinking milk from rBGH treatment, assuming no degradation and complete absorption, represents **0.09% of the normal daily production of IGF-1 in adults.**...

The available evidence shows that the use of rBGH can cause adverse health effects in cows. The evidence for potential harm to humans is inconclusive. It is not clear that drinking milk produced using rBGH significantly increases IGF-1 levels in humans or adds to the risk of developing cancer. More research is needed to help better address these concerns.

The increased use of antibiotics to treat rBGH-induced mastitis does promote the development of antibiotic-resistant bacteria, but the extent to which these are transmitted to humans is unclear.

The American Cancer Society (ACS) has no formal position regarding rBGH (ACA).

In sum, yes, rBGH is bad for the cows, but it most likely is not directly bad for people who drink the milk from cows given BGH. But indirectly it can be bad in two ways. First, the increased milk production due to rBGH leads to the previously discussed environmental problems. Second, the increased infections among dairy cows requires them to be given more antibiotics, and that can lead to antibiotic resistant bacteria that might infect human beings.

However, none of this would apply to old-fashioned farms as such farms do not use rBGH or other hormones. This is yet another reason to spend the extra money for pasture-raised dairy products.

Conclusion

Most of the claims of the anti-milk crowd do not hold up under investigation. And the claims that are valid do not apply to dairy from old-fashioned farms.

But should you consume milk or not? That question only the reader can answer for yourself. But it should be mentioned, as with the consumption of meats, the potential problems could be alleviated if everyone simply reduced their intake of milk products and what they do consume is from old-fashioned farms.

As indicated, those who are lactose intolerant can generally tolerate small amounts of milk. And if milk products were not in such great demand, then many of the questionable methods of the dairy industries would not be needed.

However, the USDA is recommending the exact opposite—that people increase their consumption of milk products. The main reason for this is the calcium content of milk, along with the role of calcium in preventing osteoporosis. Before you make a decision on whether to consume milk products or not, and in what amounts, the issue of calcium and osteoporosis needs to be discussed. That issue will be the subject of the next chapter.

Bibliography:

ACA. Recombinant Bovine Growth Hormone. https://www.cancer.org/cancer/cancer-causes/recombinant-bovine-growth-hormone.html

AFPA (American Fitness Professionals & Associates). *Tainted Milk Mustache: How Monsanto and the FDA Spoiled a Staple Food.* Page no longer available, but the home page is: http://www.afpafitness.com/

Berkeley News. Virus in cattle linked to human breast cancer., http://news.berkeley.edu/2015/09/15/bovine-leukemia-virus-breast-cancer/

Bertron P, Barnard ND, Mills M. *Journal of the National Medical Association* 1999 Mar;91(3):151-7 Racial bias in federal nutrition policy, Part I: *The public health implications of variations in lactase persistence.*

Buehring, Gertrude Case. Et. al. Exposure to Bovine Leukemia Virus Is Associated with Breast Cancer: A Case-Control Study Published: September 2, 2015.
http://dx.doi.org/10.1371/journal.pone.0134304

Cohen, Robert. The Dairy Industry Self-destructs.

Cohen, Robert. New America—The Not So Great Society –
The above pages are no longer available. But the home page for Not Milk is: http://www.notmilk.com

Cohen, Robert. Leukemia.
http://www.notmilk.com/leukemia.html

Eat Wild. News & Notes.
http://www.eatwild.com/news.html

Eat Wild. Pasture-Based Farming Enhances Animal Welfare.
http://www.eatwild.com/animals.html

Eat Wild. Pastured Products Directory - All-Grass Dairies.
http://www.eatwild.com/products/allgrassdairies.html

FARE (Food Allergy Research & Education). Facts and Statistics.
https://www.foodallergy.org/facts-and-stats

Free from Harm. Home / 10 Dairy Facts the Industry Doesn't Want You to Know.
http://freefromharm.org/dairyfacts/

Food Guide Pyramid: A Guide to Daily Food Choice –
http://www.nal.usda.gov:8001/py/pmap.htm

Iacono, G. ,et al, "Persistant Cow's Milk Protein Intolerance In Infants: The Changing Faces Of The Same Disease", *Clinical and Experimental Allergy*, 28: 817-823, 1998, quoted in Scott, Laura. Losing Your Bottle: Laura Scott takes a close look at the the white stuff and discovers that we've all been milked.-
http://www.viva.org.uk/Viva!%20Campaigns/os%20article.htm

Kradjian, Robert M. MD. *The Milk Letter: A Message to My Patients.*
http://www.afpafitness.com/MILKDOC.HTM

McBean LD, and GD Miller . *Journal of the American Dietetic Association* 1998 Jun;98(6):671-6. *Allaying fears and fallacies about lactose intolerance.*

Parsonnet, Mia, M.D. *What's in Our Food?* New York: Madison Books, 1996.

PETA (People for the Ethical Treatment of Animals). The Dairy Industry.
http://www.peta.org/issues/animals-used-for-food/factory-farming/cows/dairy-industry/

Robbins, John. *Factory Farm Alarm.*
http://www.earthsave.org/news/factfarm.htm

Rubino MJ, Donham KJ. *American Journal of Veterinarian Resource.* 1984 Aug;45(8):1553-6. Inactivation of bovine leukemia virus-infected lymphocytes in milk.
https://www.ncbi.nlm.nih.gov/pubmed/6089622

Science Blogs. Milk allergy is the most common form of food allergy found in humans, but you don't have one and neither does your baby.
http://scienceblogs.com/gregladen/2011/01/20/milk-allergy-is-the-most-commo/

Vandenplas, Yvan, et. all, *Arch Dis Child.* 2007 Oct; 92(10): 902–908. Guidelines for the diagnosis and management of cow's milk protein allergy in infants.
https://www.ncbi.nlm.nih.gov/pmc/articles/PMC2083222/

Vegan Society of the UK. *The Dairy Cow.* No longer available.

Yale Environment. As Dairy Farms Grow Bigger, New Concerns About Pollution.
http://e360.yale.edu/features/as_dairy_farms_grow_bigger_new_concerns_about_pollution

Chapter Twelve:
Calcium and Osteoporosis

As we have seen, milk, especially milk from old-fashioned cows, is an excellent source of high quality protein, vitamins and minerals, and other beneficial elements. But the primary reason the consumption of milk and other dairy products is recommended is for their high calcium content. And it is true, dairy products generally contain high amounts of calcium. Moreover, the main reason increased calcium consumption is being recommended is because of the problem of osteoporosis. But does milk consumption help to prevent osteoporosis? That claim is disputed by anti-milk advocates.

But before getting to the debate, it would be helpful to define osteoporosis and to provide some information about calcium absorption and utilization:

> **Osteoporosis is a degenerative bone disease characterized by long-term loss of calcium from the bones**, especially of the jaw, spine, pelvis, and the long bones of the legs. The bones gradually become porous, brittle, and break easily. The humped posture common in people with osteoporosis is called dowager's hump and also results from changes in the spine as the bones deteriorate and compress.... **In some cases, the first sign of osteoporosis is a bone fracture** (Somers, p.213).

> **The body gets the calcium it needs in two ways. One is by eating foods or supplements that contain calcium**. Good sources include **dairy products, which have the highest concentration per serving of highly absorbable calcium**, and dark leafy greens or dried beans, which have varying amounts of absorbable calcium. Calcium supplements often contain vitamin D; taking calcium paired with vitamin D seems to be more beneficial for bone health than taking calcium alone....
>
> **The other way the body gets calcium is by pulling it from bones. This happens when blood levels of calcium drop too low**, usually when it's been a while since having eaten a

357

meal containing calcium. **Ideally, the calcium that is "borrowed" from the bones will be replaced at a later point. But, this doesn't always happen. Most important, this payback can't be accomplished simply by eating more calcium…**

Bone is living tissue that is always in flux. Throughout the lifespan, bones are constantly being broken down and built up in a process known as remodeling. **Bone cells called osteoblasts build bone, while other bone cells called osteoclasts break down bone.**

In healthy individuals who get enough calcium and physical activity, **bone production exceeds bone destruction up to about age 30. After that, destruction typically exceeds production….**

Achieving adequate calcium intake and maximizing bone stores during the time when bone is rapidly deposited (up to age 30) provides an important foundation for the future. But it will not prevent bone loss later in life. **The loss of bone with aging is the result of several factors, including genetic factors, physical inactivity, and lower levels of circulating hormones (estrogen in women and testosterone in men)** (Harvard. Calcium).

It should also be noted that the chemical symbol for calcium is Ca, magnesium is Mg, phosphorus is P, potassium is K, and sodium is Na (salt is sodium chloride or NaCl). These symbols often appear in scientific literature on this subject.

Population Comparisons

The first argument used to claim milk calcium does not help to prevent osteoporosis is population comparisons. Simply put:

> … **osteoporosis and its resulting bone fractures are most common in countries where dairy and calcium consumption is highest**: Canada, the United States, the United Kingdom, and the Scandinavian countries (Henry).

...statistics show that countries with the lowest consumption of dairy products also have the lowest fracture incidence in their population....

Amy Lanou Ph.D., nutrition director for the Physicians Committee for Responsible Medicine in Washington, D.C., who states that:

"The countries with the highest rates of osteoporosis are the ones where people drink the most milk and have the most calcium in their diets. **The connection between calcium consumption and bone health is actually very weak, and the connection between dairy consumption and bone health is almost nonexistent**" (Save Institute).

Such statistics are true and are repeatedly pointed to in anti-milk literature. Moreover, an article from the *Journal of the National Medical Association* was quoted in the previous chapter to confirm that lactose intolerance is very high among "African-, Asian-, Hispanic-, and Native-American individuals." However, it is much lower among whites. The same article goes on to state:

Osteoporosis is less common among African Americans and Mexican Americans than among whites, and **there is little evidence that dairy products have an effect on osteoporosis among racial minorities** (Bertron, et al).

However, population comparisons are fraught with difficulties. Nutrition professor Stephanie Atkinson states in this regard:

... you can't make interracial and intercountry comparisons because of other factors—like genetics, weight-bearing exercise, exposure to sunlight, and other nutritional factors—also influence rates of osteoporosis. Calcium isn't the only factor to predict bone mass (*Nutrition Action*, April 1998, p.4).

... in countries such as India, Japan, and Peru where average daily calcium intake is as low as 300 milligrams per day (less than a third of the U.S. recommendation for adults, ages 19 to 50), the incidence of bone fractures is quite low. Of course, **these countries differ in other important bone-health factors as well—such as level of physical activity and amount of sunlight—which could account for their low fracture rates** (Harvard. Calcium).

It is thus too simplistic to compare dairy and calcium intake and osteoporosis rates between populations. There are other nutritional and non-nutritional factors to consider.

Comparison with Animals

The second argument used against the need for milk consumption among humans to prevent osteoporosis is a point mentioned in the previous chapter—no other mammal consumes the milk of another species, and no other mammal consumes milk past the age of weaning.

Henry David Thoreau (1817-62), a lifelong vegan, sums up the idea:

> One farmer says to me, "You cannot live on vegetable food solely, for it furnishes nothing to make bones with"; and so he religiously devotes a part of his day to supplying his system with the raw material of bones; **walking all the while as he talks behind his oxen, which, with vegetable-made bones, jerk him and his lumbering plow along in spite of every obstacle** (*Columbia*).

The point is—all other animals manage to develop strong bones without consuming milk past weaning. This is true even for pure herbivorous animals like elephants and the above-mentioned oxen, both of which have very strong bones. Where do such animals get their calcium?—mainly from greens of all sorts.

Meanwhile, carnivorous animals get their calcium from the bones and internal organs of the animals they eat. The latter would include undigested greens.

But this line of reasoning misses one important point—humans are not pure herbivores (plant eaters) nor pure carnivores (meat eaters). We are omnivorous (eaters of both plants and animals).

Herbivore:

An herbivore is an organism that feed exclusively or mainly on plants. **Herbivores typically have adaptations towards a specialization of eating and digesting plant matter**. This could include but is neither limited to nor has to have flatter teeth to grind plant matter, long intestines, gut microbiome to digest cellulose and other hard-to-digest parts of plants.

Carnivore:

A carnivore is an organism that feed exclusively or mainly on animal tissue. As herbivores, **they typically have adaptations towards specialization of eating animal tissue** such as sharp teeth, short gut and some way of capturing prey, such as claws, ability to sprint or venom.

Omnivore:

Omnivores are organisms that feed on both animal tissue and plants. There is no strict definition of how large portion of the diet that has to be, to be classified as omnivore. **Omnivores typically lack specializations to either animal or plants, and have more intermediate traits** (Vegan Biologist).

To put it another way, God designed human beings differently than oxen or tigers. God designed oxen to eat grasses, while He designed tigers to eat meat. But He designed human beings to eat both plant foods and animal foods. Now, vegans will dispute this and claim that human beings have more in common with herbivores than with carnivores. They claim things like the length of our digestive tract or the pH of our digestive tract reflects that of herbivores (Pavlina). But other sites claim just as strongly that human digestive systems are more reflective of carnivores than of herbivores (Raising Rabbits).

Interestingly, in an article titled "Humans Are Not Herbivores," the "Vegan Biologist" addressed this debate and comes to the following conclusion:

I've said it earlier and I say it again. This is not an argument for not being vegan. **Humans are omnivores**, but can live on a completely vegan diet with the supplementation of B12 from fermentation. **I think that trying to claim that humans are something else than omnivores are just counter productive since it's quite easily debunked and we lose credibility.** There are plenty of reasons to be vegan and still stick to what is true. **This post is mainly focused on debunking the claim that humans are herbivores and should therefore eat only plants,** but the post should qualify to debunk anyone claiming that humans are biological meat eaters and therefore should eat meat, likewise.

This discussion could have been included in Chapter Five, but it is being included here as it is often brought up in discussions on calcium and osteoporosis. The point is, comparison to pure herbivores is irrelevant, as humans are not herbivores. God designed us differently than herbivores, so we have different nutrient needs than they do.

Bioavailability of Milk Calcium

The next anti-milk claim is the most radical—that the calcium in milk is not bioavailable. In other words, the claim is the calcium in milk cannot be absorbed or used by the human body.

But many scientific studies have shown an assortment of detrimental health effects directly linked to milk consumption. And the most surprising link is that **not only do we barely absorb the calcium in cow's milk (especially if pasteurized), but to make matters worse, it actually increases calcium loss from the bones.** What an irony this is!

Here's how it happens. **Like all animal protein, milk acidifies the body pH which in turn triggers a biological correction.** You see, calcium is an excellent acid neutralizer and the biggest storage of calcium in the body is – you guessed it… in the bones. So **the very same calcium that our bones need to stay strong is utilized to neutralize the acidifying effect of milk.** Once calcium is pulled out of the bones, it leaves the body via the urine, so that the surprising net result after this is an actual calcium deficit (Save Institute).

However, those who make this claim usually do not cite scientific evidence to support it. But there is scientific evidence that shows the contrary. And interestingly, this evidence comes about as a result of lactose intolerance.

For instance, one study involving "11,619 Finnish women aged 47-56 years" found the rate of bone fractures at some, but not all, body sites to be highest in the women with lactose intolerance. It also found these same women to have lower bone mass densities (BMD).

The conclusion of the researchers was, "Long-term premenopausal calcium deficiency differentially affects bones with weight-bearing non-ankle bones being at the greatest risk of suffering reduced strength" (Honkanen R, Kroger H, et al.).

A similar study was done also in Finland with, "A random population sample of 2025 women aged 48-59...." The study found:

The mean dairy calcium intake was 558 mg [milligrams]/day in women with LI [lactose intolerance] and 828 mg/day in other women (p < 0.0001). The mean spinal BMDs were 1.097 and 1.129 g/cm2 (-2.8%) (p = 0.016) and the mean femoral BMDs were 0.906 and 0.932 g/cm2 (-2.8%) (p = 0.012) for the LI and other women, respectively.

The researcher's conclusion was, "Our results suggest that LI slightly reduces perimenopausal BMD, possibly through reduced calcium intake" (Honkanen R, Pulkkinen P, et al). So there are studies showing dairy calcium consumption to be associated with increased bone mass densities and decreased fractures. However, there are also occasionally studies that seem to show the opposite.

For instance, a study by the Department of Health Science, Kinesiology, Recreation, and Dance, University of Arkansas found, "Women who had suffered hip fracture reported higher dairy use than women who had not experienced these fractures...." And the anti-milk crowd will jump on such reports.

However, the rest of this sentence reads, "a finding that is dramatically inconsistent with the literature." So the researchers themselves indicate that this finding is different from what the majority of other studies have found.

Moreover, the next sentence states, "This finding may reflect positive behavioral changes resulting from the hip fracture event" (Turner LW, et al.). Thus what this study might have found is that those women who already had fractures began drinking more milk, so you always have to evaluate studies carefully.

The preceding are older studies that I cited in the First Edition of this book. For this Second Edition, I redid the research. The following are additional studies on this subject.

Skeletal mass is a major determinant of susceptibility to osteoporotic fracture in menopause. At menopause, the skeletal mass is the resultant of the **Peak Skeletal Mass (PSM)** reached early adulthood minus the bone mass lost through the process of **Adult Bone Loss (ABL)**. Current interventions for the maintenance of skeletal resilience in advanced age address the ABL peri- or postmenopausally. **This study indicates that the effects of milk consumption in childhood and adolescence on bone density may manifest as higher bone density decades later in menopause**. The assumed mechanism of the reported effect is through augmentation of the PSM, and acquisition of favorable nutritional habits which may influence the extent of ABL (Sandler).

There was a statistically significant graded association between **increasing lifetime intake of caffeinated coffee and decreasing BMD [bone mineral density]** at both the hip and spine, independent of age, obesity, parity, years since menopause, and the use of tobacco, alcohol, estrogen, thiazides, and calcium supplements. **Bone density did not vary by lifetime coffee intake in women who reported drinking at least one glass of milk per day during most of their adult lives**. (Barret-Conner).

The effects of milk intake on bone health are not clear in elderly Asian men with low dietary calcium intake. This study showed that **greater milk intake is associated with lower bone turnover, higher bone density, and higher bone** microarchitecture index in community-dwelling elderly Japanese men....

Results:

The median intake of milk in the 1479 participants (mean age, 73.0 ± 5.1 years) was one glass of milk per day. **Bone turnover markers showed a decreasing trend** ($p < 0.05$) and **aBMD** at TH ($p = 0.0019$) and FN ($p = 0.0057$) **and TBS [trabecular bone score]** ($p = 0.0017$) **showed increasing trends with greater milk intake** after adjusting for demographic and behavioral confounding factors. This association was attenuated after further adjusting for nutrient intake, in particular, calcium intake.

Conclusions:

Greater milk intake was associated with lower bone turnover, higher aBMD, and higher TBS in community-dwelling elderly Japanese men (Sato).

Objective: We assessed relations between postmenopausal hip fracture risk and calcium, vitamin D, and milk consumption....

Results: Women consuming ≥ 12.5 g vitamin D/d from food plus supplements had a 37% lower risk of hip fracture (RR = 0.63; 95% CI: 0.42, 0.94) than did women consuming < 3.5 g/d. **Total calcium intake was not associated with hip fracture risk** (RR = 0.96; 95% CI: 0.68, 1.34 for $\geq$ 1200 compared with < 600 mg/d). **Milk consumption was also not associated with a lower risk of hip fracture** (P for trend = 0.21).

Conclusions: An adequate vitamin D intake is associated with a lower risk of osteoporotic hip fractures in postmenopausal women. Neither milk nor a high-calcium diet appears to reduce risk. Because women commonly consume less than the recommended intake of **vitamin D,**

supplement use or dark fish consumption may be prudent (Feskanich).

Nutrition plays an important role in bone health. The two nutrients essential for bone health are calcium and vitamin D. **Reduced supplies of calcium are associated with a reduced bone mass and osteoporosis, whereas a chronic and severe vitamin D deficiency leads to osteomalacia, a metabolic bone disease characterized by a decreased mineralization of bone.** Vitamin D insufficiency, the preclinical phase of vitamin D deficiency, is most commonly found in the elderly. The major causes of vitamin D deficiency and insufficiency are decreased renal hydroxylation of vitamin D, poor nutrition, scarce exposition to sunlight and a decline in the synthesis of vitamin D in the skin.

The daily average calcium intake in Europe has been evaluated in the SENECA study concerning the diet of elderly people from 19 towns of 10 European countries. In about one third of subjects the dietary calcium intake results were very low, between 300 and 600 mg/day in women, and 350 and 700 mg/day in men. **Calcium supplements reduce the rate of bone loss in osteoporotic patients.** Some recent studies have reported a significant positive effect of calcium treatment not only on bone mass but also on fracture incidence.

The SENECA study, has also shown that vitamin D insufficiency is frequent in elderly populations in Europe. There are a number of studies on the effects of vitamin D supplementation on bone loss in the elderly, showing that **supplementations with daily doses of 400-800 IU of vitamin D, given alone or in combination with calcium, are able to reverse vitamin D insufficiency, to prevent bone loss and to improve bone density in the elderly** (Gennari).

All of the research I could find showed that either increased milk and calcium intake was beneficial for bone health or there was no effect. I could not find a single study that showed milk consumption was detrimental for bone health. I'm not saying such does not exist, but they would be outside of the mainstream of the evidence.

But this does not stop the anti-milk crowd from citing other possible reasons that milk consumption would be detrimental for bone health.

Other Nutritional Factors

Anti-milk Atkinson outlines some of the other nutritional factors to be considered besides calcium, "Higher levels of protein, sodium, and caffeine have all been associated with a higher excretion of calcium in the urine, so they may increase the risk of osteoporosis in the U.S."

Protein and Sodium:

The claim of animal protein leading to calcium loss was seen in a previous quote in this chapter. Here, Atkinson provides further claimed details on the issues of protein and sodium:

> The Recommended Dietary Allowance (RDA) for protein is 50 grams a day for women and 65 grams a day for men. **Each gram of protein raises calcium excretion by 1 to 1.5 mg**. So if a woman consumed 65 grams of protein a day—which is typical—she would lose an extra 15 to 23 mg [milligrams] of calcium a day ....
> **You lose 10 mg of calcium for every 500 mg of sodium**. So if you eat, say, 4,400 mg of sodium a day instead of the recommended 2,400 mg, you'd lose an extra 40 mg of calcium (*Nutrition Action*, April 1998, p.4).

The claim that a high animal protein intake increases calcium loss was debunked in Chapter Six. But I am repeating it here to show how persistent this myth is. But new here is a similar claim is made about sodium. And there is some evidence in this regard, but it is not clear cut.

One study compared a DASH (Dietary Approaches to Stopping Hypertension) diet with a lower level of sodium intake than a control diet. It concluded:

> ... the DASH diet significantly reduced bone turnover, which if sustained may improve bone mineral status. **A reduced sodium intake reduced calcium excretion** in both diet groups and serum OC in the DASH group. The DASH diet and reduced

367

sodium intake may have complementary, beneficial effects on bone health (Lin).

Another study compared a low sodium DASH diet that included six servings of lean meat per day (labeled LNAB) with a with a high-carbohydrate low-fat diet with a higher acid load (labeled (HCLF). It concluded:

> Fasting serum bone markers (baseline and week 14) and 24 h urinary electrolyte excretion (baseline, weeks 4, 8, 12 and 14) were measured. After the intervention period, **the LNAB group** (n 46) had a fall of 26 (sem 6) % (P < 0.0001) in urinary Na, an increase in K excretion (6.8 (sem 3.6) mmol/d; P = 0.07) and, compared with the HCLF group (n 49), **a greater reduction in urinary Ca excretion** by 0.7 (sem 0.3) mmol/d. Serum 25-hydroxyvitamin D, intact parathyroid hormone and osteocalcin did not change, and both groups had a similar increase of 23 (sem 5) % (P < 0.0001) in C-terminal telopeptide of type I collagen. The HCLF group had an 11 (sem 4) % increase (P = 0.003) in N-terminal propeptide, type I procollagen, which could indicate an increased rate of bone turnover. **The fall in urinary Ca with the lower-Na lower-acid load diet is likely to have long-term beneficial effects on bone**. As bone resorption was not different between the two dietary patterns with relatively high Ca intake, the effect on bone health of a dietary pattern with a lower acid load warrants further study on a lower Ca intake (Nowson).

Thus these studies did find a connection between sodium intake, calcium loss, and long-term bone health. But another study started with this premise but did not find that decreasing sodium intake had any effect on calcium excretion.

> **Sodium intake increases urinary calcium excretion** and may thus lead to negative calcium balance and bone loss. ... We **hypothesised that reducing sodium intake would reduce urinary calcium excretion** and have a beneficial influence in bone metabolism....

A total of 29 subjects, 14 males and 15 females, were divided into two study groups. **One group (low-sodium group (LS))** reduced sodium intake for 7 weeks by substituting low-salt alternatives for the most important dietary sources of sodium. The other group, serving as a **control group (C)**, was given the same food items in the form of normally salted alternatives....

The LS group showed a significant decline (P = 0.001) in urinary sodium/creatinine ratio **without a significant effect on urinary calcium/creatinine ratio.** In the LS group, s-PTH increased (P = 0.03). The C group showed an increase in s-PTH (P = 0.05) and in s-B-ALP, but **no differences were observed between the study groups in the changes of serum markers of calcium and bone metabolism**....

We have shown that **reducing the sodium intake** of young, healthy people with adequate calcium intake over a 7-week period **does not affect the markers of bone metabolism.** (Natri).

Thus a high sodium intake increases calcium excretion, but a low intake does not necessary lead to better bone health. Therefore, there is no reason to be too restrictive with one's sodium intake in this regard, but an excessively high intake should be avoided. What is "high" or "low" is hard to put numbers on, but the recommendation about sodium for blood pressure purposes would probably be a good recommendation in regards to calcium loss as well:

The "Dietary Guidelines for Americans 2010" addresses sodium intake in detail. **The average daily sodium intake for Americans is 3,400 milligrams per day, an excessive amount** that raises blood pressure and poses health risks. In general, **Americans should limit daily sodium consumption to 2,300 milligrams,** but this is an upper safe limit, not a recommended daily allowance. Even active people who lose lots of sodium through sweating **require no more than 1,500 milligrams of sodium per day** (SF Gate. Sodium).

Phosphorus:

The next nutrient to be considered in regards to calcium status is phosphorus.

Somers writes about phosphorus:

Recommended Dietary Allowances for phosphorus are arbitrary and are based on an estimate of the best ratio (1:1) for calcium and phosphorus. The average American diet contains 1,500 mg to 1,600 mg, or twice the adult RDA for phosphorus, and the ratio of calcium to phosphorus is often as low as 1:2...

Food additives contribute as much as 30% of dietary phosphorus. Soft drinks contain as much as 500 mg of phosphoric acid per serving and can contribute to excessive phosphorus intake if consumed regularly....

Overconsumption of phosphorus might occur in people who consume diets high in meat, convenience foods, and soft drinks and low in calcium containing foods such as non-fat milk and dark green leafy vegetables. The effects of this imbalance in the ratio of calcium to phosphorus can contribute to faulty bone maintenance and osteoporosis (pp.84-86).

Moreover, Keith Ayood, Ed.D, R.D. states:

It's a mistake to think only women need calcium as they age. Men need it too, especially because they eat larger portions of meat, which is high in phosphorus. **A high intake of phosphorus increases the body's need for calcium** (*Men's Health*, p.26).

Thus excessive phosphorus can also increase calcium loss, but meat is not the main culprit—junk foods are, especially soft drinks. And in addition to junk foods, white bread can also contain phosphorus. The reason for this is the chemicals added to it, such as monocalcium phosphate, dicalcium phosphate, and diammonium phosphate.

It should be noted that two of these three chemicals contain calcium. And the use of these chemicals do add some calcium to the bread, but it is it is insignificant compared to the amount of phosphorus added. It should also be noted that whole wheat bread generally does not contain

370

these chemicals, so that's another reason, besides the ones mentioned previously, to consume whole wheat rather than refined, white bread.

Caffeine:

Caffeine was mentioned in a previous study as increasing calcium excretion. Dr, Kenneth Cooper concurs when he writes about caffeine that it can cause, "Loss of the body's calcium through the urine, a result that could decrease bone density and lead to osteoporosis" (p.132).

Conclusion on Other Nutritional Factors:

Protein is a non-factor, but phosphorus, sodium, and caffeine can all contribute to loss of calcium. And, unfortunately, all three of these substances are consumed in excessive amounts in the American diet. It is a combination of these substances that is causing the American osteoporosis problem. But where does milk fit into this picture?

Milk contains about the same amount of phosphorus as calcium, so if milk were the only source of phosphorus in the diet, it would provide calcium and phosphorus in the ideal proportion. But, unfortunately, milk is not. As Somers points out, "meat, convenience foods, and soft drinks" also contribute phosphorus to the diet, as well as processed white bread. And it is the total amount of phosphorus in the diet that can be a problem.

But the solution would not be to not drink milk, as that would reduce one's intake of calcium. It would be to not eat an excessive amount of meat as has already been suggested and to avoid these other very unhealthy foods, which have no place in a Creationist Diet anyway.

Other Bone Beneficial Nutrients

Besides calcium, other nutrients are also needed for the proper formation and maintenance of bones. Vitamin D was mentioned in a couple of studies previously as being needed for the absorption of calcium. Vitamin D is called the "sunshine vitamin" as the body can manufacture it from sunshine.

Somers writes, "Adequate annual stores of vitamin D probably are obtained with 10 minutes of sunbathing daily during the summer months" (p.24). Since the vitamin is fat soluble, it can be stored in the body, so getting a little sun during the summer months will provide the body enough vitamin D to last through the winter.

If one does not get into the sun, or always wears sunscreen while in the sun, then dietary vitamin D is needed. Fish is the best natural food source of vitamin D, as was discussed in Chapter Seven. Fortified milk is a good source of vitamin D, but so is any other food product that is vitamin D fortified. But frankly, given that getting into the sun can be beneficial to the mood, sunshine would be the preferred method to get one's vitamin D if it is at all possible.

Magnesium is the next nutrient that is important to bone health. Magnesium is plentiful in nuts and whole grains (but not refined grains). As such, if you are following the recommendations of this book and consuming these foods, then sufficient magnesium is probably being attained from the diet.

Manganese is a trace element that is also needed for bone health. It is found in a wide variety of unrefined plant foods. Boron is also possibly important and found in unrefined foods (Somer, pp. 109, 120). In addition, "Vitamin K may help to strengthen bones" (*Nutrition Action*, April 2000, p.9). Vitamin K is found in most vegetables, but especially in dark green leafy ones. So it is not just calcium, but a variety of nutrients that are important in preventing osteoporosis.

Don't Forget Exercise!

One last point needs to be mentioned—exercise. This is something anyone concerned with the health of their bones, and their health in general, most definitely should be doing (cleared with your doctor first, of course). But note, not just any exercise will do; it has to be weight bearing. Therefore, an exercise like swimming, although all around an excellent exercise, is not good for the bones.

The best exercise for strengthening bones is strength training. Next would be "striking" exercises, i.e. any exercise where your foot or arm and hand "strikes" against something, as in the foot against the ground in walking or jogging, or the arm with racket against a ball as in tennis and racquetball.

Summary of Milk and Osteoporosis

Calcium intake is important. But how much calcium one needs is affected by other factors in the diet. The more phosphorus, sodium, and caffeine one consumes, the more calcium that is required to maintain strong bones. And the less of these substances one consumes, the less calcium is needed. Moreover, sufficient amounts of vitamin D, magnesium, manganese, vitamin K, and possibly boron are also needed.

So the best way to ensure bone health is to limit ones intake of junk foods, while consuming foods that contain these nutrients, like dairy, dark green vegetables, fish, nuts, and whole grains. And such a diet is exactly what is recommended in the Creationist Diet. Performing weight-bearing exercise regularly and getting sunshine occasionally are also important.

In sum, does milk consumption help to prevent osteoporosis? Yes. Is it necessary for doing so? No. This is exactly what would be expected given the later introduction of milk into the human diet. Thus milk is a helpful and nutritious food but not a necessary one.

Non-fat, Low Fat, or Full Fat?

Before closing this discussion on milk, one last question needs to be addressed. What is the best form of milk to drink: non-fat, low fat, or full fat? The answer to this questions depends on if you are taking the previous recommendation to consume milk from old-fashioned cows rather than factory farm cows. The reason for this is there is a significant difference between the fat in each type of cow's milk.

> The reason for confining cows in feedlots and feeding them grain rather than grass is that they produce far more milk under these unnatural conditions. If you also inject them with bi-weekly hormones, standard practice in the dairy industry, they produce even more....
>
> **But with so much emphasis on quantity, the nutritional content of our milk has suffered. One of the biggest losses has been in its CLA content.** CLA, or "conjugated linoleic acid," is a type of fat that may prove to be one of our most potent

373

cancer fighters. **Milk from a pastured cow has up to five times more CLA than milk from a grain-fed cow**....

Milk from pastured cows also contains an ideal ratio of essential fatty acids or EFAs. There are two families of EFAs—omega-6 and omega-3 fatty acids. Studies suggest that if your diet contains roughly equal amounts of these two fats, you will have a lower risk of cancer, cardiovascular disease, autoimmune disorders, allergies, obesity, diabetes, dementia, and various other mental disorders....

Besides giving you five times more CLA and an ideal balance of EFAs, **grass-fed milk is higher in beta-carotene, vitamin A, and vitamin E** (Eat Wild. Super).

CLA and Omega 3 were discussed in Chapter Six. All that was said there about old-fashioned beef being healthier than factory farm beef would apply here, including in regard to these beneficial elements in the milkfat offsetting the deleterious effects of the saturated fat. Thus again, if a scientific study does not ask what kind of cow the milk was derived from, then that study is not fully reliable.

But to answer the question posed by the subtitle, if you are consuming factory farm milk, then it would probably be best to use non-fat or at least low fat milk so as to avoid the deleterious effects of the saturated fat. However, CLA and Omega 3s are fats, while vitamins A and E are fat-soluble, so they would not be found in non-fat milk unless they are added. As such, if you are consuming old-fashioned milk, then whole milk would contain the greatest amount of these beneficial nutrients and thus would not only not be problematic but most likely beneficial. Also probably beneficial rather than problematic would be fatty dairy products like butter and cheese. But until a scientific study specifically looks the differing health effects of factory farm dairy products versus old-fashioned ones, then the beneficial effects cannot be asserted without qualification.

Conclusion on Dairy Foods

Before concluding this discussion on milk and other dairy products, the following "meta-analyses of observational studies and randomized controlled trials" is worth considering.

Results:

The most recent evidence suggested that **intake of milk and dairy products was associated with reduced risk of childhood obesity.** In adults, **intake of dairy products was shown to improve body composition and facilitate weight loss** during energy restriction. In addition, **intake of milk and dairy products was associated with a neutral or reduced risk of type 2 diabetes and a reduced risk of cardiovascular disease, particularly stroke.**

Furthermore, the evidence suggested **a beneficial effect of milk and dairy intake on bone mineral density** but no association with risk of bone fracture. Among cancers, **milk and dairy intake was inversely associated with colorectal cancer, bladder cancer, gastric cancer, and breast cancer, and not associated with risk of pancreatic cancer, ovarian cancer, or lung cancer,** while the evidence for prostate cancer risk was inconsistent. Finally, consumption of milk and dairy products was not associated with all-cause mortality.

Calcium-fortified plant-based drinks have been included as an alternative to dairy products in the nutrition recommendations in several countries. However, nutritionally, **cow's milk and plant-based drinks are completely different foods, and an evidence-based conclusion on the health value of the plant-based drinks requires more studies in humans.**

Conclusion:

The totality of available scientific evidence supports that intake of **milk and dairy products contribute to meet nutrient recommendations, and may protect against the most prevalent chronic diseases,** whereas very few adverse effects have been reported (Thorning).

Thus overall, when all of the evidence is considered, milk and other dairy products are nutrient-packed, beneficial foods. And this is without even factoring in the difference between factory farm and old-fashioned dairy.

So should you consume dairy products or not? The answer here is similar to that for meats. The Biblical evidence is strong that milk and milk products are God-given foods, so a follower of the Creationist Diet can choose to consume them if you want to. However, since dairy foods entered the human diet later than plant foods and even meats, if they are included in the diet, it should be in comparatively smaller amounts to these foods.

Bibliography:

Barrett-Connor, Elizabeth MD; Jae Chun Chang; Sharon L. Edelstein, ScM. January 26, 1994. Coffee-Associated Osteoporosis Offset by Daily Milk Consumption. The Rancho Bernardo Study. JAMA.1994;271(4):280-283.
http://jamanetwork.com/journals/jama/article-abstract/363200

Bertron P, Barnard ND, Mills M. *Journal of the National Medical Association* 1999 Mar; 91(3):151-7 Racial bias in federal nutrition policy, Part I: *The public health implications of variations in lactase persistence.*

Burckhardt P. *Ther Umsch* 1998 Nov;55(11):712-6. *Osteoporosis and nutrition* (Article in German).

Columbia Dictionary of Quotations is licensed from Columbia University Press. Copyright © 1993 by Columbia University Press. All rights reserved.

Cooper, Dr. Kenneth H. *Advanced Nutritional Therapies.* Nashville: Thomas Nelson, 1996.

Eat Wild. Super Healthy Milk.
http://www.eatwild.com/articles/superhealthy.html

Feskanich, Diane and Walter C Willett, and Graham A Colditz. Calcium, vitamin D, milk consumption, and hip fractures: a prospective study among postmenopausal women. *American Journal of Clinical Nutrition.* 2003;77:504–11
http://www.naturaleater.com/Science-articles/Calcium-milk-bone-unhelpful-feskanich.pdf

Gennari, C. *Public Health Nutrition.* 2001 Apr;4(2B):547-59. Calcium and vitamin D nutrition and bone disease of the elderly.
https://www.ncbi.nlm.nih.gov/pubmed/11683549

Henry, Susan O. *Milk: Is it Really Our Best Source for Calcium?* – http://www.afpafitness.com/MilkCal2.htm

Harvard T.H. Chan. School of Public Health. Calcium: What's Best for Your Bones and Health?

https://www.hsph.harvard.edu/nutritionsource/calcium-full-story/

Honkanen R, Kroger H, Alhava E, Turpeinen P, Tuppurainen M, Saarikoski S. *Bone* 1997 Dec;21(6):473-7. *Lactose intolerance associated with fractures of weight-bearing bones in Finnish women aged 38-57 years.*

Honkanen R, Pulkkinen P, Jarvinen R, Kroger H, Lindstedt K, Tuppurainen M, Uusitupa M. *Bone* 1996 Jul;19(1):23-8. *Does lactose intolerance predispose to low bone density? A population-based study of perimenopausal Finnish women.*

Kradjian, Robert M. MD. *The Milk Letter: A Message to My Patients.*
http://www.afpafitness.com/MILKDOC.HTM

Lin PH, et. al. *Journal of Nutrition.* 2003 Oct;133(10):3130-6. The DASH diet and sodium reduction improve markers of bone turnover and calcium metabolism in adults.
https://www.ncbi.nlm.nih.gov/pubmed/14519796

Men's Health: 101 Nutrition Secrets. By the editors of *Men's Health,* Emmaus, PA; Rodale, 1999.

Natri AM, et. al. *European Journal of Clinical Nutritition.* 2005 Mar;59(3):311-7. A 7-week reduction in salt intake does not contribute to markers of bone metabolism in young healthy subjects.
https://www.ncbi.nlm.nih.gov/pubmed/15674316

Nowson CA1, Patchett A, Wattanapenpaiboon N. *British Journal of Nutrition.* 2009 Oct;102(8):1161-70. The effects of a low-sodium base-producing diet including red meat compared with a high-carbohydrate, low-fat diet on bone turnover markers in women aged 45-75 years.
https://www.ncbi.nlm.nih.gov/pubmed/19445819

Nutrition Action HealthLetter. Vol. 25, No. 2, April 1998. "Avoiding the Fracture Zone." Interview by Bonnie Leidman of Stephanie Atkinson, pp. 1,3-7.

Nutrition Action HealthLetter, Vol. 27, No. 3, April, 2000, "Multiple Choice: How to Pick a Multivitamin, pp. 1,5-13. Also, p. 4.

Pavlina, Steve. Are Humans Carnivores or Herbivores?
http://www.stevepavlina.com/blog/2005/09/are-humans-carnivores-or-herbivores-2/

Raising Rabbits. Carnivore Digestive System.
http://www.raising-rabbits.com/carnivore-digestive-system.html

377

Robbins, John. *Spotlight on Soy.*
http://www.earthsave.org/news/spotsoy.htm
What About Dairy? Looking Behind the Mustache.
http://www.earthsave.org/news/whatdary.htm

Sandler, R B, et. al. Copyright © 1985 by The American Society for Clinical Nutrition, Inc. Postmenopausal bone density and milk consumption in childhood and adolescence.
http://ajcn.nutrition.org/content/42/2/270.short

Sato Y, et. al. Osteoporos International. 2015 May;26(5):1585-94. doi: 10.1007/s00198-015-3032-2. Epub 2015 Jan 28. Greater milk intake is associated with lower bone turnover, higher bone density, and higher bone microarchitecture index in a population of elderly Japanese men with relatively low dietary calcium intake: Fujiwara-kyo Osteoporosis Risk in Men (FORMEN) Study.
https://www.ncbi.nlm.nih.gov/pubmed/25627112

Save Institute. Debunking The Milk Myth: Why Milk Is Bad For You And Your Bones.
https://saveourbones.com/osteoporosis-milk-myth/

SF Gate. The FDA Recommended Sodium Intake.
http://healthyeating.sfgate.com/fda-recommended-sodium-intake-1873.html

Somer, Elizabeth, M.A., R.D. *The Essential Guide to Vitamins and Minerals.* New York: HarperPaperback, 1992.

Thorning TK, et.al. *Food Nutrition Resource.* 2016 Nov 22;60:32527. doi: 10.3402/fnr.v60.32527. eCollection 2016. Milk and dairy products: good or bad for human health? An assessment of the totality of scientific evidence.
https://www.ncbi.nlm.nih.gov/pubmed/27882862

Tsuchida K, Mizushima S, Toba M, Soda K. *Journal of Epidemiology* 1999 Feb;9(1):14-9. *Dietary soybeans intake and bone mineral density among 995 middle-aged women in Yokohama.*

Turner LW, Hunt S, Kendrick O, Eddy J. *Psychol Rep* 1999 Oct;85(2):423-30. *Dairy-product intake and hip fracture among older women: issues for health behavior.*

Vegan Biologist. Humans Are Not Herbivores.
https://veganbiologist.com/2016/01/04/humans-are-not-herbivores/

Section Three
Miscellaneous

Creationist Diet

Chapter Thirteen:
Summary of Creationist Diets and God-given Foods

The preceding chapters of this book have described four different variations of the Creationist Diet. Each is summarized below. Foods in square brackets are not actually mentioned in the Bible but would fit in the places indicated.

Variations of the Creationist Diet

Edenic Diet: Raw fruits and vegetables (preferably organic), raw nuts and seeds, and possibly raw grains.

Antediluvian Diet: The above foods, plus: cooked fruits, vegetables, nuts and seeds, whole grains (preferably non-GMO), legumes [including peanuts], olive oil, [nut, peanut, and seed oils]).

Noahic Diet: The above foods, plus: old-fashioned, blood-drained, fat-trimmed, clean meats; old-fashioned, blood-drained, skinless poultry; clean, low-mercury fish.

Promised Land Diet: The above foods, plus: old-fashioned milk and other dairy products, old-fashioned eggs, honey (preferably raw honey).

But which of these diets should the reader follow? Only the reader can answer that question. But a few points are worth noting.

First, these different diets are not a progression. In other words, it is not being recommended that one start with the bottom diet and work your way up, gradually eliminating foods. The point of presenting four different diets is because everyone is different. And the type of diet that works best for one person might not for another, so these are different options worth trying.

381

Second, it is advisable to stick with a diet for at least three months before deciding if it is working or not. It takes a while for the body to adapt to a new dietary regime. Also, it is possible, even likely, that when making major dietary changes you will actually feel worse initially. The reason for this is what is called variously the "detox" or "healing" phase of a new diet. The idea is; if you have been living on a junk food based diet for years, toxins have been built up in your system. While the body is eliminating these toxins, you can feel worse.

Other possible symptoms of the detox phase are increased urination and defecation as the body, especially the colon, is ridding itself of the build-up of toxins over the years. The latter might be especially true if you are switching from a meat-based diet using factory farm meats to a meat free-diet or one only using old-fashioned meats. There might also be an increase in sweating and even the formation of pimples as toxins are being released through the skin. Such symptoms are normal and usually past within a few days or weeks.

These symptoms can be lessened by gradually changing to a new diet. The place to begin would be to start including more fruits and vegetables in the diet and reducing the amount of processed junk foods.

The next easiest step would be to change from eating refined grains to whole grains. Reducing the amount of fatty factory farmed meats and dairy and replacing them with fat-trimmed, old-fashioned meats and dairy or nuts, seeds, and legumes would be the next step.

A book published by *Natural Health* magazine provides some further suggestions:

> **Make incremental changes to your diet over a period of time rather than radical changes overnight**. Making slower changes is not only easier it is more likely to be effective....
>
> If you're not sure where to start, as a first step you might identify and try to correct your worst eating habits.... **Rather than attempting to break all of your worse eating habits at once, focus on cutting back on total fats and increasing servings of fresh vegetables and fruits** (Mayell, pp.8-9).

Changing from a factory farm animal food based, junk food based diet to a more plant food based, old-fashioned meats and dairy, natural foods diet is not easy. But it is worth the effort as there are proven health benefits to such a diet.

And finally, these four different diets are not absolute dividing lines. It is possible to mix foods from the different diets. For instance, when following an Antediluvian/ vegan type of diet, you could choose to include honey or fish in the diet. As indicated previously, many vegans do in fact eat honey and even fish. And this point leads to another way of looking at the Creationist Diet.

God-given Foods

Rather than looking at specific versions of the Creationist Diet, you could simply restrict yourself to eating only or at least mostly God-given foods, while avoiding non-God-given foods. God-given foods are:

Fruits (preferably organic)
Vegetables (preferably organic)
Nuts
Seeds
Whole grains (preferably non-GMO)
Legumes
Blood-drained, fat-trimmed, old-fashioned, clean meats
Blood-drained, skinless, old-fashioned, clean poultry
Clean, low-mercury fish
Old-fashioned eggs
Honey (preferably raw honey)
Old-fashioned milk and milk products
Extra virgin olive oil
Unrefined nut, peanut, and seed oils

By sticking to these foods, you could design a very healthy diet for yourself. As for proportions of foods, a suggestion of the Creationist Diet is that one's food consumption of each kind of food should parallel the order the foods came into the human diet. In other words, the earlier a food entered the human diet, the more of it a person should consume, and the later, the less of it.

Thus a Creationist Diet should be predominately raw fruits, nuts, vegetables, seeds, and if one likes them, raw grains and sprouts, then cooked versions of these foods, particularly whole grains. These foods should constitute a significant proportion of the daily diet.

Legumes then would have a place in a Creationist Diet, but in lesser amounts than the preceding. The same would go for olive and nut oils. Old-fashioned meats can be eaten in lesser amounts, but only from clean animals. Old-fashioned dairy, eggs, and raw honey can be eaten, but again, in lesser amounts. If one wants to follow a vegan diet, then, of course, the meats and dairy, and possibly honey would be eliminated.

Olive oil is the only Biblical oil and thus should be the primary oil used, but it should be unrefined, which is to say, extra virgin and cold processed. But oils derived from nuts, peanuts, and seeds can be used as well. These foods are naturally high in fat, so it does not take a lot processing to derive oil from them. And if they are unrefined, the naturally occurring nutrients would still be present to some degree. But refined olive, nut, peanut, and seed oils are highly processed with little nutritional value and should only be used in limited amounts. But what foods should be avoided? These will be discussed next.

Not God-given Foods

Some foods that would not be considered to be God-given have already been discussed. It has already been mentioned that "enriched" grains are anything but. God gave whole grains to us to eat, not grains that have a major portion of their nutrients refined out.

Refined sugar is another food that has already been discussed. Honey and raisins are the only sweeteners mentioned in the Bible. Sweeteners like white sugar, corn syrup, and high fructose corn sugar have had all the nutrients in the original plant refined out of them, so they are not God-given.

Refined vegetable oils would be another class of non-God-given foods. These would include corn and soy oils. Corn and soy are naturally low in fat, so it takes a lot of processing to derive oil from them, and the resulting oil is devoid of nutrients. Meanwhile, safflower and canola are not even foods to begin with, so their oils could hardly be God-given. And they are plants that are low in fat, so again, a lot of processing is needed to make them into oil.

The difference between clean and unclean meats was discussed in depth. Only clean meats would be considered to be God-given. Unclean meats would not. The same goes for factory farm versus old-fashioned meats. The former would not be God-given while the latter would be.

Animal blood and fat were mentioned as being forbidden by God, so meats with the blood in it and/or with the cover fat on or processed into it would not be God-given. This would include untrimmed meats and poultry with the skin. Ground meats and processed meats like hot dogs and sausage would also not be God-given if the cover fat is ground into the item.

Lard, being pure animal fat, would not be a God-given food. Butter, however, would be God-given, if it is derived from old-fashioned cows. Moreover, given the choice, you should choose butter over margarine. Even with trans fats now banned, margarine is still a highly-processed food, while butter is a natural food mentioned in the Bible.

Deep frying was beyond the cooking methods of Biblical times and adds a large amount of unnatural fats to the food, so fried foods would not be considered to be God-given.

Eggs would be God-given if they are from chickens raised the old-fashioned way, but not if derived from factory farm chickens.

Finally, any kind of artificial food ingredients would not be God-given, as by definition such items are artificial, not natural food stuffs. These would include artificial sweeteners, flavorings, colorings, and preservatives.

With this background, the list of foods which are not God-given would be:

Refined grains
Refined sugars
Refined vegetable oils
Unclean meats
Factory farm meats, dairy, and eggs
Untrimmed meats
Processed meats
Ground meat if the cover fat is ground into it
Factory farm poultry
Poultry with the skin
All deep-fried foods
Margarine, lard
All artificial food ingredients

Of course, any food containing any of these items as ingredients would not be God-given. Thus a breakfast cereal made with refined grains, a significant amount of added sugar, and artificial colorings and flavorings would not be God-given. It would also not be such due to being highly processed.

On the other hand, oatmeal, with user-added fruit and nuts, would be a God-given breakfast. All three ingredients are God-given foods and are minimally processed. Meanwhile, an all-natural breakfast cereal made with whole grains and honey (or at least little added sugar) contains all God-given ingredients, but is still a highly-processed food. Therefore, it would be borderline if it is God-given or not.

It should be noted, it is not being said one can never eat non-God-given foods. But if eaten, they should only be eaten in limited amounts occasionally, such as for special events. Such foods would not constitute any kind of significant proportion in a Creationist Diet.

Words of Warning

Before proceeding it would be appropriate to insert here a few words of warning about diet and its relation to the Christian faith.

Paul the apostle writes:

[1]Now be receiving the one being weak in the faith, not for disputes over opinions. [2]One believes [it is permissible] to eat all [things], but the one being weak eats [only] vegetables. [3]**Stop letting the one eating despise [or, look down on] the one not eating; and stop letting the one not eating judge the one eating, for God [has] accepted him.** [4]Who are you, the one judging another's household bondservant? To his own master he stands or falls; but he will be made to stand, for God is able to make him stand. [5]One indeed judges [or, considers] a day [to be] above [another] day, but another judges every day [to be alike]; **be letting each be fully convinced in his own mind.**

[6]The one honoring [or, observing] the day, to [the] Lord he honors [it]; and the one not honoring the day, to [the] Lord he does not honor [it]. And **the one eating, to [the] Lord he eats,**

for he gives thanks to God; and the one not eating, to [the] Lord he does not eat, and he gives thanks to God. [7]For none of us lives to himself, and none dies to himself. [8]For both if we live, to the Lord we live, and if we die, to the Lord we die. So both if we live and if we die, we are the Lord's. [9]Because for this [reason] Christ also died and rose and lives, so that He should exercise lordship over both dead [people] and living [people].

[10]But why do you judge your brother? [fig., fellow believer] Or also, why do you despise [or, look down on] your brother? For we will all stand before the judgment seat of Christ. [11]For it has been written, *"[As] I live, says [the] LORD, every knee will bow to Me, and every tongue will confess to God."* [Isaiah 45:23, LXX; cp. Phil 2:10,11] (Rom 14:1-11).

There is no cause in the Christian faith for one Christian to think he or she is superior to another because of their eating habits. If the reader decides not to eat animal foods, that is fine; but don't think you are a "better" Christian than the person still eating animal foods, and vice-a-versa.

Moreover, Paul writes:

[14]I know and have been persuaded in [the] Lord Jesus that nothing [is] unclean by means of itself, except to the one considering anything to be unclean, to that one [it is] unclean. [15]But if on account of food your brother is grieved, you are no longer walking about [fig., conducting yourself] according to love; **stop ruining with your food that one on behalf of whom Christ died** (Romans 14:14-16).

Fellow Christians are more important than food. What this means is, if you are still eating meat, you shouldn't be tempting the vegetarian to eat meat. Similarly, if you know someone who is trying to lose weight, or simply to avoid junk foods, don't be offering the person cake and ice cream. Of all people, Christians should be watching out for the consciences of others.

And finally, Paul writes:

[17]For **the kingdom of God is not eating and drinking, <u>but</u> righteousness and peace and joy in [the] Holy Spirit** (Romans 14:17).

What you eat is important; that is the obvious theme of this book. But what you eat or don't eat should not become the most important aspect of your life. Keep things in perspective.

Conclusion

With those words of warning, this chapter can be summarized by noting that foods can rather easily be divided into categories of God-given foods and not God-given foods. But how does this division compare to how scientific research would classify foods? This question will be addressed in the next chapter.

Bibliography:

Mayell, Mark. *52 Simple Steps to Natural Health*. New York: Pocket Books, 1995.

Chapter Fourteen:
Foods, Heart Disease, Cancer, and Stroke

Reference has been made to many scientific studies throughout this book. In fact, this writer has spent much time doing searches and reading abstract after abstract on PubMed (www.ncbi.nlm.nih.gov/pubmed).

Among other things, I have been looking for patterns in regard to what foods are associated in epidemiological and controlled studies with increased or decreased risks for heart disease, cancer, and stroke. The following chart is how I would classify foods based on this research. Comments will follow.

Classifications of Foods

Decrease Risk (Protective):
Vegetables
Fruits
Nuts, seeds
Whole grain products
Legumes
Vegetable oils (especially olive and canola)
Yogurt (especially low/ non-fat)
Fish (except if overcooked, charred, or deep fried) and fish oils
Chicken/ turkey (with skin removed, baked not fried, and not overcooked/charred)
Garlic
Tea

Increase Risk:
Red meat, pork (if untrimmed or well-done/ charred)
Processed meats
Chicken/ turkey (with skin, or overcooked/charred, or deep fried)
Whole milk

Butter, margarine, lard
Eggs (especially greater than one/ day)
Fried foods
Refined grains
Refined sugars

Neutral (neither increase nor decrease risk):
Low-fat/ skim milk

Split evidence:
Red meat, pork (if lean, not processed or well-done/ charred)
Cheese
Alcohol

Comments

These lists should look rather familiar. With a few exceptions, the foods in the "Decrease Risk" category are the same as the God-given foods listed in the previous chapter, while the foods in the "Increase Risk" category are similar to the not God-given foods list. It would thus seem science is finally catching up with the Bible. But before discussing the few minor differences, some comments on how I developed the preceding lists will be helpful.

What I particularly like about PubMed is it enables a large number of abstracts on a subject to be read in a short time. It is always possible to find a study somewhere that would support almost any dietary claim. But what I was trying to do is determine where the "preponderance of evidence" was. In other words, what foods repeatedly showed up in the "decrease risk" category versus the "increase risk" category in a wide variety of studies.

Moreover, trying to look at three different maladies, and with the wide variety of cancers possible, made things difficult as some foods might increase the risk of one malady but decrease the risk of another. And the amount consumed can also be a confounding factor.

For instance, eggs were listed as increasing the risk of heart disease in several studies. But as previously noted, a study reported in the *Journal of the American Medical Association* concluded, "These findings suggest that consumption of up to 1 egg per day is unlikely to have substantial overall impact on the risk of CHD [coronary heart disease] or stroke among healthy men and women" (Hu FB, et al.). Similarly, some studies show eggs only increase the risk of prostate cancer at high intakes (e.g., Wilson). However, other studies showed eggs increase the risk of prostate cancer even at intake levels of less than one per day (e.g., Richman, Wu). Given this somewhat contradictory data, I included eggs in the "increase risk" category but with the notation "especially greater than one/ day." However, eggs from old-fashioned chickens could possibly be a different story.

Also, how a food is prepared can be relevant. Overcooking and frying meats are definite risk factors, as is leaving the skin on chicken. However, in the case of fish and chicken without the skin, if they are not overcooked or fried, they are associated with decreased risk. Such is not the case with red meat and pork. They are generally not associated with decreased risk even if not overcooked, though sometimes with an increased risk and sometimes without an increased risk (e.g. Rohmann, et. at). I thus put red meat and pork in the split evidence category.

However, as has been mentioned before, these studies often do not differentiate between clean meats (beef) and unclean meats (pork) and never take into account if the meat is derived from a factory farm animal or an old-fashioned farm animal, and they often do not indicate if the fat is trimmed or not. If those distinctions would be made, things would probably be different. Old-fashioned, trimmed, clean meats could very well be associated with a decreased risk. For a more detailed discussion of red meat, see the section at the end of this chapter on "meat cancer."

Dairy products are hotly debated, so I paid particular attention to them. Some studies show they decrease risk of cancer while others show they increase the risk. But such inconsistencies are only seen when dairy products are "lumped together." When they are separated based on their fat content and on whether they have been fermented or not, then I believe the preceding divisions are appropriate. For instance, one study concluded:

> "Ovarian cancer risk was positively associated with increasing consumption of **whole milk and other full-fat dairy foods**, but was not associated with consumption of **low-fat dairy foods** and was inversely related to consumption of **skimmed milk**" (Webb PM, et. al).

Thus in this study, whole milk was associated with an increased risk of ovarian cancer. But low-fat milk was "neutral." It seemed to neither increase nor decrease risk, while skim milk actually decreased the risk. But I couldn't find strong enough additional evidence to place skim milk in the "protective" category, so I put it, along with low-fat milk, in the "neutral" category. But then, a more recent study on ovarian cancer came to somewhat different conclusions:

> In analyses of the highest versus lowest cumulative average intake in adulthood, we observed **a non-significant inverse association with skim milk intake** (HR 0.76, 95% CI 0.54-1.06, p(trend) = 0.05), a non-significant inverse association with lactose intake (HR 0.87, 95% CI 0.69-1.11, p(trend) = 0.22) and **no association with consumption of whole milk, dairy calcium, or dairy fat**. Similar risk estimates were observed for dairy food/nutrient intake during high school, premenopause or postmenopause. Lactose intake in adulthood was inversely associated with risk of endometrioid EOC (HR 0.32, 95% CI 0.16-0.65, p(trend) < 0.001) (Merritt).

Such contradictions show the difficulties of doing this research. And again, such studies do not take into account if the milk is derived from factory farm or old-fashioned farm cows. If the latter, then whole milk and high fat dairy products could very well be protective. At the very least, they most likely would not increase risk.

Another interesting point was the value of yogurt. It is associated with a decreased risk of heart disease, colon cancer, and in one study breast cancer, so yogurt was the one dairy food that was "protective" enough to place in the first category. Again, it would probably be even more so if it was made from old-fashioned milk.

For cheese, however, I was not able to find a definite answer. Some studies showed it increased risk while others showed it decreased risk. It could be that the type of cheese eaten made the difference. The studies didn't specify, so I placed cheese in the "spilt evidence" category. But again, being derived from factory farm versus old-fashioned cows could make a difference and move cheese into the decrease risk category.

Also in the last category is alcohol. Light to moderate consumption (i.e. one glass/week to one glass/day) is associated with a decreased risk of heart disease and some cancers. But for other cancers, such as breast cancer, alcohol increases the risk. Moreover, at high consumption levels (greater than two drinks/day), alcohol increases the risk for heart disease (along with causing many other problems), so if one does drink, do so cautiously and moderately.

For the rest of the foods listed, the evidence was overwhelming. There is no doubt that unrefined plant foods in general, and especially vegetables and fruit, reduce the risk of all three maladies, while high-fat animal foods, refined foods, and fried foods increased the risk.

I could be more specific in terms of which vegetables and fruits are the most protective. For instance, one study on strokes concluded, "These data support a protective relationship between consumption of fruit and vegetables—particularly cruciferous and green leafy vegetables and citrus fruit and juice—and ischemic stroke risk" (Joshipura KJ, et al.). Cruciferous vegetables are broccoli, cauliflower, cabbage, and Brussel sprouts. These were mentioned previously as being particularly healthy, along with "green leafy vegetables" like kale and collards, and brightly colored vegetables like carrots. And this study would add citrus as a class of especially healthy fruits.

Comparison to God-given and not God-given Foods Lists

How does all of this scientific research compare to the foods lists of the previous chapter? As indicted, the "Decrease Risk" and "God-given foods" are very similar, and the "Increase Risk" and the "Not God-given Foods" lists are similar.

Unfortunately, as previously indicated, studies do not distinguish between clean and unclean meats. In fact, in most studies, red meat and pork are lumped together. But one point that is brought out in the studies that the Bible does not address is the issue of overcooking meats. This is definitely a risk factor. Processed meats are another definite risk factor. And, as Chapter Eight indicated, such processing would render meats far from the God-given kind.

God's decree against eating meat fat is supported in the preceding classifications. It is untrimmed meats, chicken skin, and pure animal fats like lard that don't fare very well.

The emphasis of the Bible on eating whole plant foods is seen in the lists. As for chicken and fish doing better than red meats, this would fit with the earlier discussion about factory farm meats today being fattier than meats in Biblical times. Skinless chicken probably has similar fat content to the meat of Biblical times and old-fashioned meats today.

Canola oil being protective is probably due to its monounsaturated fat content. But such can be attained from more natural oils like olive, nut, and peanut oils, and those oils (if unrefined) contain other beneficial elements, so they would be preferred.

And finally, the issue of wine and other alcoholic beverages would require a book in itself. Here, it will just be repeated what was said previously—if one does drink, do so in moderation.

Thus overall, generally speaking, the foods to be included and to be excluded in any version of the Creationist Diet have scientific support, along with the more important support of the Bible.

"meat cancer"

In response to claims that meat consumption increases the risk of cancer, I did a search of PubMed for "meat cancer." I limited the search to studies reported within the past ten years and done on humans. My search turned up 1,576 abstracts. Needless to say, I did not read all of the abstracts, but I did read through dozens of them. Below is a summary of what I found in the abstracts.

1. Some controlled studies have found increased risk of cancer with meat consumption, especially prostate cancer.

2. Other studies found no correlation between meat consumption and cancer, including prostate cancer.

3. Several studies showed a correlation with well-done, overcooked, charred meat and increased risk of cancer.

4. Numerous studies have found a correlation between processed meats and increased cancer risk, especially colorectal cancer.

5. Meat consumption was found to reduce the consumption of foods that reduce the risk of cancer, such as fruits and vegetables, nuts and seeds, whole grain products, legumes, and fish.

6. A couple of studies showed an inverse correlation between meat consumption and cancer. However, this was only when the meat eaters also had the highest consumption of fruits and vegetables.

What does this all mean? I submit the following conclusions:

1. Meat, especially processed meats, can increase the risk of some cancers, especially prostate cancer. There is also some indication meat can increase the risk of breast cancer.

2. Overcooked meat is definitely a risk. But undercooked meat has its own risks. As such, if you are going to eat meat, you have to be very careful about how it is cooked. Overcooking it can cause carcinogens; undercook it, and there's the risk of food poisoning.

3. A high intake of meat can replace foods that can reduce cancer risk. And the higher in fat a meat is, the more potentially beneficial calories it will replace.

4. Fruits and vegetables provide the greatest protection against cancer, so whatever else you eat, be sure to eat plenty of fruits and vegetables!

5. The difference between factory farm and old-fashioned meats is not addressed in any of these studies. If that distinction was held, then the results might be quite different.

For Those Who Are Already Suffering

Does any of this information apply to those already suffering with heart disease or cancer, or have already had a heart attack or stroke, or are struggling with any of a myriad of other possible health maladies? The answer of course depends on which malady you are suffering with.

But first, let me say, my heart and prayers go out to you if you are struggling with such problems. I have never had cancer, heart disease, or a stroke, but many who are close to me have. As such, I know how difficult it can be to deal with such problems, both on a physical and emotional level. I myself have struggled with many health problems in my life, as I will relate in Chapter Eighteen.

But here; in regard to cancer, I will not claim as many do for their diet plans that following a Creationist Diet will cure cancer. No diet will, despite what many might claim. Sure, you will find testimonies of people on the Internet who claim to have been healed of cancer by following a raw foods diet or vegan diet or Paleolithic diet or whatever kind of diet. But if you are able to do follow-ups, you will often find those same people later relapsed and died from their cancer. Moreover, as any cancer specialist will tell you, there are cases of people having spontaneous remissions for no apparent reason, though those who do will try to attribute it to something they did, such as a change in diet.

However, I have no doubt that following a healthy diet will enable a cancer sufferer to better deal with their situation, both in in regard to the physical symptoms of the disease and the side effects of treatment and in regard to the emotional trauma such can cause. The latter was addressed in the study on fibromyalgia that was cited in Chapter Seven. There it was said that those who ate a healthy diet had "more favorable psychosocial outcomes" such as more optimism and less depression. As noted there, that has been my experience with my own health struggles.

Now I know many who are suffering with cancer or other maladies might have little appetite or even nausea due to the symptoms of their disease or side effects of treatments like chemotherapy or radiotherapy. But I would encourage you to eat as best as you are able to keep your strength up, and try to make what you do eat be as healthy as possible.

I would also suggest you avoid as much as possible the artificial food ingredients, pesticides, GMOs, hormones, antibiotics, mercury, and other chemicals in non-God-given foods, including in commercial produce and factory farm animal foods. Your body already has enough of a toxic load on it from the treatments and enough to deal with from the disease without adding even more toxins for your body to clear.

Of all times, this is the time to spend the extra money on organic, non-GMO plant foods and old-fashioned meats, dairy, and eggs, and to eat only low-mercury, clean fish. And yes, such animal foods should be eaten if possible for the protein and other nutrients they provide, though the emphasis should be on organic fruits and vegetables. Drink fruit and vegetables juice if that is all you can tolerate, though whole produce would be best.

Now it might be tempting when diagnosed with a life-threatening disorder to just "throw in the towel," accept you are going to die, and then figure you will "will live it up" by eating lots of junk food in your remaining days. But if you do that, those remaining days will be much harder to bear, the pain will probably be worse, you'll have even less energy, and your emotional state will be worse.

As a result, you will be less able to enjoy your final days with your family and friends, but instead will be an even greater burden on them. But if you follow a healthy diet, all of this will be better, and, at the least, you will maintain some sense of control over your life. As a website about pancreatic cancer states, "Nutrition is an important part of your care. Getting the right nutrition can help you feel better and have more strength" (Pancreatic.org).

For those who have heart disease or have already had a heart attack or stroke, then yes, following a healthy diet can make a huge difference in the progress of your disease and the likelihood of a recurrence. This has been demonstrated by many studies that have been conducted in this regard. And the emotional benefit, including a sense of well-being and of being in control, would also apply here.

Then there are diseases that are directly related to diet, such as type II diabetes. This is a disease that should not be taken lightly. I have had a couple of people close to me first go blind, then have heart attacks, lose all ability to take care of themselves, and finally to die from this disease. But there is no doubt that a healthy diet can make an immense difference in forestalling all of this.

Simply put, no matter what you are suffering with, a healthy diet will enable you to better deal with it both physically and emotionally.

However, I would be remiss if I did not say that making an even greater difference would be faith in the LORD. That is the theme of my book *The LORD Has It Under Control* (see Appendix One). In it, I relate my own struggles and how faith in the sovereignty of God has pulled me through them and enabled me to deal with them.

With that serious discussion behind us, the next chapter will investigate other dietary factors to be considered in following a Creationist Diet.

Bibliography:

Hu FB, Stampfer MJ, Rimm EB, Manson JE, Ascherio A, Colditz GA, Rosner BA, Spiegelman D, Speizer FE, Sacks FM, Hennekens CH, Willett WC. *Journal of the American Medical Association*. 1999 Apr 21;281(15):1387-94. A prospective study of egg consumption and risk of cardiovascular disease in men and women.

Joshipura KJ, Ascherio A, Manson JE, Stampfer MJ, Rimm EB, Speizer FE, Hennekens CH, Spiegelman D, Willett WC. *Journal of the American Medical Association* 1999 Oct 6;282(13):1233-9. Fruit and vegetable intake in relation to risk of ischemic stroke.

Merritt, MA, et. al. *Cancer Causes Control*. 2014 Jul;25(7):795-808. Dairy food and nutrient intake in different life periods in relation to risk of ovarian cancer.
https://www.ncbi.nlm.nih.gov/pubmed/24722953

Richman, EL, *Cancer Prevention Resource* (Phila). 2011 Dec;4(12):2110-21. Egg, red meat, and poultry intake and risk of lethal prostate cancer in the prostate-specific antigen-era: incidence and survival. https://www.ncbi.nlm.nih.gov/pubmed/21930800

Rohrmann S, et. al. International Journal of Cancer. 2013 Feb 1;132(3):617-24.Meat and fish consumption and risk of pancreatic cancer: results from the European Prospective Investigation into Cancer and Nutrition. https://www.ncbi.nlm.nih.gov/pubmed/22610753

Pancreatic.org. Nutrition.
http://pancreatic.org/pancreatic-cancer/supportive-care/nutrition/

Webb PM, Bain CJ, Purdie DM, Harvey PW, Green A. *Cancer Causes Control* 1998 Dec;9(6):637-44. Milk consumption, galactose metabolism and ovarian cancer. Australia.

Wilson KM, et. al. *Cancer Prevention Resource* (Phila). 2016 Dec;9(12):933-941. Epub 2016 Sep 20. Meat, Fish, Poultry, and Egg Intake at Diagnosis and Risk of Prostate Cancer Progression.
https://www.ncbi.nlm.nih.gov/pubmed/27651069

Chapter Fifteen:
Caloric Distributions

So far in this book, no reference has been made to caloric distributions, as in what percentage of calories should come from fat, carbohydrates (carbs), and protein. The reason for this is simple— people do not eat fats, carbs, and protein; people eat foods. In other words, most people do not calculate what caloric distributions each of their meals contain. And doing so could get rather tedious very quickly. But what people eat are foods. As such, the emphasis of this book has been on which foods are healthiest and which are not so healthy.

That said, there is major debate raging today as to which is the best kind of diet in regard to caloric distribution, both for weight loss as well as for health in general. Since the 1970's, most nutritionists have been recommending people eat a low-fat diet. But of late, low-carb diets are the rage.

So where does the Creationist Diet fit into this debate? Is it a low-fat or a low-carb diet, or something in-between? Before answering this question, some definitions would be helpful.

Definitions

What is meant by "low-fat?" This is where confusion often comes in, as people often don't define terms. The "low-fat" diet recommended by the American Heart Association has 25-30% of calories from fat, with only 5-10% being from saturated fats. It then has about 15% of calories from protein, and the remaining 55-60% from carbs.

Dr. Dean Ornish's plan is a very low-fat diet. It restricts fat intake to 10%, with less than 5% being from saturated fat. Protein levels are 15-20%, and the remaining 70-75% from carbs.

Next is the term "low-carb." How low is "low?" Dr. Sears' "The Zone Diet" would be a low-carb diet. It recommends 40% carbs, 30% protein, and 30% fat, with 6% saturated fat.

Dr. Atkin's plan would be a very low-carb diet. He doesn't specify caloric distributions, but calculations on it put it at about 22% protein,

50% fat, with 25% from saturated fat, and the remaining 18% from carbs (*Nutrition Action*, p.6).

Using these different diets as guidelines, for the purposes of this book, a low-fat diet will be defined as one having 20-30% fat, 15% protein, and 55-65% carbs. A very low-fat diet will be a diet with 10-20% fat, 15% protein, and 65-75% carbs.

Conversely, a low-carb diet has 30-40% fat, 20-30% protein, and 30-40% carbs. A very low-carb diet has 50-60% fat, 20-30% protein, and 10-30% carbs.

Extremes Eliminated

Are any of these rather different dietary proportions compatible with a Creationist Diet? A low-fat diet can include some animal foods, along with nuts and seeds. But for a very low-fat diet, you almost have to follow a vegan diet. Also on a very low-fat diet, eating nuts and seeds would not be possible, or at least be very limited.

To attain a low-carb diet would necessitate the elimination of most grain foods from the diet. A very low-carb diet, along with eliminating grains, would also require eliminating fruits and "starchy" vegetables like potatoes. Only low-carb vegetables, such as leafy greens, would be permitted. Conversely, the amount of animal foods would need to be increased in both these diets to make up the calories.

Thus in a low-fat or very low-fat diet, the emphasis would be on plant-foods, whereas in the low-carb or very low-carb diets, the bulk of calories would be from animal foods. So it can be seen that these diets are very different. But would any of them fit into a Creationist Diet?

Fruits and vegetables and nuts and seeds are definitely a part of a Creationist Diet. So just these points would eliminate both a very low-fat and a very low-carb diet.

As indicated, the consumption of nuts and seeds would be very limited at a 10% fat level, so it would not fit with a Creationist Diet as these are basic foods in the Creationist Diet. On the other hand, a very low-carb diet would also not fit, as such a diet requires the elimination of fruits and certain vegetables. But fruits and all kinds of vegetables are also basic foods in the Creationist Diet. Moreover, there would be no reason to believe that the earliest humans would have been "choosy" about which vegetables they ate based on their "starch" content.

400

Low-fat Preferred

So that leaves the two more moderate diets, low-fat and low-carb. By eating little or no animal foods and only moderate amounts of nuts and seeds, one would end up with a low-fat diet. And this would be compatible with the Creationist Diet.

Conversely, by including meats and other animals foods and copious amounts of nuts and seeds, while limiting the amounts of whole grains, one could end up with a low-carb diet. But the amount of animal foods needed would be more than what has been recommended since animal foods are a "later" addition to the human diet.

Therefore, of these two choices, the low-fat diet would be the most compatible with the Creationist Diet. And most people will get "results" from such a diet. But some people claim to have tried a low-fat diet but without results. But they then try a low-carb diet and get results.

By "results" is usually meant weight loss, lowering of total and LDL ("bad") cholesterol levels, raising of HDL ("good") cholesterol, more energy, and/ or a general sense of well-being. But it should be noted, all these things take time and can be affected by other factors, such as exercise. Also, bodyweight and blood lipid levels are measurable factors, but energy levels and a sense of well-being are subjective.

For the measurable items, I would recommend having a blood test, including testing for total cholesterol, LDL cholesterol, HDL cholesterol, and triglycerides levels before making any dietary changes, and again several months into the new diet. Only with these objective standards can you know if the new diet is working, though emotional factors cannot be ignored.

An Alternative

But what about the person who doesn't get results from either a low-fat or a low-carb diet? There is an alternative—a diet that is somewhat in-between. Specifically, this would be a diet that has about 30-40% of calories from fat, but, and this is very important, the majority of these fat calories should be in the form of the "good" monounsaturated kind. And, as with the low-fat diet, only 10% of the fats should be from saturated fats. It would then have about 15-20% protein, and 40-55% carbs. Such a diet could be called a moderate-fat/ moderate carb diet.

In fact, this kind of diet was the point about the study on peanuts performed at this writer's alma mater that was referred to earlier in this book. As reported on PRNewswire:

> The study, conducted by Dr. Penny Kris-Etherton and researchers at Penn State University, showed that **a diet with peanuts and peanut butter reduced risk of heart disease by 21% while the low-fat diet reduced it by only 12%**. Dr. Kris-Etherton adds, "Our study shows that people can now include some of their favorite foods, peanuts and peanut butter, in a high-mono, heart-healthy diet and achieve even better results than with a low-fat diet."

More recently, Penn State performed a similar study with similar results, but this time using avocados as the monounsaturated fat source:

> Results from a recent nutrition study led by Pennsylvania State University show that eating **a moderate fat diet with fresh avocado may benefit cholesterol levels more than moderate fat or low fat diets without avocado**. Published in the *Journal of the American Heart Association*, the research found that healthy, overweight and obese men and women who followed a moderate fat diet that included one fresh avocado daily **had significantly improved bad cholesterol to good cholesterol ratios** compared to when eating a similar moderate fat or low fat diet without avocados....
>
> "The results of this study suggest that the monounsaturated fat, fiber, phytosterols and other dietary bioactives in avocados may provide greater benefits to cardiovascular disease risk factors compared to a calorie matched low fat diet," said Penny Kris-Etherton, Ph.D., RD, lead author of the study who is an expert in cardiovascular nutrition and Distinguished Professor at the Pennsylvania State University (PRN Newswire. Avocados).

Another study, this one from University at Buffalo, confirms the benefit of a moderate-fat diet:

> Participants who consumed a diet containing **33 percent fat (moderate fat) reduced their cardiovascular risk by 14 percent**, based on their lipid profiles, findings showed. Those consuming a diet containing **18 percent fat (low fat) reduced their lipid-based risk by nine percent**....
>
> **Carbohydrates replaced the calories from saturated fats in the low-fat diet, while monounsaturated fats replaced saturated fats in the moderate-fat diet**. Chemical analysis of the diets validated the composition of the two diets.
>
> During the weight-loss period, **both groups lowered their total and LDL cholesterol, but the low-fat group also experienced a 12 percent drop in HDL cholesterol**. Triglycerides dropped in both groups, as well. However, during the weight-maintenance phase, there was a reversal of the weight-loss induced drop in triglycerides and a reduction in HDL cholesterol compared to baseline in the low-fat group, but not in the moderate-fat group.
>
> "These results show that although weight loss does improve the lipid profile, **a moderate-fat, weight-loss diet reduces risk more than a low-fat, weight-loss diet**, so dieters don't need to cut out all the fat to improve their risk profile," Pelkman said. "**Monounsaturated fats can be a healthy part of a weight-loss diet**" (Science Daily. Moderate).

In addition to peanuts and avocadoes, nuts, seeds (and nut and seed oils and butters), olive oil, peanut oil, fish, and grass-fed beef also contain the healthy monounsaturated fats. A diet emphasizing these foods could be the most heart-protective of all. And such a diet would fit perfectly well with the Creationist Diet.

Summary on Diet Proportions

The parameters of the Creationist Diet would disallow "extremes" in caloric proportions, such as very low-fat or very low-carb diets.

403

However, the proportions of the various God-given foods can be manipulated to give a low-carb, a low-fat, or a moderate-fat diet. Which one of these the reader should follow would be a matter of personal experimentation. But it will be said; the Creationist Diet does fit best with either of the latter two (low-fat and moderate-fat), and not too well with the former (low-carb). But before deciding which type of diet to follow, there are a few other matters worth considering.

Metabolic Syndrome Basics

Metabolic syndrome is another condition to consider before deciding what caloric proportions would be best for you. Other names for it are: Dysmetabolic syndrome, Hypertriglyceridemic waist, Insulin resistance syndrome, Obesity syndrome, Syndrome X, Nonalcoholic fatty liver disease (NAFLD), with the severest form being called nonalcoholic steatohepatitis (NASH) (NIH; Names. Zivkovic).

Metabolic syndrome is characterized by five risk factors. If you have three or more of these, you probably have metabolic syndrome.

- increased blood pressure (greater than 130/85 mmHg)
- high blood sugar levels (insulin resistance)
- excess fat around the waist
- high triglyceride levels
- low levels of good cholesterol, or HDL (Healthline. Metabolic Syndrome).

Metabolic syndrome is rather common. "The American Heart Association (AHA) reports that 23 percent of adults currently have metabolic syndrome" (Healthline. Metabolic Syndrome).

This percentage is not surprising given that most Americans are overweight and do not exercise, while "The risk of having metabolic syndrome is closely linked to overweight and obesity and a lack of physical activity" (NIH. Metabolic Syndrome).

The obvious answer to this condition would be to lose weight and to exercise. But what type of diet is best for those with metabolic syndrome? Unfortunately, that is not an easy question to answer. But some parameters can be ascertained.

> **There is no consensus as to what diet or lifestyle approach is the right one for NAFLD and NASH patients**, largely because of a lack of scientific evidence. It is likely that **there will be no one correct approach for all NAFLD patients**, and diets will therefore need to be tailored to individual needs. **The inclusion of n−3 [omega 3] fatty acids, high-MUFA [monounsaturated fatty acids] foods, fruit, vegetables, and low-GI [glycemic index], high-fiber foods and reduced intakes of saturated fats, simple carbohydrates, and sweetened drinks may be universally recommended to NAFLD patients.** More studies are needed to clarify the specific effects of different diets and dietary components on the health of NAFLD patients. The general recommendations described in this review may be a useful guide for determining the appropriate diet for individual patients now, while evidence-based recommendations from future clinical trials are assembled (Zivkovic).

No caloric distribution is specifically mentioned, but the types of foods recommended would fit best with a moderate-fat Creationist Diet. Note also that the recommended foods are all God-given foods, while non-God- given foods are contradicted.

Diabetes and Hypoglycemia

Related to the preceding would be diabetes and hypoglycemia. Diabetes is high blood sugar or hyperglycemia, while hypoglycemia is the opposite, low blood sugar. But despite being opposites, the goal for both conditions is the same—keep blood sugar levels from fluctuating too high or too low. But eating a low-fat/ high-carb diet would play havoc with blood sugar. I first thought of this potential blood sugar problem with high-carb diets back in college, when I was majoring in Nutrition Science (Penn State; '83).

We were studying diabetes, and I remember clearly the professor saying, "We used to put diabetics on low-carb, high-fat diets, but they

405

were dropping like flies from heart disease." So now she was saying the recommendation was for a high complex carb diet.

I remember thinking, "If diabetics have a problem with carbs, then why put them on a high-carb diet?" I just wished I had spoken up and asked the professor that question back then. It made no sense to me then and still does not today. But I'm not recommending a low-carb diet for those with blood sugar problems. The reason such a diet caused people to "drop like flies" was because it was high in saturated fats. A moderate-fat diet with an emphasis on unsaturated fats will work just as well at controlling blood sugar but with a decreased not elevated heart disease risk. It is also nowhere near as restrictive as a low-carb diet. Also, consider the following:

New research adds clarity to the connection between a high fat diet and type 2 diabetes. The study finds that **saturated fatty acids but not the unsaturated type can activate immune cells to produce an inflammatory protein, called interleukin-1beta** (Science Daily. Link).

The most recent position statement on nutrition from the **American Diabetes Association recommends** an individualized approach to nutrition that is based on the nutritional assessment and desired outcomes of each patient and that takes into consideration patient preferences and control of hyperglycemia and dyslipidemia. To achieve these nutritional goals, **either low-saturated-fat, high-carbohydrate diets or high-monounsaturated-fat diets can be advised**. A meta-analysis of various studies comparing these two approaches to diet therapy in patients with type 2 diabetes revealed that **high-monounsaturated-fat diets improve lipoprotein profiles as well as glycemic [blood sugar] control** (Garg.).

Based on these data, we tested the efficacy of diets with various **protein—carbohydrate—fat ratios** for 5 weeks on blood glucose control in people with untreated type 2 diabetes. The results were compared to those obtained in the same subjects after 5 weeks on a **control diet** with a protein—carbohydrate—fat ratio of **15:55:30**. **A 30:40:30 ratio diet** resulted in a moderate but significant decrease in 24-hour integrated glucose area and % total glycohemoglobin (%tGHb). A 30:20:50 ratio diet resulted in a 38% decrease in 24-hour glucose area, a reduction in fasting glucose to near normal and a decrease in %tGHb from 9.8% to 7.6%. The response to a 30:30:40 ratio diet was similar (BioMed).

Thus my misgivings about a high card diet for diabetes from college have been proven true—a moderate-fat/ moderate-carb diet is best for controlling blood sugar levels and for heart health.

Testosterone Levels

Chapter Four discussed that saturated fats and monounsaturated fats increases testosterone levels. This is seen in the followings study:

Preexercise T was significantly positively correlated with percent energy fat, SFA (g · 1,000 kcal−1 · day−1), and MUFA (g · 1,000 kcal−1 · day−1) and was significantly negatively correlated with the percent energy protein, the PUFA/SFA ratio, and the protein-to-carbohydrate ratio....

Our results demonstrated that dietary protein, fat, SFA, MUFA, PUFA/SFA ratio, and protein-to-carbohydrate ratio were all significantly correlated with preexercise T [testosterone] concentrations. However, none of these dietary variables were significantly correlated with C [cortisol] concentrations. These data are consistent with the findings of several other investigations that have reported a decrease in T in individuals consuming a diet containing ~20% fat compared with a diet containing ~40% fat (7, 9, 13, 25). Vegetarians also consume less fat, SFA, and a higher PUFA/SFA ratio compared with omnivores, and vegetarians exhibit lower concentrations of T compared with omnivores (3, 11, 12, 15, 24). These data suggest that alteration in dietary energy and/or dietary composition has the potential to modify T concentrations (Voltek).

To be clear, this study is saying a higher amount of fat, saturated fatty acids (SFA), and monounsaturated fatty acids (MUFA) increased testosterone levels, but a higher amount of protein and polyunsaturated fatty acids (PUFA) decreased testosterone levels. But in regards to protein:

> Also, **the source from which the protein is derived may influence T concentrations**. Raben et al. compared the effects of two diets differing only in the source of protein in male athletes. Results showed a **reduced resting and post-exercise increase in T concentrations in athletes consuming protein derived mainly from vegetable sources compared with a diet with protein derived mainly from animal sources** (Volek).

Thus it is only plant sourced protein that reduces testosterone levels, not animal sourced protein. The tendency of soy to decrease testosterone levels might be a factor here. And this is another possible reason (along with little or no cholesterol intake) why vegetarians and especially vegans tend to have lower testosterone levels than omnivores.

But in regard to caloric distribution, concerns about keeping testosterone levels elevated would point towards a moderate-fat or low-carb diet as being more ideal than a low-fat diet.

Exercise and Carb Intake

The next question is, what level of carbohydrate intake is best for exercise performance? Consider the following:

> In spite of your body's improved use of fat and ketones after you have been on a low-carb regimen for several weeks, **it's an undeniable fact that fat will never be your body's first choice of fuel during moderate and intense workouts lasting more than a couple of minutes**. If carbs are available, your body will use them over fats, especially as your workout gets more intense. **It simply comes down to how the body works,** and **using carbs is more fuel efficient** -- that is, you get more energy out of carbs for a given quantity of oxygen (5.05 vs. 4.7

calories per gram for carbs and fats, respectively). Carbs are like using a higher-octane fuel, resulting in more miles to the gallon.

If you want to exercise intensely and you eat a low-carb diet, you will simply not be able to perform at the highest level possible. However, if you're eating enough calories to cover your body's basal needs and your exercise use, **you can easily get by with 40% or less of your calories coming from carbs.** Eating more carbs than that will not necessarily benefit exercise (it is NOT a case of "some is good, so more is better"). I do believe that **most people who are training overdo their carb intake**, given the limited amount and intensity of training that they do. For example, you really don't need to eat a huge pasta dinner the night before you do a 5K (3.1 mile) run (Colberg-Ochs).

We investigated the effects of adaptation to a ketogenic low-carbohydrate (CHO), high-fat diet (LCHF) during 3 wk of intensified training on metabolism and performance of world-class endurance athletes. We controlled three isoenergetic diets in elite race walkers: High CHO availability (8.6 g.kg- 1.d-1 CHO, 2.1 g.kg- 1.d-1 protein; 1.2 g.kg- 1.d-1 fat) consumed before/during/after training (HCHO, n = 9): identical macronutrient intake, periodised within/between days to alternate between low and high CHO availability (PCHO, n = 10); LCHF (<50 g.d-1 CHO; 78% energy as fat; 2.1 g.kg- 1.d-1 protein; LCHF, n = 10)....

In contrast to training with diets providing chronic or periodised high-CHO availability, and despite a significant improvement in VO2peak, **adaptation to the topical LCHF diet negated performance benefits in elite endurance athletes**, in part, due to reduced exercise economy (Burke. *Journal*).

During the period 1985-2005, studies examined the proposal that adaptation to a low-carbohydrate (<25 % energy), high-fat (>60 % energy) diet (LCHF) to increase muscle fat utilization during exercise could enhance performance in trained individuals by reducing reliance on

409

muscle glycogen. As little as 5 days of training with LCHF retools the muscle to enhance fat-burning capacity with robust changes that persist despite acute strategies to restore carbohydrate availability (e.g., glycogen supercompensation, carbohydrate intake during exercise). Furthermore, a 2- to 3-week exposure to minimal carbohydrate (<20 g/day) intake achieves adaptation to high blood ketone concentrations.

However, **the failure to detect clear performance benefits during endurance/ultra-endurance protocols, combined with evidence of impaired performance of high-intensity exercise via a down-regulation of carbohydrate metabolism** led this author to dismiss the use of such fat-adaptation strategies by competitive athletes in conventional sports. Recent re-emergence of interest in LCHF diets, coupled with anecdotes of improved performance by sportspeople who follow them, has created a need to re-examine the potential benefits of this eating style. Unfortunately, **the absence of new data prevents a different conclusion from being made**. Notwithstanding the outcomes of future research, there is a need for better recognition of current sports nutrition guidelines that promote an individualized and periodized approach to fuel availability during training, allowing the athlete to prepare for competition performance with metabolic flexibility and optimal utilization of all muscle substrates. Nevertheless, **there may be a few scenarios where LCHF diets are of benefit, or at least are not detrimental, for sports performance** (Burke. *Sports*).

So the best currently available evidence is a low-carb diet does not improve exercise performance and could very well be detrimental to it.

Moreover, there is a popular belief that exercising in a fasting state will cause the body to burn fat for fuel rather than carbs. It is therefore recommended that people do cardio first thing in the morning before breakfast. But the research does not bear out this claim:

Skeletal muscle gene response to exercise depends on nutritional status during and after exercise, but it is unknown whether muscle adaptations to endurance training are affected by nutritional status during training sessions. Therefore, this study investigated the effect of an endurance training program (6 wk, 3 day/wk, 1–2 h, 75% of peak $\dot{V}o2$) in moderately active males. **They trained in the fasted (F; n = 10) or carbohydrate-fed state (CHO; n = 10) while receiving a standardized diet** [65 percent of total energy intake (En) from carbohydrates, 20%En fat, 15%En protein]....

Although there was a decrease in exercise-induced glycogen breakdown and an increase in proteins involved in fat handling after fasting training, **fat oxidation during exercise with carbohydrate intake was not changed** (De Bock).

Thus low-carb is not the way to go. But what percentage of carbs is best for exercise performance? Consider the following:

Six male football [soccer] players competed in a 90 min game (4-a-side) on two occasions following an exercise and diet (either high- approximately 65% or low- approximately 30% carbohydrate intake) regimen designed to manipulate muscle glycogen concentrations. Movement and technical parameters of performance and selected physiological responses were measured. Pre-game muscle glycogen concentrations following the high carbohydrate diet (mean +/- SD) (395.6 +/- 78.3 mmol x kg(-1) dw) were significantly higher than following the low carbohydrate diet (287.1 +/- 85.4 mmol x kg(-1) dw). **The results of the movement analysis showed that the players performed significantly more (approximately 33%) high intensity exercise in the game played following the high carbohydrate diet.** No significant differences were found, between the two dietary conditions, in any of the measured technical variables....

The main finding from this study was that the **carbohydrate content of the diet influenced the amount of high intensity exercise performed** during a small-sided football game. This suggests that to optimise performances, in not only football but possibly also other multiple sprint sports of similar duration, **a high carbohydrate diet should be administered in preparation for intense training and competition** (Balsom).

This study was designed to examine the effects of alterations in dietary carbohydrate (CHO) intake on the performance of high-intensity exercise lasting approximately 10 min (EXP 1) and 30 min (EXP 2). Trained subjects exercised to exhaustion on four occasions on a cycle ergometer at 90% of maximal oxygen consumption (VO2max; EXP 1, n = 5) and 80% of VO2max (EXP 2, n = 7). The first two tests were familiarisation trials and were carried out following the subjects' normal diet. Normal training was continued but standardised during the periods of dietary control. The subsequent two tests were performed 2 weeks apart after 7 days of dietary manipulation. **The two diets were a 70% and a 40% CHO diet,** isoenergetic with each subject's normal diet and administered in a randomised order. At both exercise intensities, **time to exhaustion following the high CHO and low CHO diets was not different** [mean (SD) EXP 1: 11.56 (3.78) min and 8.95 (2.35) min, P = 0.22; EXP 2: 26.9 (7.4) min and 26.5 (6.5) min, P = 0.90]....

No differences in oxygen uptake, heart rate (EXP 2) or ratings of perceived exertion (both experiments) were found between conditions. These results indicate that **moderate changes in diet composition during training do not affect the performance of high-intensity exercise in trained individuals when the total energy intake is moderately high** (Pitsiladis).

Thus in the first study, a 30% carb levels reduced exercise performance, while in the second study a 40% carb level did not. As such, it would appear that a 40% carb level is the minimum for optimal exercise performance. However, there is not much advantage to going much higher for the average person or even athlete. The only exception might be ultra-endurance athletes such as marathoners and tri-athletes.

Strength Training and Protein Intake

The next issue to consider is protein intake. What type of exercise someone does, if any, affects their protein needs. Strength athletes require more protein than sedentary individuals and even more than endurance athletes, and both types of athletes need more than the Recommend Daily Allowance (RDA) of 0.8 grams/ kilogram [0.36 grams/ pound]. But the exact recommendations vary:

Although there remains some debate, recent evidence suggests that **dietary protein need increases with rigorous physical exercise**. Those involved in **strength training** might need to consume as much as **1.6 to 1.7 g [grams] protein x kg [kilogram]** (-1) [0.72 to 0.77 grams/ pound] x day(-1) (approximately **twice the current RDA**) while those undergoing **endurance training** might need about **1.2 to 1.6 g x kg**(-1) x [0.55 to 0.72 g/lb] day(-1) (approximately 1.5 times the current RDA)" (Lemon, *International*).

... since the 1970s, an increasing number of studies have appeared that indicate dietary protein needs are elevated in individuals who are regularly physically active. Together, these data suggest that the RDA for those who engage in regular **endurance exercise** should be about **1.2-1.4 g protein/kg [0.55 to 0.64 g/lb]** body mass/d (150-175% of the current RDA) and **1.7-1.8 g protein/kg body [0.77 to 0.82 g/lb] mass/d (212-225% of the current RDA) for strength exercisers** (Lemon, *Nutrition*).

While protein needs of both endurance and power athletes are greater than that of non-athletes, they're not as high as commonly perceived. The Academy of Nutrition and Dietetics, Dietitians of Canada and the American College of Sports Medicine recommend the following for power and endurance athletes, based on body weight:

• **Power athletes (strength or speed): 1.2 to 1.7 grams/kilogram a day**
• **Endurance athletes: 1.2 to 1.4 grams/kilogram a day** (Protein and the Athlete)

The average adult needs 0.8 grams per kilogram (2.2lbs) of body weight per day.

• **Strength training athletes need about 1.4 to 1.8 grams per kilogram** (2.2lbs) of body weight per day

• **Endurance athletes need about 1.2 to 1.4 grams per kilogram** (2.2lbs) of body weight per day (Sports Nutrition)

Consequently, growing evidence indicates that **strength athletes should ingest quantities of protein at the upper end of the range of 1.5 to 2.0 g/kg per day**, as well as ingest protein or amino acids either before, during, or after exercise (or at more than one of these times) in order to optimize training adaptations (Campbell).

• We don't know how much protein is required to optimize all of the potential pathways important to athletes.

• We know that **a protein intake of 1.4 g/lb (3.0 g/kg) isn't harmful and may have benefits that are too small to be measured in research.**

• As long as eating lots of protein doesn't keep an athlete from eating too few of the other nutrients (carbs/fats), there's no reason to not eat a lot. And there may be benefits. (Protein Requirements).

The range for strength athletes is 1.2-3.0 grams of protein per kilogram of bodyweight. That works out to 0.54-1.4 grams/ pound. That is a large range. But many strength athletes (such as powerlifters and bodybuilders) would scoff at the lower end and would claim 1.0-1.5 grams/ pound is needed.

The range for endurance athletes is 1.2-1.6 grams / kilogram. That works out to 0.54-0.73 grams per pound, less than commonly perceived and far less than the claims of strength athletes. But to put these numbers into a percentage of calories is difficult given the wide range of calories an athlete might consume

The average for non-athletes, at least the standard used on food labels, is 2,000 calories/ day. But athletes would consume more, and in the case of large strength athletes and ultra-endurance athletes, much more, as much as 5,000-10,000 calories/ day.

But to use a number somewhat in-between these extremes and using the 1.0-1.5 gram/ pound claims of strength athletes, a 180-pound strength athlete would need from 180-270 grams of protein. At four calories/ gram, this would require 360-1,080 calories worth of protein. At 3000 calories, an amount such an athlete would easily consume, this would be 25-36% of calories. Meanwhile, if the same sized person were an endurance athlete, he or she would need 97-131 grams or 13-17% of calories from protein.

To round off these numbers, it would put the protein recommendation at 15-35% of calories. The upper end of this range is far higher than is generally recommended, but again, it is what many strength athletes have found to be beneficial.

And it should be noted that the last quote reiterates that claims of a high protein intake being deleterious are not true. But I should state, there is some evidence that a very high protein intake reduces testosterone levels, but that is for an intake of 44% of calories, much higher than the 15-35% being recommended here.

It should also be noted that consumption of protein and carbs immediately before and after a workout is beneficial for muscle growth and recovery from the workout. I address pre- and post-workout nutrition at length in my *Starting and Progressing in Powerlifting* book (see Appendix's One), so I will not repeat that information here. But it will be said, it would be best if athletes consume a snack or meal 1-2 hours before a workout and a major meal or some kind of post-workout drink immediately after a workout. That way, they will consume both protein and carbs in adequate amounts at a time when the body needs them most.

Recommended Caloric Proportions

With this information, recommended caloric proportions would be:

Carbs: 40-60%
Protein: 15-35%
Fat: 20-40% (with <10% of calories from saturated fat)

Endurance athletes should aim for the higher end of the carb range, while ultra-endurance athletes, like marathoners and triathletes, might

415

need to go even higher. But strength athletes should aim for the higher end of the fat range for the testosterone boost fat provides and of the protein range for the muscle building properties of protein.

For non-athletes who do not have blood sugar problems, the higher levels of carbs and lower levels of fat would be recommended. But for those with blood sugar problems or who have not had "success" with low-fat diets before, then the lower levels of carbs and higher levels of fat should be tried. For everyone else, it is simply recommended to experiment within these ranges to see what works best for you.

By manipulating the proportions of God-given foods, it is possible to attain these differing caloric distributions. As such, the Creationist Diet can provide for athletes, or anyone who exercises, as well as for people with blood sugar problems.

Of course, if your doctor recommends a diet with specific caloric distributions for a given health condition, by all means follow his or her advice. But don't be afraid to ask your doctor exactly why he or she is recommending that specific diet.

Bibliography:

Balsom PD, Wood K, Olsson P, Ekblom B. *International Journal of Sports Medicine* 1999 Jan;20(1):48-52. Carbohydrate intake and multiple sprint sports: with special reference to football [soccer]. https://www.ncbi.nlm.nih.gov/pubmed/10090462

BioMed. Control of blood glucose in type 2 diabetes without weight loss by modification of diet composition. http://nutritionandmetabolism.biomedcentral.com/articles/10.1186/1743-7075-3-16

Burke LM, et.al. *Journal of Physiology.* 2016 Dec 23. Low Carbohydrate, High Fat diet impairs exercise economy and negates the performance benefit from intensified training in elite race walkers. https://www.ncbi.nlm.nih.gov/pubmed/28012184

Burke LM. *Sports Medicine.* 2015 Nov;45 Suppl 1:S33-49. Re-Examining High-Fat Diets for Sports Performance: Did We Call the 'Nail in the Coffin' Too Soon? https://www.ncbi.nlm.nih.gov/pubmed/26553488

Campbell et al. 2007; Kerksick et al. 2008; Lemon 2001; Protein intake in relation to performance.

http://www.humankinetics.com/excerpts/excerpts/protein-intake-in-relation-to-performance

De Bock, K., et. al. Journal of Applied Physiology Published 1 April 2008 Vol. 104 no. 4, 1045-1055. Effect of training in the fasted state on metabolic responses during exercise with carbohydrate intake. http://jap.physiology.org/content/104/4/1045.short

Colberg-Ochs, Sheri, Dr. Does Low-Carb Eating Compromise Your Ability to Exercise? http://www.shericolberg.com/exercise-columns16.asp

Garg, A. *American Journal of Clinical Nutrition.* 1998 Mar;67(3 Suppl):577S-582S.High-monounsaturated-fat diets for patients with diabetes mellitus: a meta-analysis. https://www.ncbi.nlm.nih.gov/pubmed/17490960

Healthline. Metabolic Syndrome. http://www.healthline.com/health/metabolic-syndrome#Overview1

NIH (National Institutes of Health). Other Names for Metabolic Syndrome. https://www.nhlbi.nih.gov/health/health-topics/topics/ms/names

NIH. What is Metabolic Syndrome? https://www.nhlbi.nih.gov/health/health-topics/topics/ms

Nutrition Action HealthLetter. Vol. 27, No. 2, March 2000, "Syndrome X: The Risks of High Insulin"," pp.1,3-8.

Pitsiladis YP, Maughan RJ. *European Journal of Applied Physiology.* 1999 Apr;79(5):433-42; The effects of alterations in dietary carbohydrate intake on the performance of high-intensity exercise in trained individuals. https://www.ncbi.nlm.nih.gov/pubmed/10208253

PRN Newswire. New Research Looks Closer at Effects of a Moderate Fat Diet that Includes Eating Avocados Daily. http://www.prnewswire.com/news-releases/new-research-looks-closer-at-effects-of-a-moderate-fat-diet-that-includes-eating-avocados-daily-300029721.html

Protein Requirements for Strength and Power Athletes. http://www.bodyrecomposition.com/muscle-gain/protein-requirements-for-strength-and-power-athletes.html/

Science Daily. Link between high-fat diet and type 2 diabetes clarified. https://www.sciencedaily.com/releases/2011/04/110411121539.htm

Creationist Diet

Science Daily. Moderate-fat Diet Is Kinder To Heart Than Low-fat Diet, Study Shows.
https://www.sciencedaily.com/releases/2004/02/040202070609.htm
Sports Nutrition - Protein Needs for Athletes.
http://sportsmedicine.about.com/od/sportsnutrition/a/Protein.htm
Volek, Jeff S. et.al., *Journal of Applied Physiology*. Published 1 January 1997 Vol. 82 no. 1, 49-54 DOI. Testosterone and cortisol in relationship to dietary nutrients and resistance exercise.
http://jap.physiology.org/content/82/1/49
Zivkovic, Angela M, J Bruce German, and Arun J Sanyal. © 2007 American Society for Clinical Nutrition. Comparative review of diets for the metabolic syndrome: implications for nonalcoholic fatty liver disease.
http://ajcn.nutrition.org/content/86/2/285.full

Chapter Sixteen:
Comparison with Other Diets

How does the Creationist Diet compare to other types of diets? This chapter will answer this question.

The USDA Pyramid

How does the Creationist Diet compare to what the United States Department of Agriculture (USDA) recommended with their 1992 "Food Pyramid?" (It was actually a triangle, but why be technical?) The "pyramid" recommended (starting at the "base" and going up):

Bread, Cereal, Rice, and Pasta - 6-11 servings (serving = 1 slice of bread, 1 ounce of ready to eat cereal, ½ cup of cooked cereal, rice, or pasta).

Fruits and Vegetables - 5-9 servings (2-4 of fruits and 3-5 of vegetables; serving = 1 medium apple, banana, orange, ½ cup of chopped, cooked, or canned fruit, ¾ cup of fruit juice, 1 cup of raw leafy vegetables, ½ cup of other vegetables, cooked or chopped raw, ¾ cup of vegetable juice)

Meat, Poultry, Fish, Dry Beans, Eggs, and Nuts - 2-3 servings (serving = 2-3 ounces of cooked lean meat, poultry, or fish, ½ cup of cooked dry beans, 1 egg, or 2 tablespoons of peanut butter count as 1 ounce of lean meat).

Milk, Yogurt, and Cheese - 2-3 servings (serving = 1 cup of milk or yogurt, 1½ ounces of natural cheese, 2 ounces of process cheese)

Fats and oils - use sparingly (*Pyramid*).

There are many similarities between this dietary plan and the Creationist Diet. But what changes would need to be made to make it

419

Creationist Diet

even more so? First off, fruits and vegetables should be at the "base" of the pyramid to emphasize their importance. Second, the grains should be indicated to be only *whole* grains, while so-called "enriched" grains shouldn't count as a serving.

Nuts and seeds would need to be put into a separate group. This would emphasize their importance. The same would go for fish. But legumes (dry beans) would be kept in the same group as meats. This way, for those avoiding meat, the legumes would be an alternative. The dairy group would be about the same.

Lastly, trying to give a range for number of servings is not appropriate, especially for the bread and cereal group. How many servings of grains someone consumes would be determined by whether they are following a low-fat, moderate-fat, or low-carb diet. There is simply too much individual variation to give recommendations.

With these changes, following would be how a "food pyramid" for the Creationist Diet would be designed, starting at the base and going up. Foods at the based should be consumed in the greatest amounts, and then in decreasing amounts as one moves up levels.

Foods in square brackets are not actually mentioned in the Bible, but would fit in the places indicated.

Level One: Raw fruits and vegetables, raw nuts and seeds, (grains/ sprouts). - daily

Level Two: Cooked fruits, vegetables, nuts and seeds, along with cooked whole grains, potatoes (white and sweet) - daily

Level Three: Legumes, [including peanuts]; clean trimmed old-fashioned meats and skinless poultry - daily.

Level Four: Fish - at least twice weekly

Level Five: Dairy products – daily (optional)

Level Six: Oils and sweeteners (olive oil, [nut and seed oils], honey) - in limited amounts.

Or to look at it another way, the primary food groups should be:

Fruits and vegetables (raw and cooked)
Nuts and seeds (raw and roasted)
Whole Grains
Legumes
Meats and Poultry
Fish
Dairy Products
Oils and sweeteners

A variety of foods should be chosen from each of these groups (optional on the animal foods). Again, I hesitate to recommend specific amounts, but 8-10 servings of fruits and vegetables would be a good number to shoot for. At least one serving of nuts or seeds per day would also be good, along with a few servings of whole grains, plus at least two servings of fish a week. For additional protein, two or more servings of meats, dairy, and/ or legumes daily.

The USDA's MyPlate

"MyPlate" is the USDA's newest food guide for Americans, having been designed in 2011. The website is www.ChooseMyPlate.gov. The home page states:

> MyPlate illustrates the **five food groups** that are building blocks for a healthy diet using a familiar image – a place setting for a meal. Before you eat, think about what goes on your plate, in your cup, or in your bowl.

The accompanying picture is of plate divided into four parts and a cup. The four parts are labeled: **Fruits, Vegetables, Grains, Protein,** while the cup is labeled: **Dairy**. The Vegetables and Grains sections are somewhat larger than the Fruits and Protein sections, and all four are larger than the Dairy section. The idea is, you are supposed to eat foods from each of these five food groups in about these proportions.

To comment: focusing on these five groups is a good idea. The best part is having half of the plate devoted to fruits and vegetables, with vegetables in slightly larger amounts than fruits. As mentioned

421

repeatedly in this book, eating more fruits and vegetables is the single most important change a person can do to improve their diet. But given the sugar content of fruit, their intake needs to be limited somewhat.

But then the proportions of grains and protein foods would again depend on what kind of diet a person is following, though about a fifth of the diet from each would be a good starting point.

Having dairy off to the side in somewhat lesser amounts is a good way of picturing the good but nonessential nature of dairy foods.

But to return to the MyPlate website, the "What is MyPlate" page then states:

> MyPlate is a reminder to find your healthy eating style and build it throughout your lifetime. **Everything you eat and drink matters**. The right mix can help you be healthier now and in the future. This means:
>
> • Focus on variety, amount, and nutrition.
> • Choose foods and beverages with less saturated fat, sodium, and added sugars.
> • Start with small changes to build healthier eating styles.
> • Support healthy eating for everyone.
> • Eating healthy is a journey shaped by many factors, including our stage of life, situations, preferences, access to food, culture, traditions, and the personal decisions we make over time. All your food and beverage choices count. MyPlate offers ideas and tips to help you create a healthier eating style that meets your individual needs and improves your health.

All of these recommendations are sound and in accordance with a Creationist Diet. There is such a variety of healthy God-given foods available in the USA, there is no reason for a healthy diet to be monotonous. And the value of limiting saturated fat, sodium, and added sugars has been discussed in this book. And yes, we should support each other in trying to follow a healthy diet, and there are wide variations in each person's eating habits due to many factors. These factors need to be taken into account as a person begins to improve their diet. And generally speaking, making gradual changes is easier than making wholesale changes all at once.

The "What is MyPlate" page continues:

Focus on making healthy food and beverage choices from all five food groups including fruits, vegetables, grains, protein foods, and dairy to get the nutrients you need.

This is the rub. What are "healthy choices?" These are explained on separate pages for each food group. The Fruit page states:

What foods are in the **Fruit Group**?

Any fruit or 100% fruit juice counts as part of the Fruit Group. Fruits may be **fresh, canned, frozen, or dried**, and may be whole, cut-up, or pureed.

How much fruit is needed daily?

The amount of fruit you need to eat depends on age, sex, and level of physical activity. Recommended daily amounts are shown in the table below.

The recommended amount of fruit is 1-2 cups, with specifications on what constitutes a cup.

To comment, the main problem here is the inclusion of fruit juice. Fruit juice is highly processed, and commercial fruit juice especially so. It is generally filtered, so little nutritional content remains beyond the sugar. Such juices would not be included in a Creationist Diet. But if you juice the fruit yourself, such as squeezing oranges into orange juice while retaining the pulp, that would be better. Although, there would still be more of a blood sugar spike than from eating an orange. But elsewhere, the MyPlate website does state, "Focus on whole fruits." That is good, but it should have been mentioned on this page also.

The **Vegetables Group** page states:

Any vegetable or 100% vegetable juice counts as a member of the Vegetable Group. Vegetables may be **raw or cooked; fresh, frozen, canned, or dried/dehydrated**; and may be whole, cut-up, or mashed.

423

Based on their nutrient content, vegetables are organized into **5 subgroups:** dark-green vegetables, starchy vegetables, red and orange vegetables, beans and peas, and other vegetables.

Dividing vegetables into these five groups is a good idea, as each group contains different nutrients, although this might get a bit confusing for some people.

The recommended amount of vegetables is 1-3 cups, with again, specifications on what constitutes a cup.

The **Grains Group** page states:

Any food made from wheat, rice, oats, cornmeal, barley or another cereal grain is a grain product. Bread, pasta, oatmeal, breakfast cereals, tortillas, and grits are examples of grain products.

Grains are divided into 2 subgroups, Whole Grains and Refined Grains. Whole grains contain the entire grain kernel — the bran, germ, and endosperm. Examples of whole grains include whole-wheat flour, bulgur (cracked wheat), oatmeal, whole cornmeal, and brown rice. Refined grains have been milled, a process that removes the bran and germ. This is done to give grains a finer texture and improve their shelf life, but it also removes dietary fiber, iron, and many B vitamins. Some examples of refined grain products are white flour, de-germed cornmeal, white bread, and white rice.

Most refined grains are enriched. This means certain B vitamins (thiamin, riboflavin, niacin, folic acid) and iron are added back after processing. **Fiber is not added back to enriched grains**. Check the ingredient list on refined grain products to make sure that the word "enriched" is included in the grain name. Some food products are made from mixtures of whole grains and refined grains.

This is all good information, but there are far more nutritional differences between whole and refined grains than just the fiber content, as has been detailed in this book. This ignoring of this great difference is why the MyPlate site states elsewhere, "Make half your grains whole

424

grains." Half is hardly good enough given the incredible difference between the two kinds of grains. And this would be one big difference between MyPlate and the Creationist Diet. There is also no mention of consuming organic and non-GMO plant foods that is an important aspect of the Creationist Diet.

The **Protein Foods Group** page states:

> **All foods made from meat, poultry, seafood, beans and peas, eggs, processed soy products, nuts, and seeds** are considered part of the Protein Foods Group. Beans and peas are also part of the Vegetable Group....
>
> **Select a variety of protein foods** to improve nutrient intake and health benefits, including **at least 8 ounces of cooked seafood per week**. Young children need less, depending on their age and calorie needs. The advice to consume seafood does not apply to vegetarians. Vegetarian options in the Protein Foods Group include beans and peas, processed soy products, and nuts and seeds. **Meat and poultry choices should be lean or low-fat**.

These recommendations are all good. But it does brush by that vegetarians are losing out on an incredibly healthy food by not eating fish. But most of all, there is not a hint of the incredible difference between factory farm meats and old-fashioned meats. That is a very important aspect of the Creationist Diet that is missed here.

The **Dairy Group** page states:

> **All fluid milk products and many foods made from milk are considered part of this food group**. Most Dairy Group choices should be **fat-free or low-fat**. Foods made from milk that retain their calcium content are part of the group. Foods made from milk that have little to no calcium, such as cream cheese, cream, and butter, are not. Calcium-fortified soymilk (soy beverage) is also part of the Dairy Group.

The recommendation for non or low-fat dairy is par for the course for government recommendations. But it ignores once again the great difference between factory farm dairy and old-fashioned dairy. It was

425

discussed earlier that the fat in old-fashioned dairy would probably not be problematic.

But overall, the recommendations of MyPlate are similar to the Creationist Diet. The main differences are again the Creationist Diet not including fruit juice or refined grains and that non-organic, GMO plant foods and factory farm animal foods are included in MyPlate.

2015-2020 Dietary Guidelines for America

Every five years, the USDA issues its "Dietary Guidelines for America." It is from these much more detailed guidelines that the Food Pyramid, MyPlate, and other simplified USDA recommendations over the years are developed. The most recent edition was released in December of 2015 and is called "2015-2020 Dietary Guidelines for America."

Given that these guidelines represent the basis for all other governmental dietary recommendations, it would be good to look into them in detail. We will do so by looking at each section in turn.

The Guidelines' website is designed as an online book, with an introduction, three chapters, and 14 appendixes. The quotes are from various pages on the website:
https://health.gov/dietaryguidelines/2015/guidelines/

Introduction:

The Introduction to the Guidelines begin with a description of the state of health of Americans in regards to "chronic diet-related diseases," and this state is not good.

About half of all American adults—117 million individuals—have one or more preventable chronic diseases, many of which are related to poor quality eating patterns and physical inactivity. These include cardiovascular disease, high blood pressure, type 2 diabetes, some cancers, and poor bone health. **More than two-thirds of adults and nearly one-third of children and youth are overweight or obese.**

It is not surprising that these health difficulties are related to the poor eating patterns and lack of exercise on the part of the majority of Americans.

The Introduction then overviews the methodology used in developing the Guidelines. In a nutshell, the best available scientific studies were reviewed and analyzed. That means these Guidelines are not *ad hoc*, but based on the best available research. It is apparent that every step was taken to ensure these Guidelines are evidence-based and not based on opinions or personal experiences. And there is no evidence they were influenced by special interest groups, despite many claims to the contrary. In this writer's opinion, the USDA has done its job in thoroughly and honestly reviewing the research.

Once the research is evaluated, it needs to be developed into specific guidelines. Then recommendations need to be made for implementing those guidelines. Therefore, there are three steps to the Guidelines:

1. Review of the scientific evidence.
2. Development of the actual Guidelines.
3. Implementation of the Guidelines.

General Guidelines:

The first chapter of the Guidelines is "Key Elements of Healthy Eating Patterns." This is a summary of the available scientific research. It begins:

> Over the course of any given day, week, or year, individuals consume foods and beverages in combination—an eating pattern. **An eating pattern is more than the sum of its parts; it represents the totality of what individuals habitually eat and drink,** and these dietary components act synergistically in relation to health. As a result, the eating pattern may be more predictive of overall health status and disease risk than individual foods or nutrients.

The term "eating pattern" is used throughout the Guidelines. It indicates that what is being evaluated and recommended is not specific foods to eat for one meal or a day but what people eat over a long period of time, a pattern.

427

Creationist Diet

It is very true that it is not what people eat on occasion but regularly that has greatest effects on their health. That is why I called my other book on nutrition and the Bible *God-given Foods Eating Plan*. The idea behind an "eating pattern" or "eating plan" is the same: long-term eating habits. But I used "diet" in the title of this book, as it is the more common term. This chapter then presents some general guidelines:

Individuals should aim to meet their nutrient needs through healthy eating patterns that include **nutrient-dense foods**. Foods in nutrient-dense forms contain essential vitamins and minerals and also dietary fiber and other naturally occurring substances that may have positive health benefits.

By "nutrient-dense forms" the USDA means foods that do not have the density of their nutrients diluted by the presence of added sugars, added refined carbs, added refined vegetables oils, and/ or large amounts of added or naturally occurring saturated fats. There are also recommendations to limit sodium and trans fats.

Previously in this book, the recommendation has been to consume whole, natural foods as closely as possible to the forms in which God gave them to us. These two recommendations are basically the same. They are both saying to eat mostly unprocessed, whole, natural foods.

The USDA then gives the following specific recommendations for the unhealthy aspects of foods:

- Consume less than 10 percent of calories per day from **added sugars**
- Consume less than 10 percent of calories per day from **saturated fats**
- Consume less than 2,300 milligrams (mg) per day of **sodium**

The scientific evidence for the problems caused by excess added sugars (and refined carbs in general), saturated fat, and sodium has been presented previously in this book. I am sure the USDA had access to far more research than I did in writing this book, but we came to similar conclusions.

Most authorities would agree that excessive added sugar and refined carb intake is unhealthy, but some are now question the restrictions on sodium and saturated fat. I won't repeat here all that was said before, but I will say, there is some evidence that some people could consume higher amounts of sodium without adverse effects and that too low of an intake of sodium is unhealthy. But the average per day intake of Americans of 3,440 mg per day cited on this website and previously in this book is more than is necessary and can be unhealthy for many people as such amounts can elevate blood pressure.

Even more so, many today try to claim that saturated fats are not unhealthy. But as was explained previously, such people are misreading the evidence. What it actually shows is there is no benefit to replacing saturated fats with processed carbs, which is what most people do by eating processed low-fat foods. But there is benefit to replacing saturated fats with unsaturated fats, which is what the Guidelines recommend. I also believe there is benefit to replacing saturated fat with unprocessed carbs, but the evidence is not there as yet as with unsaturated fats.

Guidelines for Specific Food Groups:

Chapter One next gives guidelines for each food group. It begins with vegetables:

Healthy eating patterns include **a variety of vegetables from all of the five vegetable subgroups—dark green, red and orange, legumes (beans and peas), starchy, and other.** These include all **fresh, frozen, canned, and dried options in cooked or raw forms, including vegetable juices.** The recommended amount of vegetables in **the Healthy U.S.-Style Eating Pattern** at the 2,000-calorie level is **2½ cup-equivalents of vegetables per day**. In addition, weekly amounts from each vegetable subgroup are recommended to ensure variety and meet nutrient needs.

Note that "Healthy U.S.-Style Eating Pattern" is what the USDA is calling its recommended diet. The word "diet" is being avoided as most people think "weight loss" when they hear "diet," which is usually something that is followed for a period of time and then abandoned. But

429

Creationist Diet

an eating pattern or plan is the ongoing way people eat over a lifetime, regardless of bodyweight goals. That is why I was leery about using the word "diet" in the title of this book and changed to "eating plan" for my other book. But the word "diet" can mean, "the kinds of food that a person, animal, or community habitually eats" (Oxford), so it is appropriate.

That said; vegetable intake is without a doubt the most important aspect of a healthy eating plan, so the USDA is very correct in recommending the consumption of a copious amount of a wide variety of vegetables. But I have a couple of minor caveats.

The first would be the inclusion of canned vegetables. There is always some loss of nutrients when foods are canned, and salt is usually added. The second would be vegetable juices. Processing vegetables into juice is just that, processing, with the concurrent loss of nutrients, and if store-bought, often the addition of an excessive amount of sodium.

The next food group is fruits:

Healthy eating patterns include **fruits, especially whole fruits**. The fruits food group includes **whole fruits and 100% fruit juice**. Whole fruits include **fresh, canned, frozen, and dried forms**. The recommended amount of fruits in the Healthy U.S.-Style Eating Pattern at the 2,000-calorie level is **2 cup-equivalents per day**. One cup of 100% fruit juice counts as 1 cup of fruit. Although fruit juice can be part of healthy eating patterns, it is lower than whole fruit in dietary fiber and when consumed in excess can contribute extra calories. Therefore, at least half of the recommended amount of fruits should come from whole fruits. **When juices are consumed, they should be 100% juice, without added sugars**. Also, when selecting canned fruit, choose options that are lowest in added sugars.

After vegetables, fruit is the next most important item to include in a healthy eating plan. But again, I would caution about canned fruits and fruit juices. They are less healthy than their fresh fruit counterparts.

As discussed previously, some people are leery about fruits due to their sugar content, but the presence of copious amounts of vitamins, minerals, and antioxidants makes fruits beneficial not deleterious. And the high fiber and water content of whole fruits moderates the blood sugar response from the sugar. But fruit juices can cause blood sugar problems, as the fiber has been removed. The same goes for dried fruits due to the loss of the fluid content. And even with whole fruits, due to the sugar content, they cannot be eaten as freely as vegetables, which is why the USDA recommends a somewhat smaller amount of fruit than of vegetables.

The next food group is grains:

Healthy eating patterns **include whole grains and limit the intake of refined grains and products made with refined grains, especially those high in saturated fats, added sugars, and/or sodium, such as cookies, cakes, and some snack foods.** The grains food group includes grains as single foods (e.g., rice, oatmeal, and popcorn), as well as products that include grains as an ingredient (e.g., breads, cereals, crackers, and pasta). **Grains are either whole or refined.** Whole grains (e.g., brown rice, quinoa, and oats) contain the entire kernel, including the endosperm, bran, and germ. **Refined grains differ from whole grains in that the grains have been processed to remove the bran and germ, which removes dietary fiber, iron, and other nutrients.** The recommended amount of grains in the Healthy U.S.-Style Eating Pattern at the 2,000-calorie level is **6 ounce-equivalents per day. At least half of this amount should be whole grains ...**

This whole paragraph contains very sound advice, until the last sentence. After describing the immense difference between whole grains and refined grains, the USDA only recommends that "at least half" of grains consumption should be whole grains. "All" of at least "almost all" would be more in line with what was just said.

That said; some would disagree with this recommendation in that they think any form of grains, whether whole or refined, is unhealthy. These are mainly those who advocate low-carb or Paleolithic types of diets. But such people ignore the wealth of scientific research that whole grain consumption is beneficial, as has been cited in this book.

There are also many today who have jumped on the gluten-free bandwagon and thus avoid wheat, rye, and barley. But as previously discussed, for the vast majority of people, that is a misguided fad. Only a very small percentage of the population actually has a problem digesting gluten. As such, for most people, such self-imposed dietary restrictions are unnecessary.

The next food group is dairy:

Healthy eating patterns include **fat-free and low-fat (1%) dairy, including milk, yogurt, cheese, or fortified soy beverages** (commonly known as "soymilk")....

The recommended amounts of dairy in the Healthy U.S.-Style Pattern are based on age rather than calorie level and are 2 cup-equivalents per day for children ages 2 to 3 years, 2½ cup-equivalents per day for children ages 4 to 8 years, and **3 cup-equivalents per day for adolescents ages 9 to 18 years and for adults.**

There are two different groups of people who would disagree with this recommendation. The first would be the "no milk" crowd. These people think that dairy consumption of any type and in any form is unhealthy, as they claim it is "unnatural" for adult mammals to consume dairy. Such concerns have already been addressed. Moreover, as the Guidelines detail, dairy foods contain a wealth of nutrients, namely, "calcium, phosphorus, vitamin A, vitamin D (in products fortified with vitamin D), riboflavin, vitamin B12, protein, potassium, zinc, choline, magnesium, and selenium."

The second opposing group would be those who do not think saturated fat is problematic. Therefore, they would disagree with the recommendation to consume low-fat or fat-free versions of dairy; instead recommending whole milk products. But again, the actual evidence shows that saturated fat is unhealthy. However, it has been discussed that the fat in grass-fed dairy is probably not unhealthy. Consequently, there is not a need to consume low or non-fat if consuming grass fed dairy. But the value of low-fat and fat-free dairy is it contains the same amounts of nutrients at a much lower caloric "cost" than their whole fat counterparts, so more of these foods can be consumed without excessive caloric consumption.

The next food group is protein foods:

Healthy eating patterns include **a variety of protein foods in nutrient-dense forms**. The protein foods group comprises a broad group of foods from both animal and plant sources and includes several **subgroups: seafood; meats, poultry, and eggs; and nuts, seeds, and soy products**. Legumes (beans and peas) may also be considered part of the protein foods group as well as the vegetables group....

Protein also is found in some foods from other food groups (e.g., dairy). The recommendation for protein foods in the Healthy U.S.-Style Eating Pattern at the 2,000-calorie level is **5½ ounce-equivalents of protein foods per day**.

This guideline to consume protein from a variety of sources is very well-founded. Each of the mentioned classes of foods contain different nutrients, so consuming some of each provides a well-rounded nutrient intake. The USDA goes on to provide some more important guidelines about these foods.

When selecting protein foods, nuts and seeds should be unsalted, and meats and poultry should be consumed in lean forms. Processed meats and processed poultry are sources of sodium and saturated fats, and intake of these products can be accommodated as long as sodium, saturated fats, added sugars, and total calories are within limits in the resulting eating pattern...

These guidelines are due to the benefits of restricting saturated fat and sodium. But it is interesting that the USDA seems a little lenient in regards to processed meats. But what they are demonstrating is that even these less healthy forms of meat can be included in a healthy eating plan, as long as they are in limited amounts and the high sodium and saturated fat content are allotted for in the overall eating plan.

This section goes on to recommend consuming at least eight ounces of seafood a week due to its omega 3 (EPA and DHA) content. Cautions are also given about mercury, with recommendations to consume fish that is less likely to be contaminate with it, namely "salmon, anchovies, herring, shad, sardines, Pacific oysters, trout, and Atlantic and Pacific mackerel (not king mackerel, which is high in methyl mercury)." The same recommendation has been made previously in this book.

My only caveat in this group would be with the recommended amount of 5-1/2 ounces a day total. As discussed previously, there is strong evidence that strength athletes need far more protein than non-athletes. But then elsewhere in the Guidelines, the USDA recommends that all people engage in at least an hour of strength training each week, so a higher protein intake would be warranted for all such persons.

The next food group is oils:

> **Oils are fats that contain a high percentage of monounsaturated and polyunsaturated fats and are liquid at room temperature.** Although they are not a food group, oils are emphasized as part of healthy eating patterns because they are **the major source of essential fatty acids and vitamin E. Commonly consumed oils extracted from plants include canola, corn, olive, peanut, safflower, soybean, and sunflower oils. Oils also are naturally present in nuts, seeds, seafood, olives, and avocados.** The fat in some tropical plants, such as **coconut oil, palm kernel oil, and palm oil, are not included in the oils category** because they do not resemble other oils in their composition. Specifically, they contain a higher percentage of saturated fats than other oils....
>
> The recommendation for oils in the Healthy U.S.-Style Eating Pattern at the 2,000-calorie level is 27 g (about 5 teaspoons) per day.

Some of the recommended oils would not fit in a Creationist Diet as they are unnatural, namely corn, canola, and safflower. It takes lots of processing to attain oil from these low in fat items, and the latter two are not really foods to begin with. Much more natural is attaining oil from high fat foods like olives and nuts and seeds.

Now some would disagree with the caution about tropical oils due to the saturated fat content. This disagreement is not only because some do not believe saturated fat is unhealthy, but they claim the type of saturated fat in these food is different from that in animal foods. In fact, some even claim almost magical benefits from these fats. But there is little evidence to support such claims.

Other Dietary Components:

After looking at the various food groups, the Guidelines next look at "Other Dietary Components," starting with added sugars:

Added sugars include syrups and other caloric sweeteners. **When sugars are added to foods and beverages to sweeten them, they add calories without contributing essential nutrients.** Consumption of added sugars can make it difficult for individuals to meet their nutrient needs while staying within calorie limits. **Naturally occurring sugars, such as those in fruit or milk, are not added sugars.**...

Healthy eating patterns limit added sugars to **less than 10 percent of calories per day**... When added sugars in foods and beverages exceed 10 percent of calories, a healthy eating pattern may be difficult to achieve.

As indicated, the main problem with consuming foods with added sugars is it makes it impossible to consume sufficient nutrients without consuming too many calories, as added sugars contain no nutrients themselves other than calories in the form of carbs. That is why added sugars are called "empty calories." But naturally occurring sugars in fruit and dairy always come packed with a wealth of nutrients. There is also growing evidence that added sugars contribute to health problems independent of the weight gain they can cause. Therefore, the guideline of limiting added sugars to less than 10% of calories is sound.

The next dietary component is saturated fats:

Intake of saturated fats should be limited to less than 10 percent of calories per day by replacing them with unsaturated fats and while keeping total dietary fats within the age-appropriate AMDR [Acceptable Macronutrient Distribution Ranges] ...

Strong and consistent evidence shows that **replacing saturated fats with unsaturated fats, especially polyunsaturated fats**, is associated with reduced blood levels of total cholesterol and of low-density lipoprotein-cholesterol (LDL-cholesterol). Additionally, strong and consistent

435

evidence shows that replacing saturated fats with polyunsaturated fats is associated with a reduced risk of CVD events (heart attacks) and CVD-related deaths.

Some evidence has shown that **replacing saturated fats with plant sources of monounsaturated fats, such as olive oil and nuts**, may be associated with a reduced risk of CVD. However, the evidence base for monounsaturated fats is not as strong as the evidence base for replacement with polyunsaturated fats. … **Replacing total fat or saturated fats with carbohydrates is not associated with reduced risk of CVD**. Additional research is needed to determine whether this relationship is consistent across categories of carbohydrates (e.g., **whole versus refined grains; intrinsic versus added sugars**), as they may have different associations with various health outcomes. Therefore, saturated fats in the diet should be replaced with polyunsaturated and monounsaturated fats.

These points were mentioned previously but bear elaboration given the controversy surrounding them. Again, replacing saturated fats with unsaturated fats is beneficial, no matter what some might claim; but there is no benefit to replacing saturated fats with processed carbs. The only question remaining is if replacing saturated fats with unprocessed carbs would be beneficial. I personally think that it would be, but the question needs further investigation.

The next food component is trans fats:

Individuals should limit intake of trans fats to as low as possible by limiting foods that contain synthetic sources of trans fats, such as partially hydrogenated oils in margarines, and by limiting other solid fats. A number of studies have observed an association between increased intake of trans fats and increased risk of CVD. This increased risk is due, in part, to its LDL-cholesterol-raising effect.

There is no question remaining—trans fats are unhealthy and should be avoided as much as possible. That is why they are being banned in the USA. In the meantime, they are easily avoided by avoiding processed foods, as they are the main source of trans fats. The small amounts of naturally occurring trans fats is some animal foods is not problematic. As the USDA states, "Because natural trans fats are present in dairy products and meats in only small quantities and these foods can be important sources of nutrients, these foods do not need to be eliminated from the diet."

The next food component is cholesterol:

The Key Recommendation from the 2010 Dietary Guidelines to limit consumption of dietary cholesterol to 300 mg per day is not included in the 2015 edition, but this change does not suggest that dietary cholesterol is no longer important to consider when building healthy eating patterns....

In general, foods that are higher in dietary cholesterol, such as fatty meats and high-fat dairy products, are also higher in saturated fats. The USDA Food Patterns are limited in saturated fats, and because of the commonality of food sources of saturated fats and dietary cholesterol, the Patterns are also low in dietary cholesterol.

Strong evidence from mostly prospective cohort studies but also randomized controlled trials has shown that eating patterns that include lower intake of dietary cholesterol are associated with reduced risk of CVD, and moderate evidence indicates that these eating patterns are associated with reduced risk of obesity. ... **More research is needed regarding the dose-response relationship between dietary cholesterol and blood cholesterol levels.** Adequate evidence is not available for a quantitative limit for dietary cholesterol specific to the Dietary Guidelines.

This is another controversial area that some would now disagree with that was addressed previously. But basically, there is a relationship between dietary cholesterol and blood cholesterol, but it is difficult to quantify.

The next dietary component is sodium:

The scientific consensus from expert bodies, such as the IOM, the American Heart Association, and Dietary Guidelines Advisory Committees, is that **average sodium intake, which** is currently 3,440 mg per day (see Chapter 2), is too high and should be reduced. Healthy eating patterns **limit sodium to less than 2,300 mg per day** for adults and children ages 14 years and older....

This is again a controversial issue, but the evidence still supports restricting sodium at least to some degree.

The final dietary component is alcohol:

The Dietary Guidelines does not recommend that individuals who do not drink alcohol start drinking for any reason. If alcohol is consumed, it should be in moderation— up to one drink per day for women and up to two drinks per day for men—and **only by adults of legal drinking age.** There are also many circumstances in which individuals should not drink, such as during pregnancy.

Alcohol contains calories but no nutrients. It is thus another form of empty calories. For that reason alone, its intake should be limited. But the potential problems from excessive intake go far beyond excessive calorie consumption. There is some evidence that moderate alcohol consumption can be beneficial, but the potential risks far outweigh the possible benefits. That is why the USDA says to not start drinking if you are not already doing so. I concur.

Current Eating Patterns:

Chapter Two of the Guidelines is "Shifts Needed To Align With Healthy Eating Patterns." It begins by looking at what American are currently eating, and the picture is not good:

About three-fourths of the population has an eating pattern that is **low in vegetables, fruits, dairy, and oils.**

More than half of the population is meeting or **exceeding total grain and total protein foods recommendations,** but, as discussed later in the chapter, are **not meeting the recommendations for the subgroups** within each of these food groups.

Most Americans **exceed the recommendations for added sugars, saturated fats, and sodium**.

In addition, the eating patterns of many are **too high in calories**....

Only 20 percent of adults meet the **Physical Activity Guidelines** for aerobic and muscle-strengthening activity.

The mention of "subgroups" in the second line is due to Americans not consuming sufficient whole grains, seafood, and legumes. All of these poor habits contribute to the fact that, "more than two-thirds of all adults and nearly one-third of all children and youth in the United States are either overweight or obese." This in turn leads to many of the health problems experienced by Americans, such as heart disease, cancer, and diabetes. This poor eating pattern also leads to nutritional deficiencies in the current American diet:

Although the majority of Americans consume sufficient amounts of most nutrients, some nutrients are consumed by many individuals in amounts **below the Estimated Average Requirement or Adequate Intake levels**. These include **potassium, dietary fiber, choline, magnesium, calcium, and vitamins A, D, E, and C. Iron** also is under-consumed by adolescent girls and women ages 19 to 50 years. Low intakes for most of these nutrients occur within the context of unhealthy overall eating patterns, **due to low intakes of the food groups—vegetables, fruits, whole grains, and dairy—that contain these nutrients**.

Thus Americans are consuming too much of detrimental elements of food while not consuming sufficient amounts of the beneficial elements of foods.

The rest of this chapter of this online book describes the changes needed in people's eating plans to correct these deficiencies. But most of them are self-evident—Americans need to consume more fruits and vegetables, whole grains instead of refined grains, while reducing overall grain consumption, replace some red meat consumption with seafood and legumes, and to exercise more. These recommendations have all been previously made in this book.

Moreover, the basic recommendation of the Creationist Diet to consume less processed foods and more unprocessed foods would go a long way towards a reduction in the overconsumption of sugars, saturated fats, sodium, and calories. As the Guidelines puts it:

> **Achieving a healthy eating pattern means shifting typical food choices to more nutrient-dense options**—that is, foods with important nutrients that aren't packed with extra calories or sodium. **Nutrient-dense foods and beverages are naturally lean or low in solid fats and have little or no added solid fats, sugars, refined starches, or sodium.**

The Guidelines provide specifics in these regards, as has this book. The chapter concludes with the following summary:

> The U.S. population, across almost every age and sex group, consumes eating patterns that are **low** in vegetables, fruits, whole grains, dairy, seafood, and oil and **high** in refined grains, added sugars, saturated fats, sodium, and for some age-sex groups, high in the meats, poultry, and eggs subgroup.

Everyone Has a Role in Supporting Healthy Eating Patterns:

The third and last chapter of the Guidelines is titled, "Everyone Has a Role in Supporting Healthy Eating Patterns." It begins

> … collective action is needed to **create a new paradigm** in which healthy lifestyle choices at home, school, work, and in the community are easy, accessible, affordable, and normative.

What follows are recommendations for changing people's and society's attitudes towards food.

This is attitude shift is sorely needed. Much of this country's poor eating pattern is due to habit and tradition, most of which is relatively new, having originated in the past century or less. And I am all for the government encouraging businesses and other organizations to provide healthy foods and opportunities for exercise. However, I would be absolutely opposed to the government forcing such entities to do so via governmental regulations or taxation. As much as I desire for people to follow healthy habits, it should ultimately their choice. But I agree with the next point to encourage people to choose the healthy options:

> **Education** to improve individual food and physical activity choices can be delivered by a wide variety of nutrition and physical activity professionals working alone or in multidisciplinary teams.

Such education is exactly what I try to provide in this and my other book on nutrition and the Bible, with my *FitTips* newsletter, and on my fitness website (see Appendixes One and Two). But in addition to this general education, personal one-on-one education can be beneficial:

> **Professionals can work with individuals in a variety of settings** to adapt their choices to develop a healthy eating pattern tailored to accommodate physical health, cultural, ethnic, traditional, and personal preferences, as well as personal food budgets and other issues of accessibility. **Eating patterns tailored to the individual are more likely to be motivating, accepted, and maintained over time**, thereby having the potential to lead to meaningful shifts in dietary intake, and consequently, improved health.

Appendixes:

This online book concludes with 14 appendixes. Most of these provide data related to the main chapters, such as providing lists of the amounts of various nutrients in various foods and details on what constitutes a serving of the various food groups.

The appendix that provides some new information is: "Appendix 7. Nutritional Goals for Age-Sex Groups Based on Dietary Reference Intakes and Dietary Guidelines Recommendations." It is here that the USDAs guidelines for "Acceptable Macronutrient Distribution Ranges" (AMDR) is given. They are arranged by age and gender.

But as discussed in the previous chapter, it is hard to make blanket recommendations for macronutrient levels, as everyone is different. It is thus good that the Guidelines only put this in an appendix and use wide ranges.

What is Not Discussed:

That concludes my review of what is presented in the Guideline's online book. But I have to mention some points that are not discussed, but which I believe are very important and are discussed elsewhere in this book.

The first issue is organic produce versus commercial produce. The Guidelines do not mention this, but it is an important issue. Many have found health benefits by eliminating such chemicals from their diets.

Second, there is no mention of consuming only non-GMO foods. But this is again an important issue with far-reaching ramifications.

Third, there is no mention of artificial food ingredients, except for artificial sweeteners, which the Guidelines call "high-intensity sweeteners" and state about:

> High-intensity sweeteners that have been approved by the U.S. Food and Drug Administration (FDA) include saccharin, aspartame, acesulfame potassium (Ace-K), and sucralose. Based on the available scientific evidence, **these high-intensity sweeteners have been determined to be safe for the general population**. This means that there is reasonable certainty of no harm under the intended conditions of use because the estimated daily intake is not expected to exceed the acceptable daily intake for each sweetener.

But again, many have found health benefits by eliminating such chemicals from their diets.

And finally, there is no mention about the manner in which cattle and other livestock are raised. This is probably why the Guidelines state:

> Strong evidence from mostly prospective cohort studies but also randomized controlled trials has shown that **eating patterns that include lower intake of meats as well as processed meats and processed poultry are associated with reduced risk of CVD in adults**. Moderate evidence indicates that these eating patterns are associated with reduced risk of obesity, type 2 diabetes, and some types of cancer in adults.

442

However, as has been previously asserted using the terms "factory farm meats" versus "old-fashioned meats," these detrimental aspects of a high meat intake are only due to the way the vast majority of cattle and other livestock are raised and fed in America. The animals are confined to small stalls, with little movement possible, kept indoors, with no sunshine, and fed grains, usually GMO corn or soy, and given hormones and antibiotics.

Such practices produce a meat that is far different than that found in organic, pasture-raised, grass-fed, hormone-free, antibiotic-free cattle. I would contend that if studies would be done comparing these two types of meat, it would be found that only the former carry adverse health effect, while the latter would be proven to be beneficial.

Along these lines, the Guidelines state, "Meat, also known as red meat, includes all forms of beef, **pork**, lamb, veal, goat, and non-bird game (e.g., venison, bison, and elk)." But I contend that there is a difference between "pork" (meaning all forms of pig meat) and the rest of the meats mentioned. Pig meats are Biblically unclean while the rest are Biblically clean meats, and I believe there is a reason God made this distinction. Pigs are not fit for human consumption while the rest of these animals are.

Conclusion:

I would probably agree with over 90% of the Guidelines. They present evidence-based, sound dietary recommendations. Therefore, I would highly recommend the reader read through the website for the 2015-2020 Dietary Guidelines for America and put the Guidelines into practice. Just take note of the few minor disagreements between the Guidelines and the Creationist Diet.

Creationist Diet vs. the SAD

The Creationist Diet would differ significantly from the Standard American Diet, which, has the fitting acronym of SAD. The SAD contains a high proportion of highly processed foods. It is also very low in fruits and vegetables, whole grain breads and cereals, and fish, while being too high in fat, mainly in the form of fatty meats, fried foods, and refined vegetables oils, and too high in sugar and other processed carbs.

Creationist Diet

The **standard American diet**—that is, the typical diet of the majority of Americans—is **high in meat, dairy, fat, sugar as well as refined, processed, and junk foods.** The shift in Western diets to include more animal sourced foods and more sugar and corn syrup happened especially quickly after World War II.

The standard American diet includes **low intake of fruit and vegetables.** A 2010 report from the U.S. Centers for Disease Control showed that overall, only one state improved on vegetable and fruit consumption compared to such consumption ten years earlier. A study showing compliance with 2005 U.S. Department of Agriculture dietary guidelines showed **only ¼ of Americans ate at least one fruit serving a day, while only about 1 in 10 ate the recommended minimum amount for vegetables.** The average amount of **kale** each American eats per week is about **half a teaspoon.** Americans eat so few foods rich in antioxidants, that beer represents the fifth largest source of antioxidants in the standard American diet. **Based on a scale up to 100 measuring percentage of calories from foods rich with phytonutrients, the standard American diet rates about 11** (Nutrition Facts).

According to the USDA, nearly 1,000 calories a day (out of a 2775 daily calorie diet) is attributed to added fats and sweeteners! In comparison, **dairy, fruits and vegetables only contribute 424 calories.** Our priorities for food are simply out of balance....

In fact, 38 percent of adults in the U.S. report consuming fruits less than one time daily, and less than 22 percent report eating vegetables daily. While adolescents do fare better in the vegetable category, this may be attributable to unhealthy fried vegetables (i.e. French fries) and other processed vegetables available at school....

As of 2000, Americans were consuming nearly 200 pounds of grain per year, the vast majority from wheat flour....

In 2000, according to the USDA, each individual in the U.S. consumed over 150 pounds of sugar. Over half of that came from corn. Just because high-fructose corn syrup is made from corn, of course, doesn't mean that it is a healthy sweetener....

This chart shows that **63 percent of calories Americans are consuming today are coming from processed foods. Convenience foods are packed with preservatives, added oils, sugars and refined grains** — none of which is healthy for the body, as these foods definitely do more harm than good....

Over the last hundred years, our taste buds have changed; **today everything needs to be super-sweet**, even foods we don't tend to think as sweet....

According to this graph from the CDC, Americans over the age of two are averaging **over 3,400 milligrams of sodium each day** — that is more than double the recommended level and nearly seven times what our bodies actually need. Sodium does help our bodies function, but in reality the vast majority of us need less than 500 milligrams per day.

Just like our taste for sweet foods have increased, so has our taste for salt. While the salt shaker sitting on your table doesn't help matters, it's only responsible for approximately 25 percent of our sodium intake. The other **75 percent comes from processed foods and restaurants** (Dr. Axe).

Without giving it a second thought, many Americans eat a diet that is both **nutrient-poor and calorie-dense.** We choose foods simply because they are "convenient" without giving much thought to the fact that they are full of nutritionally bankrupt ingredients such as **sugar, starch, damaged fats, sodium, and chemical additives.** In fact, we have gotten **so used to eating these processed fake foods that we consider it okay; some people even think it's healthy.** This is ideal for the food industry but not for the average American. Sadly, this way of eating is killing us (NJ Nutritionist).

1. According to Jeff Novick, RD:
* 66% of American adults are overweight or obese
* 42 % of American children are overweight or obese

2. According to David Pimental, Ph.D., Professor at Cornell:

445

* **Americans eat an average of 3800 calories per day.**
* **They should eat only 2500 calories per day.**

3. According to Jeff Novick, RD:
Americans eat:
* **~ 20% of their calories from white flour**
* **37% from fat, 23% from white sugar, 15% from protein**
(leaving only ~ 5% from complex carbohydrates, which should make up the vast majority of our calories.)

4. According to Joel Fuhrman, M.D.:
* **Only 7% of calories consumed by Americans are from fruits and vegetables.**
* **Half of all vegetables consumed are potatoes.**
* **Half of all potatoes consumed are in the form of chips and fries.**
* 42% of calories consumed by Americans come from dairy and animal products
* **51% of calories consumed by Americans come from highly processed and refined carbohydrates and extracted oils.**

5. According to David Pimental, Ph.D.:
* **The average American drinks 600 cans of soda per year.**
(This is 90,000 calories totaling 50 lbs. of sugar per person per year.) (Spooky).

Gorging on bacon, skimping on nuts? These are among food habits that new research links with deaths from heart disease, strokes and diabetes....
"Good" foods that were under-eaten include: nuts and seeds, seafood rich in omega-3 fats including salmon and sardines; fruits and vegetables; and whole grains.
"Bad" foods or nutrients that were over-eaten include salt and salty foods; processed meats including bacon, bologna and hot dogs; red meat including steaks and hamburgers; and sugary drinks.

The research is based on U.S. government data showing there were about **700,000 deaths in 2012 from heart disease, strokes and diabetes** and on an analysis of national health surveys that asked participants about their eating habits. Most didn't eat the recommended amounts of the foods studied.

The 10 ingredients ["bad" foods] combined contributed to about 45 percent of those deaths, according to the study (Time. Americans).

The Standard American Diet is truly SAD. And the Creationist Diet would differ from it in just about every respect. First and foremost, just following the most basic dictate of the Creationist Diet of eating foods in the most natural form possible would be a radical change from what Americans are currently eating. To put it another way, the dependence on processed foods is the single biggest problem in the SAD.

This dependence is the main reason for the high intake of sugar, salt, and refined vegetable oils. And the intake of soda is a major problem with the SAD. None of that would fit with a Creationist Diet.

Next is the low intake of fruits and vegetables in the American diet, and when they are eaten, being in the form of French fries and potato chips. Neither of those foods would fit with a Creationist Diet. Instead, in the Creationist Diet, there is a great emphasis on eating whole fruits and fresh vegetables. Just consuming more produce would cause a vast improvement in the SAD.

Switching from refined to whole grains would be the next big difference. Then there would be a de-emphasis on animal foods, with the animal foods being consumed being from old-fashioned meats and dairy.

Simply put, it would be a radical change for Americans to switch form the SAD to a Creationist Diet. But doing so would make a dramatic difference in the health of Americans.

The Mediterranean Diet

The Mediterranean Diet is a popular diet plan and one that is often praised as being particularly healthy. What does it look like?

The Mediterranean diet is based on the traditional foods that people used to eat in countries like Italy and Greece back in the year 1960.

Researchers noted that these people were exceptionally healthy compared to Americans and **had a low risk of many killer diseases.**

Numerous studies have now shown that the Mediterranean diet can cause weight loss and help prevent heart attacks, strokes, type 2 diabetes and premature death....

Eat: Vegetables, fruits, nuts, seeds, legumes, potatoes, whole grains, breads, herbs, spices, fish, seafood and extra virgin olive oil.

Eat in Moderation: Poultry, eggs, cheese and yogurt.

Eat Only Rarely: Red meat.

Don't Eat: Sugar-sweetened beverages, added sugars, processed meat, refined grains, refined oils and other highly processed foods (Authority Nutrition. Mediterranean).

The Mediterranean diet emphasizes:

- Eating primarily plant-based foods, such as **fruits and vegetables, whole grains, legumes and nuts**
- Replacing butter with healthy fats such as **olive oil** and canola oil
- **Using herbs and spices instead of salt** to flavor foods
- Limiting red meat to no more than a few times a month
- **Eating fish and poultry at least twice a week**
- Enjoying meals with family and friends
- Drinking red wine in moderation (optional)
- Getting plenty of exercise...

The Mediterranean diet traditionally includes **fruits, vegetables, pasta and rice.** For example, residents of Greece eat very little red meat and average **nine servings a day of antioxidant-rich fruits and vegetables.**

Grains in the Mediterranean region are typically whole grain and usually contain very few unhealthy trans fats, and

448

bread is an important part of the diet there. However, throughout the Mediterranean region, **bread is eaten plain or dipped in olive oil** — not eaten with butter or margarines, which contain saturated or trans fats.

Nuts are another part of a healthy Mediterranean diet (WebMD).

At this point, you probably already know that **the Mediterranean diet is good for your health**. Research proves over and over again that **people who put an emphasis on produce, fish, whole grains, and healthy fats not only weigh less, but also have a decreased risk for heart disease, depression, and dementia. So what are you waiting for?** (Health. 10 Things).

Fruits, vegetables, nuts, whole grains, legumes, fish, and olive oil. Those foods are staples of both the Mediterranean Diet and the Creationist Diet. Both diet plans also limit the intake of refined grains, refined sugar, refined oils, processed meats, and processed foods in general. There is thus much in common between the two diet plans.

The main differences are the emphases on consuming old-fashioned meats and dairy rather than factory farm versions of these foods and organic rather commercial produce in the Creationist Diet. Such is generally not mentioned in connection with the Mediterranean Diet.

It is important to note that much research has been done on the Mediterranean Diet and its various components, and this research has proven it is a very healthy way of eating. Since the Creationist Diet is similar to the Mediterranean Diet, then this research would also support the Creationist Diet as being a healthy eating plan. So again, what are you waiting for?

The DASH Diet

The DASH Diet is another popular and highly praised dietary plan. The acronym DASH stands for Dietary Approaches for Stopping Hypertension (high blood pressure). But along with being beneficial for high blood pressure, this diet has proven to be beneficial in other ways.

The healthy **DASH diet plan was developed to lower blood pressure without medication** in research sponsored by the US National Institutes of Health. The first DASH diet research showed that it could lower blood pressure as well as the first line blood pressure medications, even with a sodium intake of 3300 mg/day! Since then, **numerous studies have shown that the DASH diet reduces the risk of many diseases, including some kinds of cancer, stroke, heart disease, heart failure, kidney stones, and diabetes**. It has been proven to be an effective way to lose weight and become healthier at the same time. It is full of fabulous, delicious, real foods. All of these benefits led to the **#1 diet ranking by *US News & World Report* in 2011, 2012, 2013, and 2014**....

The DASH diet is based on the research studies: Dietary Approaches to Stop Hypertension, and has been proven to lower blood pressure, reduce cholesterol, and improve insulin sensitivity. Blood pressure control with the DASH diet involves more than just the traditional low salt or low sodium diet advice. **It is based on an eating plan proven to lower blood pressure, a plan rich in fruits, vegetables, and low-fat or nonfat dairy. It emphasizes whole grains** and contains less refined grains compared with a typical diet. It is rich in potassium, magnesium, calcium, and fiber....

The DASH diet eating plan is a diet rich in fruits, vegetables, low fat or nonfat dairy. It also includes mostly whole grains; lean meats, fish and poultry; nuts and beans. It is high fiber and low to moderate in fat. It is a plan that follows US guidelines for sodium content, along with vitamins and minerals. In addition to lowering blood pressure, **the DASH eating plan lowers cholesterol and makes it easy to lose weight**. It is a healthy way of eating, designed to be flexible enough to meet the lifestyle and food preferences of most people. It can be considered to be **an Americanized version of the Mediterranean diet**, and to be easier to follow, since it has more specific guidelines (What is the DASH Diet?).

The new guidelines for preventing heart disease and strokes, from The American Heart Association and The

American College of Cardiology recommend the DASH diet, which "**emphasize[s] fruits, vegetables, whole grains, low-fat dairy products, poultry, fish and nuts**."

Why has the DASH diet been ranked as the best diet, **the healthiest diet, and the best diet for diabetes, 7** years in a row? The expert panel of physicians assembled by *US New & World Report* chose DASH because **it is proven to improve health**, has a balance of healthy food groups, and **it actually works**. It has been proven to lower blood pressure and cholesterol, and is associated with lower risk of several types of cancer, heart disease, stroke, heart failure, kidney stones, reduced risk of developing diabetes, and can slow the progression of kidney disease.

The DASH diet is **a plant-focused diet, rich in fruits and vegetables, nuts, with low-fat and non-fat dairy, lean meats, fish, and poultry, mostly whole grains, and heart healthy fats. You fill up on delicious fruits and vegetables, paired up with protein-rich foods to quench your hunger.** This makes a plan that is so easy to follow....

While the DASH diet was originally developed as an eating style to help lower blood pressure, **it has been found to be a fabulous plan for weight loss**....

Because it **has an emphasis on real foods**, heavy on fruits and vegetables, balanced with the right amount of protein, DASH is the perfect weight loss solution. **It is filling and satisfying.** Because it is healthy, **you can follow it for your whole life. And it is a plan that you can feed your entire family,** with larger portion sizes for those who don't need to watch their weight. It helps you easily lose weight, even though you feel as if you are not on a diet, and it actually makes you healthier! (DASH Diet Eating Plan).

Thus the DASH diet "emphasizes fruits, vegetables, whole grains, low-fat dairy products, poultry, fish and nuts." It also "has an emphasis on real foods." By that is meant whole natural foods rather than processed foods. All of these points are in accordance with the Creationist Diet, with the exception of less of an emphasis on *low-fat* dairy. But that is because, if dairy is consumed on the Creationist Diet, it should be old-fashioned dairy, for which the fat is not problematic. But it was also said in this book that if factory farm dairy is consumed, then low or non-fat would be best. There is also an emphasis on meats being old-fashioned in the Creationist Diet, and plant foods being organic and non-GMO.

But those finer points aside, just as with the Mediterranean Diet, the DASH Diet and the Creationist Diet are very similar. Thus the evidence for benefits and the praise that the DASH Diet has received would also apply to the Creationist Diet.

These comparisons to the USDA's dietary recommendations and to the Mediterranean and DASH diets are important. They show that what the Creationist Diet advocates is not radical. It is actually rather mainstream and is supported by much scientific evidence, in addition to being supported by the Bible.

The Paleolithic Diet

Mention of the Paleolithic Diet began this book, so how does the Creationist Diet compare with the Paleolithic Diet?

A paleo diet is a dietary plan based on foods similar to what might have been eaten during the Paleolithic era, which dates from approximately 2.5 million to 10,000 years ago.

A paleo diet typically includes **lean meats, fish, fruits, vegetables, nuts and seeds** — foods that in the past could be obtained by hunting and gathering. **A paleo diet limits foods that became common when farming emerged about 10,000 years ago. These foods include dairy products, legumes and grains**....

Farming changed what people ate and established dairy, grains and legumes as additional staples in the human diet. This **relatively late** and rapid change in diet, according to the hypothesis, outpaced the body's ability to adapt. This mismatch is believed to be a contributing factor to the prevalence of obesity, diabetes and heart disease today (Mayo).

Thus the Paleo Diet is based on the theory of evolution while the Creationist Diet is of course based on the theory of creation. As indicted in the Introductory Page "Creation Theory," there is a huge difference between these two theories of origins. The two most important differences for our discussion is the time scale and the intelligence of early humans.

In evolution theory, humans have been evolving for millions of years, from much less intelligent creatures to today's intelligent *homo sapiens*. But in Creation Theory, humans were created just a few thousand years ago and were created with the same intellectual capacity as today's humans.

Thus on an evolutionary viewpoint, pre-humans were around for a couple of millions years before they became intelligent enough to figure out that if you plant a seed in the ground, it will grow into a plant with edible stuff on it. It also took that long for humanoids to figure out how to harness fire and domestic animals. But from a creationist viewpoint, human beings were intelligent from the start and figured out these things very quickly. Therefore, farming, the use of fire, and domestication of animals occurred early in human history. As a result, grains, dairy, legumes, and cooked foods are not near as late of foods as they are in the evolutionary scheme. These differing mindsets lead to the main differences between the Paleo and Creationist Diets.

What to eat [on a Paleo Diet]:
Fruits, Vegetables, Nuts and seeds.
Lean meats, especially grass-fed animals or wild game.
Fish, especially those rich in omega-3 fatty acids, such as salmon, mackerel and albacore tuna.
Oils from fruits and nuts, such as olive oil or walnut oil.

What to avoid:
Grains, such as wheat, oats and barley
Legumes, such as beans, lentils, peanuts and peas
Dairy products
Refined sugar, Salt, Potatoes, Highly processed foods in general (Mayo).

453

Creationist Diet

The recommended regime, known as the paleo or caveman diet, urges people to get in sync with their evolutionary roots by **eating only what our ancient ancestors ate: meat and fish, fruits and vegetables, eggs and nuts**. Off the menu for the paleo eater are cereal grains, dairy products, legumes, refined sugar, and processed foods. **Which means no white bread, chicken nuggets, potato chips, Cocoa Puffs, gummy bears, or Velveeta cheese** (National Geographic).

It can be seen, there are many similarities between the Paleo Diet and the Creationist Diet. Both diet plans recommend the consumption of copious amounts of fruits, vegetables, nuts and seeds. Both diet plans recommend lean meats, "especially grass-fed animals or wild game," along with fatty fish. Both diet plans also recommend avoiding processed foods, with all of the foods mentioned in the last sentence of the last quote also not being included in a Creationist Diet.

The biggest differences are in regard to dairy products, legumes, potatoes, and grains. Dairy products can have a place in the Creationist Diet. Again, this is because on a creationist timescale, humans learned how to domestic and milk animals much earlier than on an evolutionary timescale. But even on a creationist timescale, this was probably after the Tower of Babel incident, and only some of the scattered people groups began consuming dairy. Thus dairy would be "natural" for those groups who did so early and not quite as natural for those that did so later. Thus the Creationist Diet and the Paleo Diet would be similar for these latter groups.

But legumes and potatoes are a different story. An assumption of evolution is humans did not "discover" fire until late in their evolution. But on a creationist timescale, humans discovered fire shortly after the Fall, so foods such as legumes and potatoes that are best consumed cooked would have been possible very early. As such, these foods have a place in the Creationist Diet but not in a Paleo Diet.

A similar situation exists for grains. Whole grains have a substantial place in the Creationist Diet while they are eliminated in the Paleolithic Diet. Paleolithic Diet advocates claim grains are the cause of many of today's degenerative diseases. But is it because of eating grains as the Paleolithic diet advocates claim, or is it because of eating *refined* grains?

The vast difference between whole and refined grains has been documented in this book, but such is ignored by Paleo Diet advocates. Consequently, they blame modern day health problems on grains in general, ignoring that most of the grains being consumed are refined. Related to this is their blaming the USDA's dietary recommendations in general for today's healthy problems.

The basic premise of the paleolithic diet is that human beings evolved over millions of years eating mostly meat and fish, and fresh fruits, vegetables, and nuts. **Grains, legumes, dairy products, and potatoes** were not part of the diet, having only been introduced since the advent of agriculture, several thousand years ago. That was not enough time for our bodies to adapt to the concentrated sources of glucose and foreign protein and toxin content found in these foods, and **we are paying for it with cancer, heart disease, diabetes, stroke, and auto-immune diseases.**

Studies done this century on **hunter-gatherers that live pre-agricultural lives show the complete absence of any of the above mentioned diseases.** Furthermore, when these hunter-gatherers adopt a "Western" diet - one high in grains, carbohydrates, and dairy products, as well as various unnatural fats (like hydrogenated oils, vegetable oils, and seed oils), they suddenly have high rates of the various diseases. Thus, **the USDA food pyramid, which is based on grains, can actually do one who follows it more harm than good** (Katz).

But, as indicated previously, most Americans do not actually follow the recommendations of the USDA, be they from the older pyramid, the newer MyPlate, or the detailed Guidelines. Thus to blame these diseases on the USDA's recommendations is disingenuous.

What Americans are consuming is the SAD. Again, the problem with the SAD is it is way too low in fruits and vegetables and way too high in saturated fats, sugars and other "empty calories" obtained from refined and processed foods. In other words, it is not the foods the USDA recommends that are causing the health problems Americans experience today, but junk foods, both by being unhealthy in themselves and by replacing more healthy foods.

455

As the book by *Natural Health* magazine puts it:
The SAD diet is appropriately named because of its long-term effects. **Eating too much animal food, fat and oil, and sugar, and too few complex carbohydrates such as fruits and vegetables and fruits, whole grains, and legumes, contributes to the development of degenerative diseases.** These include Western societies' major killers: heart disease, cancer, obesity, and strokes. It also includes a host of annoying if not fatal conditions, such as constipation, hemorrhoids, gout, osteoporosis, and tooth decay (Mayell, p.3).

Thus the Paleolithic diet advocates are correct in saying diet plays a role in many western diseases. But they are blaming the wrong diet. It is not the what the USDA recommends but what Americans are actually eating that is the problem.

Conclusion

All of the diets discussed in this chapter (except the SAD) advocate consuming more fruits and vegetables. They all recommend consuming nuts, seeds, fatty fish and only lean meats. They all recommend eliminating or at least reducing the intake of refined grains, refined sugar, refined oils, and processed foods in general.

There are differences on some finer points, but just following these common recommendations would do wonders in improving the health of the average American. These steps would also be helpful in losing body fat, something else many Americans need. That subject will be addressed in the next chapter.

Bibliography:
2015-2020 Dietary Guidelines for America.
https://health.gov/dietaryguidelines/2015/guidelines/
Authority Nutrition. Mediterranean Diet 101: A Meal Plan and Beginner's Guide.
https://authoritynutrition.com/mediterranean-diet-meal-plan/
Choose My Plate.

https://www.choosemyplate.gov

Dr. Axe. 9 Charts That Show Why America is Fat, Sick & Tired.
https://draxe.com/charts-american-diet/

DASH Diet Eating Plan, The.
http://dashdiet.org/default.asp

Food Guide Pyramid: A Guide to Daily Food Choice.
No longer available.
http://www.nal.usda.gov:8001/py/pmap.htm

Health. 10 Things to Know About the Mediterranean Diet.
http://www.health.com/health/gallery/0,,20793870,00.html

Katz, Tamir. *Tamir's* Paleolithic Diet and Exercise Page.
No longer available.
http://pages.hotbot.com/health/tbk3/index.html.

Mayo Clinic. Paleo diet: What is it and why is it so popular?
http://www.mayoclinic.org/healthy-lifestyle/nutrition-and-healthy-eating/in-depth/paleo-diet/art-20111182

Mayell, Mark. *52 Simple Steps to Natural Health*. New York:
Pocket Books, 1995.

NJ Nutritionist. The Standard American Diet is SAD.
http://njnutritionist.com/the-standard-american-diet-is-sad

Nutrition Facts. Standard American Diet. Michael Greger M.D. ·
Last Updated on January 2, 2017.
http://nutritionfacts.org/topics/standard-american-diet/

Oxford Dictionary. As found on Microsoft *Word 365*.

Paleolithic Diet Information:
http://pages.hotbot.com/health/tbk3/diet.html

Spooky Facts About the Standard American Diet.
http://alaskaveg.org/SpookyFacts/SpookyFacts.pdf

Time. Americans Are Eating Too Much Bacon and Too Few Nuts:
Study.
http://time.com/4694883/bacon-nuts-soda-heart-disease-study/

WebMD. Mediterranean diet: A heart-healthy eating plan.
http://www.mayoclinic.org/healthy-lifestyle/nutrition-and-healthy-eating/in-depth/mediterranean-diet/art-20047801?pg=1

What is the DASH Diet?
http://dashdiet.org/what_is_the_dash_diet.asp

Creationist Diet

Chapter Seventeen:
Lifestyle Changes for Maintained Body Fat Loss

"95% of people who lose weight regain it"

The above statistic is often repeated. I even did so in the First Edition of this book without researching the issue. And because of this statistic, many people who lose weight and regain it get discouraged and give up trying to lose weight, and many don't even bother trying to do so. However, this statistic is just as false as other commonly cited mythological statistics, like "We only use 10% of our brains" or "50% of marriages end in divorce."

Losing Weight and Keeping It Off

For this Second Edition of this book, I actually did some research in this regard, and I found the rate of people who lose weight and keep it off is actually much higher than the commonly claimed 95% failure/ 5% (1 out of 20) success rate. This has been demonstrated by actual research into this matter:

There is a general perception that almost no one succeeds in long-term maintenance of weight loss. However, research has shown that **approximately 20% of overweight individuals are successful at long-term weight loss** when defined as losing at least 10% of initial body weight and maintaining the loss for at least 1 y[ear] (Wing).

Data were analyzed from the 1999-2002 National Health and Nutrition Examination Survey (NHANES). This study examined U.S. adults aged 20-84 years who were overweight or obese at their maximum weight (body mass index >/=25) and had experienced substantial weight loss (weighed 10% less than their maximum weight 1 year before they were surveyed) (n=1310)....

Compared to their weight 1 year ago, **7.6% had continued to lose weight** (>5%), **58.9% had maintained their weight** (within 5%), **and 33.5% had regained weight** (>5%) (Weist).

Mitchell's study focused on Take Off Pounds Sensibly (TOPS), a national, low-cost, weight loss program led by peer-volunteers and costing just $92 a year...

The study included roughly 75,000 participants, and focused on those who renewed their annual memberships consecutively for up to seven years. **Mitchell found that 50 percent of them had clinically significant weight loss in their first year in TOPS, and 62 percent of those who stayed with the program maintained that after seven years** (Science Daily. Low-cost).

Thus in the first analysis, one-fifth of individuals were able to lose weight and keep it off, while in the second and third studies, two-thirds were able to do so. The large difference between these percentages show the difficulty in determining such a statistic. But they are all still far greater than the 5% success rate that is commonly believed.

But where did the 95% failure statistic come from?

It is a depressing article of faith among the overweight and those who treat them that 95 percent of people who lose weight regain it -- and sometimes more -- within a few months or years.

That statistic has been quoted widely over the last four decades, in Congressional hearings, diet books, research papers and seminars. And it is the reason so many people approach dieting with a sense of hopelessness.

But in fact, obesity researchers say, no one has any idea how many people can lose weight and keep it off. Now, as researchers try to determine how many people have succeeded, they are also studying the success stories for lessons that might inspire others to try.

"'That 95 percent figure has become clinical lore,'" said Dr. Thomas Wadden, a professor of psychiatry at the University of Pennsylvania. **There is no basis for it, he said, "'but it's part of the mythology of obesity.''**

Dr. Kelly D. Brownell, the director of the Yale Center for Eating and Weight Disorders, said the number was **first suggested in a 1959 clinical study of only 100 people.** The finding was repeated so often that it came to be regarded as fact, he said (New York Times. 95%).

It's a widely quoted statistic: 95 percent of people regain lost weight. Such a statistic makes you wonder if you should even bother with the workouts and the healthy eating. Before you turn your treadmill into a sanctuary for unfolded laundry and hang-dry only clothing, you should know a few facts about why people regain weight and exactly where that astonishing statistic originated.

The year is 1959 and a small study out of the Yale Center for Eating and Weight Disorders concludes that 95 percent of people regain weight within a few months to a year of losing it. The study included only 100 participants and made a catchy headline that rapidly became a centerpiece in the mythology of obesity.

In 1999, two doctors set out to determine if this discouraging fact was indeed a fact. Dr. Wena Ring and Dr. James O. Hill conducted an analysis of the National Weight Control Registry and **quickly identified more than 2,000 success stories of weight loss and maintenance.** This surprising information spurred them to compile more detailed data and survey the successful dieters. **They found that on average, most dieters maintained a loss of 67 pounds for five years and 12 to 14 percent maintained long-term losses of more than 100 pounds – proving that the 95 percent failure rate was poorly founded** (Fox News. Why)

Thus that 95% figure is a myth, but it might have come from a small study way back in the middle of the last century. Another possibility is confusion with another statistic:

Nearly 65 percent of dieters return to their pre-dieting weight within three years, according to Gary Foster, Ph.D., clinical director of the Weight and Eating Disorders Program at the University of Pennsylvania. The statistics for dieters who lose weight rapidly, according to Wellsphere, a website sponsored by Stanford University, is worse. **Only 5 percent of people who lose weight on a crash diet will keep the weight off** (Livestrong).

Thus it is only those who lose weight via a crash diet who are 95% likely to regain the weight, while in this study about a third of those who lost weight more gradually were able to keep the weight off.

But whether a success rate of one-fifth, one-third, or two-thirds, any of these figures are more encouraging than the commonly believed one-twentieth success rate. As such, overweight individuals should not get discouraged over inflated failure rates but instead should be encouraged that losing weight and keeping it off is possible.

That said; the last quote hints at one important point in losing weight and keeping it off—crash diets are much less effective for long-term weight loss maintenance than losing weight gradually. The following abstracts and quotes point to other common factors among those who achieve long-term weight loss maintenance:

The National Weight Control Registry [NWCR] provides information about the strategies used by successful weight loss maintainers to achieve and maintain long-term weight loss. National Weight Control Registry members have lost an average of 33 kg [72.75 pounds] and maintained the loss for more than 5 y[ears].

To maintain their weight loss, members report engaging in high levels of physical activity (approximately 1 h/d [hour/day]), eating a low-calorie, low-fat diet, eating breakfast regularly, self-monitoring weight, and maintaining a consistent eating pattern across weekdays and weekends.

Moreover, **weight loss maintenance may get easier over time**; after individuals have successfully maintained their weight loss for 2-5 y, the chance of longer-term success greatly increases. **Continued adherence to diet and exercise strategies, low levels of depression and disinhibition, and medical triggers for weight loss are also associated with** long-term success. National Weight Control Registry members provide evidence that **long-term weight loss maintenance is possible and help identify the specific approaches associated with long-term success** (Wing).

Participants in TOPS attend weekly meetings during the weight loss and weight maintenance phases of the program, and **the maintenance phase continues indefinitely.**
Mitchell said that unlike many commercial and academic programs, **there is a minimal difference between the weight-loss and weight-maintenance phases of the TOPS program, reinforcing weight management behaviors** (Science Daily, Low-cost).

Researchers have published one of the first studies of its kind to follow **weight loss maintenance for individuals over a 10-year period.** The results show that **long-term weight loss maintenance is possible if individuals adhere to key health behaviors....**
The participants had lost at least 30 pounds and had kept it off for at least one year when they were enrolled in the National Weight Control Registry (NWCR). The participants were then followed for 10 years....
Thomas says, "On average, participants maintained the majority of their weight loss over this extended follow-up period, and better success was related to **continued performance of physical activity, self-weighing, low-fat diets, and avoiding overeating.**"
Other findings from the study show that **more than 87 percent of the participants were estimated to be still maintaining at least a 10 percent weight loss at years five and 10.** The researchers found that a larger initial weight loss and longer duration of maintenance were associated with better long-term outcomes. **Conversely, they found that decreases in physical activity, dietary restraint and self-weighing along with increases in fat intake were associated with greater weight regain** (Science Daily. Study shows).

Thus physical activity, a low-calorie/ low-fat diet, regular meals (especially breakfast), regular self-weighing, and maintaining the new eating pattern were all factors in keeping the weight off, along with the weight loss and weight maintenance diets being similar.

The National Weight Control Registry also provides incentives for people to lose weight and to keep it off.

The National Weight Control Registry (NWCR) is, to the best of our knowledge, the largest study of individuals successful at long-term maintenance of weight loss. **Despite extensive histories of overweight, the 629 women and 155 men in the registry lost an average of 30 kg [66 pounds] and maintained a required minimum weight loss of 13.6 kg [30 pounds] for 5 y[ears].**

A little over one-half of the sample lost weight through formal programs; the remainder lost weight on their own. **Both groups reported having used both diet and exercise to lose weight and nearly 77% of the sample reported that a triggering event had preceded their successful weight loss.** Mean (+/-SD) current consumption reported by registry members was 5778 +/- 2200 kJ/d, with **24 +/- 9% of energy from fat, Members also appear to be highly active:** they reported expending approximately 11830 kJ/wk through physical activity.

Surprisingly, 42% of the sample reported that maintaining their weight loss was less difficult than losing weight. Nearly all registry members indicated that weight loss led to improvements in their level of energy, physical mobility, general mood, self-confidence, and physical health (Klem).

"This study shows that if an overweight person is able to maintain an initial weight loss -- in this case for a year -- the body will eventually 'accept'' this new weight and thus not fight against it, as is otherwise normally the case when you are in a calorie-deficit state," says Associate Professor Signe Sorensen Torekov from the Department of Biomedical Sciences and Novo Nordisk Foundation Center for Basic Metabolic Research.

The research has recently been published in the *European Journal of Endocrinology*…

The main finding in the study revealed that after one year of successful weight loss maintenance, the researchers were able to demonstrate that postprandial levels of two appetite inhibiting hormones (GLP-1 and PYY) increased (=appetite inhibition) from before-weight loss level -- in contrast to the hunger hormone ghrelin, which increased immediately after weight loss but returned to normal levels (= low hunger) after one year…

"The interesting and uplifting news in this study is that if you are able to maintain your weight loss for a longer period of time, **it seems as if you have 'passed the critical point,' and after this point, it will actually become easier for you to maintain your weight loss** than is was immediately after the initial weight loss (Science Daily. Obese people).

Thus there are many benefits to losing weight and keeping it off, and it gets easier as time goes on. Note also the mention of a "triggering event." This is often a health-scare that causes a person to start to concern themselves with getting their weight under control. But it would be far better to get control of your weight before developing health problems due to being overweight.

Don't "Go on a diet"

Personally, I do not like the phrase, "go on a diet." If you go on something, it implies that sometime in the future you will go off it. This is when dieters will go back to their old eating habits—the ones that got them overweight in the first place.

What is needed is to make permanent lifestyle changes, as the preceding quotes indicate. If you decide you want to lose body fat, then you need to accept you can never go back to eating the way you are now. Also, exercise must become a permanent part of your lifestyle.

The number one reason people regain weight is the diet mentality. The word "diet" earned its reputation as a four-letter word because it has become associated with a period of deprivation and what some would classify as torture. **For many, "diet" means a set span of time during which you must exercise superhuman willpower to resist delicious temptation and overwhelming pains of hunger at the end of which you can finally reward yourself with junk food favorites.**

Very few individuals perceive the concept that healthy eating is not finite – it's a lifelong commitment. Fad diets don't work, because you can't sustain that way of eating forever. **Choose a healthy eating plan that incorporates whole, nutritionally balanced foods** (Fox News. Why).

.

What this means is, there should be very little difference between the weight loss diet and the weight maintenance diet, except for the latter having slightly more calories. In other words, you should be eating the same type of foods while losing weight that you can eat the rest of your life; but once you reach your goal weight, you will need to increase your food intake slightly to keep from losing more weight.

That said; let's begin with a very simple and important fact—to lose body fat you must consume fewer calories than you expend. There is no other way. To lose body fat, you need to reduce caloric intake and/ or increase caloric expenditure. Dr. Ted Mitchell, director of the Cooper Wellness program in Dallas, Texas summarizes these points nicely:

To lose weight, do three simple things:
1) Eat less.
2) Exercise more.
3) Most important: Do it forever!
It's that last one that gets everyone (p.4).

But that last point need not "get" you if you change your lifestyle rather than "go on a diet." And that is what the Creationist Diet is all about—giving the reader guidance in developing a dietary plan you can follow for a lifetime.

That said, let's look at the first two points in more depth.

Reduced Intake

Using the equation: reduced intake plus increased expenditure equals body fat loss, we'll start with the first half—reduced intake. Reduced intake can be accomplished in numerous ways. You could lose weight on the *Big Mac* diet. After a week or two of eating nothing but *Big Macs*, I would suspect that you wouldn't even be able to look at the greasy thing let alone eat it. Thus, caloric intake would fall and you would lose weight. However, this would be a very unhealthy way of doing things. (Incidentally, a *McDonalds's Big Mac* contains more calories than a *Dairy Queen* Banana Split, 590 versus 510).

In other words, any diet that restricts you to eating one or two foods or classes of food will reduce intake. Unfortunately, nutritionally this would be unwise, as the body requires nutrients from a wide variety of foods to be adequately nourished. Also, such diets are so restrictive that they cannot be used for extended periods of time. Such problems with restrictive diets were discussed in Chapter Three and were indicated in the quotes earlier in this chapter.

In addition, with crash diets the dieter never learns new eating habits. As a result, when the dieter tires of these programs, a return to the old fattening eating habits is the only way known. What is needed is to make necessary dietary changes that can be continued indefinitely while ensuring adequate nutrient intake.

The best way to accomplish this would be to follow some of the suggestions already discussed in this book, such as limiting the consumption of "empty calories"—foods high in caloric density but low in nutrient density, i.e. junk foods. Notice, I said limit, not eliminate. You can continue to eat limited amounts of your favorite junk foods occasionally. The key words here are limited and occasionally. Again, we're looking for a dietary program that can continue for a lifetime.

Although, it would be best to avoid "trigger foods" altogether, at least for a while. These are foods that a person cannot seem to stop eating at a reasonable amount or which if when they are eaten once in a limited amount, the person keeps craving them for the next several days. Stop consuming such foods until they are no longer a problem. You might even find that after not consuming such foods for a while, you no longer desire them.

By eliminating or even just limiting the consumption of junk foods, the caloric intake of the average person will drop significantly, and you'll lose body fat.

To clarify what is meant by junk foods, examples include: potato chips and other greasy and salty snack foods, cakes, cookies, pies, pudding, gelatin desert, ice cream, sherbet, soda and other sugary beverages, candy, fried foods, and most fast foods. In other words, foods listed previously in the "non-God-given foods" category.

Added Sugars and Fats

What most of the foods in the preceding paragraph have in common is a high percentage of their calories come from added sugars and/ or added fats. Most also contain a large amount of sodium. The first two contain no nutrients except for calories, so restricting their intake will reduce calories without reducing nutrient intake.

Reducing these two food ingredients is sound nutritional advice for reasons other than just weight loss. Heart attacks, strokes, cancer, diabetes and hypoglycemia have been linked to diets high in these substances. Therefore, a low-fat and low-refined carb diet can and should be followed for a lifetime.

Fat levels can easily be reduced by following some of the previous recommendations in this book: trimming the cover fat off meats, removing the skin off of poultry, consuming baked or broiled chicken and fish rather than fried versions thereof, not consuming processed meats and ground meats that have the cover fat or skin ground into them, and not consuming processed foods that have refined oils added to them.

Dr. Ted Mitchell has an important warning here though:
But be careful. When you hear experts discuss low-fat diets they're not saying it's OK to go crazy eating **fat-free cookies, ice cream, cakes and other foods that have been reformulated to get some of the fat out**. While these products have been altered to reduce their fat content, **the fat often is replaced with sugar, making them calorie-rich** (p.4).

In other words, just because a food is promoted as being low in fat, this doesn't mean it won't cause you to add body fat, as "fat-free" foods are often sugar-laden, but sugar is another substance that needs to be restricted to lose body fat. But does eating excessive added fat and sugar really cause increased body fat?

Consider the following:
An Indiana University study compared the diet composition of 40 lean and 38 obese men and women. Subjects were asked to fill out a detailed food questionnaire for three days. The result: **There was virtually no difference in the number of calories consumed by lean versus obese participants.** The researchers also believe there was no significant difference in the activity levels of the two groups.

What did differ was diet composition. **The obese men got an average of 33 percent of their calories from fat, while the lean men took in 29 percent as fat. Obese women got 36 percent of their calories from fat, whereas lean women's intake was 29 percent.** Further, obese men and women tended to get **a higher percentage of their sugar from added and refined sugar. They also consumed less fiber than their lean counterparts** (*Burn*, p.10).

This study was conducted to determine the relationships among the specific components of dietary fat and carbohydrate and body fatness in lean and obese adults. ... **No differences were found between lean and obese subjects for energy intake or total sugar intake, but obese subjects derived a greater portion of their energy from fat** (33.1 +/- 2.6% and **36.3** +/- 2.3% for obese men and women, respectively, vs **29.1** +/- 1.3% and **29.6** +/- 2.0%, lean men and women, respectively). Percent of fat intake for saturated, monounsaturated, and polyunsaturated fats was not different among groups. **Obese subjects derived a greater percentage of their sugar intake from added sugars than lean subjects** (38.0 +/- 3.5% vs 25.2 +/- 2.0%, respectively, for men; 47.9 +/- 8.0% vs 31.4 +/- 3.4%, respectively, for women). **Dietary fiber was lower for obese men (20.9 +/- 1.8 g) and women (15.7**

+/- 1.1 g) than for lean men (27.0 +/- 1.8 g) and women (22.7 +/- 2.1 g)

Obesity is maintained primarily by a diet that is high in fat and added sugar and relatively low in fiber. Alterations in diet composition rather than energy intake may be a weight control strategy for overweight adults (Miller).

What is interesting about the preceding two studies is both found no association between obesity and energy intake. That seems to contradict what was said previously about energy in and energy out. But what it shows is it is not just the number of calories that matter but the form of those calories. And the most fattening form of calories is added fats and added sugars. Both are associated with increased body fat, while fiber is associated with lower body fat. But it should be noted that total sugar intake was not associated with obesity.

What this is showing is that people who consume more processed foods tend to be heavier, while those who consume less processed foods tend to have less body fat. Thus the sugar in the leaner people's diets was probably from fruit and dairy while the sugar in the heavier people's diets was from junk foods. In other words, fruit and dairy doesn't cause people to gain body fat, but junk food does.

Similarly, it is not the naturally occurring fat in meat and dairy that leads to body fat gain but the added fats in processed foods and fried foods. This would also include processed meats and ground meat which have the cover fat ground into them, such as fast food hamburger.

This is borne out in the following study:

Epidemiologic analyses have shown numerous associations between consumption of refined grains, added sugars, and fats and higher rates of obesity and diabetes in both the United States and elsewhere. As the present review demonstrates, such low-cost, energy-dense diets are indeed consumed by lower-income people, who are also more likely to be overweight.

Diets of lower–socioeconomic status households provide cheap, concentrated energy from fat, sugar, cereals, potatoes, and fatty meats, but they offer little in the way of whole grains, fish, vegetables, and fruit.

Likewise, low-income consumers are more likely to be **frequent users of fast-food** as opposed to full-service restaurants and are more likely to live in areas with less physical access to healthier foods. In contrast, **costly diets consumed by more-affluent people are likely to be associated with less obesity and better health outcomes** (Oxford).

Thus the main problem when it comes to being overweight is the consumption of processed junk foods, while the solution is to eat whole natural foods in the form that God intended us to eat them—exactly what the Creationist Diet recommends.

However, the point of this study is that a junk food diet is much less expensive than a whole foods diet. And that is true. If the reader takes the information in this book to heart and stops consuming non-God-given foods and instead consumes only God-given foods, then your food budget almost certainly will rise significantly.

But you will need to stop and ask yourself if you would really be saving money by continuing to eat junk food when it leads to you having less energy, which would include less energy for work and all other aspects of life, and in time, it leads to you incurring expensive health problems, with the concurrent loss of productivity, quality of life, and shortened lifespan that health problems cause? Only you the reader can answer that question for yourself.

But that question aside, to be clear on this section, calories do count. Eating an excessive amount of healthy unprocessed foods will cause a gain of body fat. It is just that body fat gain is much more likely with unhealthy processed foods containing added sugars and fats. But why do people overeat such foods? To that question we now turn.

The Satiety Value of Foods

The previous section asserted that consuming fruit would not lead to an increase in body fat. This is true, despite the fact that fruits contain a large percentage of naturally occurring sugars. The reason for this is that along with numerous vitamins, minerals, and antioxidants, fruit also contains fiber and water, and the preceding studies found that consuming foods with a high fiber content are associated with lower body fat, as are foods with a high water content, as we will see shortly.

Therefore, when your sweet tooth starts throbbing, reach for a piece of fruit instead of a candy bar. Fruit is just as sweet but is more filling. It would take three apples to equal the calories in one candy bar, and the apples would be more satisfying. And this leads to an important point—the satiety value of foods.

Satiation and satiety are central concepts in the understanding of appetite control and both have to do with the inhibition of eating. **Satiation** occurs during an eating episode and brings it to an end. **Satiety** starts after the end of eating and prevents further eating before the return of hunger (Bellisle).

Despite this technical distinction, generally speaking, satiation and satiety are used interchangeably, with both referring to how filling a food is and how long it keeps a person feeling full. Many studies have been done in this regard.

One such study was performed at my alma mater. It demonstrated the value of eating foods high in water content for their satiety value. A report on Penn State's website about the study begins by stating, "Drinking water before or with your meals is a healthy habit, but Penn State research has shown that it won't satisfy your hunger or help you eat less to control your weight." Thus the old "trick" of drinking water to curb appetite doesn't really work. But the Penn State researchers found something that does work:

[Dr. Barbara] Rolls and her research team have shown that eating **foods with a high water content**—pasta dishes with additional vegetables, smoothies, soup, fruits and vegetables—can **offer a way to cut back on calories and still feel full and satisfied**.

It is thus water in food, not in a glass, that can provide satiety value. This difference was proven by the following experiment:

They [24 volunteers] were served a first course 17 minutes before lunch that consisted of **either a chicken rice casserole,** the same casserole with a glass of water, or a bowl of chicken rice soup. Even though the soup and the casserole-served-with-water contained exactly the same ingredients in the same amounts, **the soup was more effective in curbing appetite and reducing the calories the women consumed during lunch.**

The researchers further suggest:

... **pasta salad bulked up with zucchini, carrots and other veggies**, which have a high water content, can provide a portion double the size for the same calories as a salad made without the veggies. **Chili augmented with lots of veggies and beans** can expand the serving size of that dish while still maintaining a low calorie count. **Sprouts, lettuce and tomato can round out the satisfaction that a sandwich provides** without increasing calories (*Reduce Calories*).

What this research shows is it is the energy density of a food that matters in satiety, not the fat content, as many people believe. In other words, when eating the same number of calories, the more caloric dense a food is, the less satisfying it is. And conversely, the less caloric dense a food is, the more satisfying it is.

For instance, a 100-calorie serving of *Peanut M&Ms* would be just ten of them. Meanwhile, three cups of air-popped popcorn also only contain 100 calories. But eating three cups of popcorn is more satisfying than just a few *M&Ms*. Similarly:

If your sweet tooth calls for cherry, you may be better off reaching for the actual fruit. You can eat a whole cup of fresh cherries for fewer calories than just two *Twizzler Cherry Twists* (Shape).

The real cherries would not only be more nutritious, but they would also be more satiating than the candy alternative. This is confirmed by the "Satiety Index."

On his website, Rick Mendosa discusses the Satiety Index:

Susanne Holt, PhD, has developed the Satiety Index, a system to measure different foods' ability to satisfy hunger. A fixed amount (240 calories) of different foods was fed to participants who then **ranked their feelings of hunger every fifteen minutes** and were allowed to eat freely for the next two hours. **Of all the foods tested, potatoes were the most satisfying.**

Mendosa explains the methodology and general trends of the study:

Using **white bread as the baseline of 100,** 38 different foods were ranked. In other words, **foods scoring higher than 100 are more satisfying than white bread and those under 100 are less satisfying....**

Holt found that some foods, like croissants, are only half as satisfying as white bread, while **boiled potatoes are more than three times as satisfying, easily the most satisfying food tested. But potatoes in a different form—French fries—did not score well.** This type of information can have important implications for those wanting to lose weight.

The chemical components of a food is one of the factors that determines how it ranks on the index. "Beans and lentils, for example, contain anti-nutrients which delay their absorption so they make you feel full for longer," says Holt. "Roughly speaking, **the more fiber, protein and water a food contains, the longer it will satisfy.** But you have to look at each foodstuff individually—and that is why we think our index will be so useful." **Another thing that makes a food satisfying is its sheer bulk. "You can eat an awful lot of popcorn without taking in a lot of calories,"** says Holt. "It may not weigh much, but it makes your stomach feel full just because it takes up so much space.... **As a group, fruits ranked at the top with a satiety index 1.7 times more satisfying, on average, than white bread.**

There are exceptions, but generally speaking "bulkier" foods will be more satisfying than more caloric-dense foods. This is an important point for dieters. It is not how much fat or carbohydrates in a food that matters as much as how much it will fill you up. And, not surprisingly, many God-given foods rank high on the satiety index.

Fruits, vegetables, and legumes are mostly ranked high on the index, and whole grains generally rank higher than their refined counterparts. For a listing of all the foods that have been tested so far, see the following webpage: www.mendosa.com/satiety.htm

A related index is the Fullness Factor (FF). It uses mathematical calculations based on the nutrient content of foods to determine its FF. The developers comment on the results of the calculations:

Foods that contain large amounts of fat, sugar, and/or starch have low Fullness Factors, and are much easier to overeat. Foods that contain large amounts of water, dietary fiber, and/or protein have the highest Fullness Factors. These high-FF foods, which include **most vegetables, fruits, and lean meats, do a better job of satisfying your hunger**...

Although all of the items in the above table are solid foods, the Fullness Factor can also be calculated for liquids, including soups and drinks. **Most liquid foods will have above average Fullness Factors, due to their high water content.** Liquid foods do, in fact, have a relatively high satiating effect, at least for the short term. **However, low viscosity liquids (such as water, juice, or soft drinks) will empty from your stomach quickly, and may leave you hungry again in a relatively short time.** Keep this in mind if you are using the Fullness Factor to select foods for weight loss (Nutrition Data).

The first sentence of this extended quote answers the question that introduced this section. Foods with large amounts of fat, sugar, and starch (i.e., processed carbs) are easy to overeat. This is why a person can easily eat a whole bag of chips or a pint of ice-cream. But try to eat a pound of carrots, and you might find yourself struggling by the last carrot. And again, God-given foods like fruits, vegetables, and lean meats have a high FF.

Moreover, *Runner's World* magazine reports about:
... a study published in the *Journal of the American Medical Association.* **Those who ate the most fiber weighed an**

average of 8 pounds less than those ate who ate the least amount of fiber. Try to consume at least 30 grams a day from **whole grain cereals and breads, vegetables, and beans** (Bauman, p.28).

Based on this information, *Men's Health* magazine presented a list of "10 foods guaranteed to keep you full for longer." They are: white potatoes, eggs, oatmeal, beans, fish, soup, apples, beef, salad, and popcorn. All of these foods are high in fiber, protein, and/ or water content, and not surprisingly, all of these foods are God-given foods.

Runner's World reports about another method to help reduce food intake:

> Researchers [at Brazosport Memorial Hospital in Lake Jackson, TX] asked seven women to **eat slowly, chew thoroughly, and push away their plates at every meal once their food no longer tasted delicious.** Meanwhile, six other women were instructed to also eat and chew slowly, but received no hints on monitoring their taste buds. After a year, the first group of women **lost an average of 9 pounds,** and those in the control group gained about three pounds....
>
> **Once you've consumed enough food, your body sends a subtle "stop-eating signal" by dampening your taste sensations** (Bauman, p.26).

So it would seem paying attention to the taste of food can actually help you to eat less. It would make eating more enjoyable as well.

Salt and Appetite

It was mentioned in passing in Chapter One that you are more likely to overeat salted versus unsalted nuts, and it was said, "The salt seems to encourage overeating." These claims were borne out in a new study, as part of preparations for a planned mission to Mars of all things. And it is not just nuts, but any salted food is more likely to be overeaten than its unsalted counterpart.

In the study, two groups of potential astronauts on two different occasions were kept in an enclosed environment and fed a controlled diet, with the only difference between the two diets being their salt content. The results were surprising in that the extra salt did not make the potential astronauts thirstier, but it did make them hungrier.

Answering the age-old question of why you can't have just one chip, **a new study shows that salty snacks don't make you thirsty at all. Instead, they stimulate appetite** (Daily News. Why).

Higher salt didn't increase their thirst, but it did make them hungrier. Also the human "cosmonauts" receiving a salty diet **complained about being hungry** (MDC Insights).

Thus, along with keeping salt intake low for blood pressure purposes, it is wise to do so if you are trying to reduce your food intake.

Increased Expenditure

Moving to the other half of the equation—increased expenditure—this, of course, means exercise. I know that is a four-letter word to some, but it need not be. There is such a wide variety of exercise modalities available that anyone can find something they enjoy doing.

Exercise is advantageous to a body fat loss program for two reasons. First is the calories burned during the activity itself. Second and more important is regular exercise, by increasing muscle mass, will increase the resting metabolic rate (RMR). This is the number of calories spent just living. By increasing the rate in which your body burns calories, you will burn up more calories in a normal day.

To force this adaptive process, you must exercise at least 30 minutes three times/week, preferably longer. Although, going over six hours per week would be unnecessary. In other words, try to work up to about one hour, six-times/ week. How important is it to include exercise in a body fat loss program? Consider the following study done at Queen's University in Klingston, Ontario:

In what might be called the dieting equivalent of throwing the baby out with the bathwater, the study showed 12 obese

477

women each losing more than 20 pounds in 16 weeks. Unfortunately, **lean tissue and skeletal muscle made up a significant part of those lost pounds.**

Yet in the same study, 12 other obese women followed a similar diet and lost the same amount of weight, and **virtually all of it was from fat.** What was the difference? Simple. **The second group exercised aerobically five times a week in addition to restricting their caloric intake** (*Burn*, p.38).

Thus exercise protects lean tissue while encouraging body fat loss. That is why exercise is so important to include in a body fat loss program. And it is not just aerobic exercise; strength training is also important to include in a body fat loss program. This was demonstrated by yet another study done at this writer's alma mater:

> 23 female collegiate tennis players **weight trained two to three times per week....** Result: The athletes **dropped from 23 percent to 18 percent body fat.** A significant change, especially given that there was no dietary restrictions placed on the study subjects" (*Burn*, p.38).

Moreover:

> [An] University of Maryland study looked at 15 sedentary post-menopausal women aged 50-69. The women **worked out three times a week for 16 weeks....** By the end of the study, the women **increased their resting metabolic rates....** The increase amounted to **about 50 calories a day**, enough to burn five pounds of fat if it were continued for a year (*Burn*, pp.39-40).

A similar study was reported in the *Journal of Applied Physiology*:

> **Two separate experiments were performed to determine the effect of acute resistive exercise on postexercise energy expenditure in male subjects previously trained in resistive exercise.**
>
> In experiment 1, after measurement of their **resting metabolic rate (RMR)** at 0700 h and their ingestion of a

standardized meal at 0800 h, seven subjects (age range 22–40 yr) beginning at 1400 h completed a 90-min weight-lifting protocol. **Postexercise metabolic rate (PEMR)** was measured continuously for 2 h after exercise and compared with a preexercise baseline. RMR was measured the following morning 15 h after completion of the workout.

In experiment 2, six different men (age range 20–35 yr) completed a similar experimental protocol as well as a control condition on a separate day in which metabolic rate was measured for 2 h after a period of quiet sitting.

For both experiments, PEMR remained elevated for the entire 2-h [two hour] measured recovery period, with the average oxygen consumption for the last 6 min elevated by 11–12%. **RMR measured the morning after exercise was 9.4% higher in experiment 1 and 4.7% higher in experiment 2 than on the previous day**....

Strenuous resistive exercise may elevate PEMR for a prolonged period and may enhance postexercise lipid oxidation (Melby).

The Livestrong website provides additional information:

Aerobic exercise, particularly vigorous aerobic exercise, boosts your calorie burn rate for hours after you finish your workout. Vigorous aerobic exercise elevates your heart rate to approximately 80 percent sub-maximal, for at least 20 minutes. A study published in "Medicine and Science in Sports and Exercise" examined young male subjects who exercised vigorously on exercise bikes for 45 minutes. After completing their workouts, **their metabolisms increased for an average of 14 hours, and they burned an average of 190 additional calories** above their resting metabolic levels.

A weight-lifting regimen has both short-term and long-term effects on your metabolism. The effects are greatest when you lift heavy, free weights. After you finish a strenuous workout, your body begins to restore glycogen and other enzymes, such as adenosine triphosphate [ATP], within your muscles. Also, your body begins to repair damaged muscle tissue. Because your workout has depleted the energy-producing components from your muscles, your body must burn more energy from the food you eat. **As you create more active muscle tissue from lifting weights, you also increase your resting metabolic rate** (Hutchins).

Medical Daily summarizes the situation well:

Aerobic activity from walking running, cycling, and swimming can speed up your metabolism and help you lose weight. Because **muscle tissue burns more calories than fat tissue**, incorporating **muscle-strength training** into your routine two or more days a week will increase your metabolic rate (Olson).

Thus with both aerobic exercise and strength training, more calories are burned than just those burned during the exercise. And with strength training, the gained muscle mass leads to an elevated RMR. Therefore, both forms of exercise are important in a body fat loss program. Moreover, both forms of exercise must become a permanent part of your lifestyle, not just something you do for a couple of weeks or until you have lost your desired pounds.

Exercising several hours a week, every week is needed for the calories burned during exercise and to maintain the elevation of the resting metabolic weight and added muscle mass. These factors will help to keep body fat from creeping back on. The same applies to maintaining a low processed foods diet. Re-adding processed foods can lead to a slow return of unwanted pounds.

Once you have reached your desired level of body fat, you will need to slightly increase your caloric intake to prevent further body fat loss. However, it would be recommended to add these calories in the form of healthy God-given foods, such as those discussed throughout this book.

Body Fat versus Bodyweight

Throughout this chapter, I have generally used the term "body fat" rather than bodyweight, as changes in bodyweight can be misleading if they include changes in both the amount of fat on one's body and the amount of muscle. The importance of this was indicted in the preceding quotes about losing muscle when losing weight if exercise is not utilized and gaining muscle leading to an increased RMR. This distinction is also important when gauging your progress.

Dr. Meinz explains:
If you lose ten pounds of fat, but because of physical activity, gain seven pounds of muscle, the liar scale will say you only lost *three little pounds*! **The scale can't tell you what the weight loss is made up of.** You're wearing smaller clothes, you're looking great in the mirror, and all your friends want to know your secret—but the scale says you're a failure. And if you believe the scale you *will* be a failure (pp., 53-54; italics in original).

The reason you'll be "wearing smaller clothes" if you lose fat while gaining muscle is because muscle is denser than fat. In other words, a pound of muscle is smaller than a pound of fat. As such, simply noticing at how your clothes fit or looking at yourself in the mirror can be helpful in gauging how well your body fat loss program is going in addition to weighing yourself on a scale.

But if you need to have an objective way of recording your fat loss, there are ways to measure how much body fat you have. Body fat is expressed in percentages. Normal levels are as follows:

Men under thirty: 14-20%
Men over thirty: 17-23%
Women under thirty: 17-24%
Women over thirty: 20-27% (Tanita, p.2).

A simple method to measure body fat percent is with skin-fold calipers. These measure the amount of "pinchable" flab on various parts of the body. The measurements are then compared to a chart that then gives the fat percent. Digital calipers are available which automatically show the body fat percentage.

A more sophisticated method is a water tank. Since muscle is denser than fat, then the more muscle a person has the more they will sink. Conversely, the more body fat someone has, then the more they will float. Such measurements can be rather expensive though.

481

A newer, and less expensive way is to use a "body fat scale." Such a scale will not only give you your bodyweight, but also your body fat percent. Body fat scales work on the principle that fat and muscle hold different amounts of water, hence their electrical conductivity differs. You stand on sensors and they send a small but unnoticeable electrical charge through your body, and the rate of conductivity is measured, then the fat percent given. But the measurements can be affected by hydration levels, so they can be a bit off. This can be alleviated somewhat by weighing yourself at the same time and under the same conditions each day.

It would also be helpful to take your body measurements at the start of a body improvement program and periodically thereafter. Measure your waist, hips, chest, shoulders, arms, forearms, thighs, and calves. Changes in these areas can indicate if you are going muscle or fat, as most people add fat in their waist or hips but muscle in the other areas.

So noticing how your clothes fit, looking at yourself in the mirror, measuring your body fat percent using calipers, a water tank, or a body fat scale, and using a tape measure are all good methods at gauging your progress in addition to using a traditional scale.

Conclusion on Losing Body Fat

In sum, do not go on a diet—change your lifestyle. Reducing the number of calories in your diet, especially by reducing the amount of added fats and sugars, along with reducing salt intake, and including exercise will allow for a slow (1-2 pounds/ week), sustained, permanent body fat loss. Crash diets will give more rapid weight loss but with just as rapid weight re-gains. Also, they will send you on a roller coaster ride of weight-loss, weight-regain, with possible health damaging effects.

Gaining Weight

The emphasis in our society is on losing weight, as a majority of Americans are overweight. But there are people who want to gain weight. These include not just those who are naturally skinny but also strength athletes like bodybuilders, football players, and powerlifters.

Can you gain weight on a Creationist Diet? Definitely yes. The only Creationist Diet I would not recommend for someone trying to gain weight would be the very restrictive Edenic Diet. But even if you are following an Antediluvian/ vegan diet, you could gain weight, though it would be easier with a diet plan that includes animal foods. Thus the Noahic or Promised Land versions would be even better.

That said, to gain weight you would want to do the opposite of some of what has been suggested in this chapter about losing body fat. It was said that the most filling foods are ones that are bulky, especially due to a high water content. Therefore, to gain weight, you would want to consume foods that are not so bulky, or to put it another way, ones that are low on the Satiety Index. Such foods are generally caloric dense.

The best such vegan foods are nuts, seeds, nut and seed butters, olive oil and nut oils, avocadoes, and dried fruits. These should be emphasized if you are trying to gain weight. And for those eating animal foods, meats and dairy would be very helpful in this regard and would enable even greater muscle gains.

Otherwise, a gain weight diet would not differ much from the regular Creationist Diet other than in larger amounts of foods being eaten. Of course, to gain muscle, not fat, you would need to be engaging in some form of strength training.

Meals per Day

Is it better to eat several small meals a day or two or three larger ones? This writer has long believed the former, that it is better to have 4-6 smaller meals a day. And I would say such a routine would be better if someone is trying to gain, lose, or maintain weight.

If you are trying to lose weight, eating several times a day, every few hours, will help prevent the feelings of hunger that often accompany diets. Of course, the meals must be small to keep total calories down.

If you are trying to gain weight, then eating several times a day would enable more calories to be consumed without having to "pig-out" at each meal and ending up with that "stuffed" feeling.

And even if you are trying to maintain weight, then eating several meals a day will keep blood sugar on an even keel, preventing hunger pains that can lead to overeating at the next meal. Moreover, if you are following a vegan or near vegan diet, they tend to be a rather bulky, so several meals a day might be necessary to consume sufficient calories.

A small hint, since increased consumption of fruits and vegetables is probably the most important thing you can do to improve your health, make it a "rule" to always eat at least one, preferably two servings of produce at each meal. That way, if you're eating five meals a day, you'll consume at least the minimum number of servings the USDA recommends for fruits and vegetables.

However, there is much debate in regard to meal frequency, with some recent studies indicating fewer not more meals are best.

The idea that eating more frequent, smaller meals raises metabolism is a persistent myth. It is true that digesting a meal raises metabolism slightly and this phenomenon is known as the thermic effect of food.

However, **it is the total amount of food consumed that determines the amount of energy expended during digestion. Eating 3 meals of 800 calories will cause the same thermic effect as eating 6 meals of 400 calories.** There is literally no difference.

Multiple studies have compared eating many smaller vs. fewer larger meals and concluded that there is no significant effect on either metabolic rate or total amount of fat lost...

It seems quite clear that the myth of frequent, small meals is just that... a myth.

There are no health benefits to eating more often, it doesn't raise metabolism and it doesn't improve blood glucose control. If anything, fewer meals is healthier.

So I'm going to propose a radical new idea for timing your meals...

1. When hungry, eat.
2. When full, stop.
3. Repeat indefinitely (Authority Nutrition).

Probably the best advice is the following:

In the end, being able to stick with your diet is more important than the actual diet you choose, according to a 2014 study published in the *Journal of the American Medical Association.* That's because if you follow any approach correctly, be it intermittent fasting or eating six small meals a day, you'll cut calories. You'll lose weight.

"Every person has a dieting personality. You have to find the diet that works best for you," Applegate says. "Don't be discouraged if one doesn't work." Your diet should work with your lifestyle, body and preferences. It should be something you can see yourself doing, and happily, over the long term.

And remember: Even though when you eat is important, **far more imperative is what you eat.** "Eat protein, fruits, vegetables, whole grains and healthy fats at every meal," Belury says. "That's what leads to weight loss, whether you want to eat one or six times a day" (US News).

On the Other Mythological Statistics

Before closing this chapter, it would be good to not leave hanging the two other mythological statistics that were cited at the beginning of this chapter. The first was, "We only use 10% of our brains." A faculty member of Washington State University states about this myth:

Somehow, somewhere, someone started this myth and the popular media keep on repeating this false statement. Soon, everyone believes the statement regardless of the evidence. I have not been able to track down the exact source of this myth, and **I have never seen any scientific data to support it.** According to the believers of this myth, if we used more of our brain, then we could perform super memory feats and have other fantastic mental abilities - maybe we could even move objects with a single thought. Again, **I do not know of any data that would support any of this** (Neuroscience).

And a writer for Psychology Today writes:

When I was a lowly graduate student—doing my PhD thesis on the brains of boas and pythons—I had the great fortune of having dinner with two Nobel prize winning brain scientists, David Hubel and Torsten Wiesel.

Not wanting to waste the opportunity, I asked the great men: where did the idea that we only use 10% of our brains come from, and is it true?

They smiled, shook their heads, and said that they weren't sure where the idea originated. But both agreed that **the 10% theory was a myth.** Nature, they observed, does not waste resources that way because there is a name for species that are inefficient: fossils.

Our brains consume about 20% of the energy our bodies use, and to invest that much energy in a function that is only 10% efficient makes no evolutionary sense. **If the 10% theory were true, we would either have much smaller brains or would be extinct.**

Neuroscientist Barry Beyerstein pointed out that **scans of metabolic activity in the brain reveal that all parts of the brain are active all of the time, and there is significant activity even during sleep** (as anyone who has ever dreamt knows) (Psychology Today).

The other mythological statistic was, "50% of marriages end in divorce." Following is real information in this regard:

Let me say it straightforwardly: **Fifty percent of American marriages are not ending in divorce. It's fiction. A myth. A tragically discouraging urban legend.**

If there's no credible evidence that half of American marriages will end up in divorce court, where did that belief originate?...

A spokesperson for the U.S. National Center for Health Statistics told me that the rumor appears to have originated from a misreading of the facts. It was true, he said, if you looked at all the marriages and divorces within a single year, you'd find that there were twice as many marriages as divorces. **In 1981, for example, there were 2.4 million marriages and 1.2** million divorces. **At first glance, that would seem like a 50-percent divorce rate.**

Virtually none of those divorces were among the people who had married during that year, however, and **the statistic failed to take into account the 54 million marriages that already existed, the majority of which would not see divorce.**

Another source for the 50-percent figure could be those who were trying to predict the future of divorce. Based on known divorce records, **they projected that 50 percent of newly married young people would divorce.** University of Chicago sociologist and researcher Linda Waite told USA Today that **the 50-percent divorce stats were based more on assumptions than facts.**

So what is the divorce picture in America? Surprisingly, **it's not easy to get precise figures** because some states don't report divorces to the National Center for Health Statistics, including one of the largest: California (Truth or Fiction?).

Overall, the divorce rate shot up after World War II, then declined, only to rise again in the 1960s and 1970s, and then leveled off during the 1980s, but in trying to give meaning to these statistics great care must be taken. According to the National Marriage Project, **the "overall divorce rate" peaked at 22.6 divorces per 1,000 marriages in 1980, 20.9 in 1990, and 18.8 in 2000....**

Half of All Marriages End in Divorce? True or False? **The 50 percent statistic is very misleading, if not completely wrong ...**

Part of the difficulty with divorce statistics is that the rates measure divorces in different ways (Divorce Source).

Despite hand-wringing about the institution of marriage, marriages in this country are stronger today than they have been in a long time. The divorce rate peaked in the 1970s and early 1980s and has been declining for the three decades since.

About 70 percent of marriages that began in the 1990s reached their 15th anniversary (excluding those in which a spouse died), up from about 65 percent of those that began in the 1970s and 1980s. **Those who married in the 2000s are so far divorcing at even lower rates. If current trends continue, nearly two-thirds of marriages will never involve a divorce**, according to data from Justin Wolfers, a University of Michigan economist (who also contributes to The Upshot) (New York Times. The Divorce).

Bibliography:

Authority Nutrition. Optimal Meal Frequency – How Many Meals Should You Eat Per Day? https://authoritynutrition.com/how-many-meals-per-day/

Bauman, Alisa, ed. "Health and Fitness." *Runners World*. May 2000, pp.26-28.

Bellisle, F., et. al. *Journal of Nutrition*. 2012 Jun;142(6):1149S-54S. Sweetness, satiation, and satiety. https://www.ncbi.nlm.nih.gov/pubmed/22573779

Burn Fat Faster. by *Runner's World*. Emmaus, PA: Rodale, 1996. Effect of acute resistance exercise on postexercise energy expenditure and resting metabolic rate

Daily News. Why you ate the whole bag: Salt makes you hungry, not thirsty, study says. http://www.nydailynews.com/life-style/salt-hungry-not-thirsty-study-article-1.3069506

Divorce Source. U.S. Divorce Rates and Statistics. http://www.divorcesource.com/ds/main/u-s-divorce-rates-and-statistics-1037.shtml

Fox News Health. Why people regain weight. http://www.foxnews.com/health/2013/07/22/why-people-regain-weight.html

Hutchins, Michael. Does Exercise Raise Your Metabolic Rate for Several Hours After the Workout? Last Updated: Feb 07, 2014. http://www.livestrong.com/article/430970-how-long-do-i-have-to-do-cardio-to-burn-600-calories/

Klem ML, et. al. *American Journal of Clinical Nutrition*. 1997 Aug;66(2):239-46. A descriptive study of individuals successful at long-term maintenance of substantial weight loss. https://www.ncbi.nlm.nih.gov/pubmed/9250100

Livestrong. The Percentage of People Who Regain Weight After Rapid Weight Loss and the Risks of Doing So. http://www.livestrong.com/article/438395-the-percentage-of-people-who-regain-weight-after-rapid-weight-loss-risks/

MDC Insights. Mission Control for the body's salt and water supplies. https://insights.mdc-berlin.de/en/2017/04/mission-control-bodys-salt-water-supplies/

Melby, C. Scholl, G. Edwards, R. Bullough. *Journal of Applied Physiology.* Published 1 October 1993 Vol. 75 no. 4, 1847-1853. http://jap.physiology.org/content/75/4/1847.short

Meinz, David L. *Eating by the Book.* Virginia Beach, VA: Gilbert Press, 1999.

Mendosa, Rick. What Really Satisfies? http://www.mendosa.com/satiety.htm

Men's Health. 10 foods guaranteed to keep you full for longer. http://www.menshealth.co.uk/lose-weight/the-satiety-index-9767

Miller, Wayne C., et al. Article in *Journal of the American Dietetic Association* 94(6):612-5 · July 1994. https://www.researchgate.net/publication/15002813_Dietary_fat_sugar_and_fiber_predict_body_fat_content

Mitchell, Ted, MD. *HealthSmart: How fat-free foods can make you fat. Weekend USA.* February 11-13, 2000, p.4.

New York Times. 95% Regain Lost Weight. Or Do They? http://www.nytimes.com/1999/05/25/health/95-regain-lost-weight-or-do-they.html

New York Times. The Divorce Surge Is Over, but the Myth Lives On. https://www.nytimes.com/2014/12/02/upshot/the-divorce-surge-is-over-but-the-myth-lives-on.html?_r=0

Neuroscience for Kids. Do We Use Only 10% of Our Brains? https://faculty.washington.edu/chudler/tenper.html

Nutrition Data. Fullness Factor. http://nutritiondata.self.com/topics/fullness-factor

Olson, Samantha, Medical Daily. 3 Meals A Day vs. 6 Meals A Day: Which Healthy Diet Plan Works For Better Metabolism, Sleep, And Energy? June 12, 2015. http://www.medicaldaily.com/3-meals-day-vs-6-meals-day-which-healthy-diet-plan-works-better-metabolism-sleep-and-337778

Oxford Academic. *Epidemiology Review* (2007) 29 (1): 160-171. The Real Contribution of Added Sugars and Fats to Obesity. https://academic.oup.com/epirev/article/29/1/160/443157/The-Real-Contribution-of-Added-Sugars-and-Fats-to

Psychology Today. Do We Only Use 10% of Our Brain? https://www.psychologytoday.com/blog/long-fuse-big-bang/201503/do-we-only-use-10-our-brain

Reduce Calories, Stave Off Hunger With Water-Rich Foods—Not Water. September 23, 1999. University Park, PA. http://www.psu.edu/ur/NEWS/news/foodwater.html

Science Daily. Low-cost weight loss program has long-term results, study shows. https://www.sciencedaily.com/releases/2015/06/150604084717.htm

Science Daily. Obese people can maintain stable weight loss. https://www.sciencedaily.com/releases/2016/04/160414095406.htm

Science Daily. Study shows keys to successful long-term weight loss maintenance. https://www.sciencedaily.com/releases/2014/01/140106115351.htm

Shape. What Does 100 Calories Really Look Like? http://www.shape.com/healthy-eating/healthy-recipes/what-does-100-calories-really-look

Tanita manual for the "TBF-551 Body Fat Monitor/ Scale." Tanita Corp. Arlington Heights, IL.

Truth or Fiction? Fifty Percent of American Marriages Are Ending in Divorce-Fiction! https://www.truthorfiction.com/divorce/

US News. Intermittent Fasting vs. 6 Small Meals a Day: What's Best for Weight Loss? http://health.usnews.com/health-news/health-wellness/articles/2015/06/16/intermittent-fasting-vs-6-small-meals-a-day-whats-best-for-weight-loss

Weiss, EC, et. al. *American Journal of Preventative Medicine.* 2007 Jul;33(1):34-40. Weight regain in U.S. adults who experienced substantial weight loss, 1999-2002. https://www.ncbi.nlm.nih.gov/pubmed/17572309

Wing RR, Phelan S. *American Journal of Clinical Nutrition.* 2005 Jul;82(1 Suppl):222S-225S. Long-term weight loss maintenance. https://www.ncbi.nlm.nih.gov/pubmed/16002825

Chapter Eighteen
Author's Diet/ Practical Tips

For the most part, so far in this book, I have avoided referring to my own diet. The reason for this is I do not want to hold up myself and my diet as being the "example" that everyone else should follow.

This book tries to present dietary guidelines from the Scriptures and scientific studies and then leaves it to the reader to decide for yourself what is the best dietary strategy for you to follow.

But in case the reader is curious by now as to what type of diet this writer is following, this final chapter will discuss my personal diet plan. Along the way, I will present practical tips for following a Creationist Diet and tell a few personal stories. But first, some personal information and background would be helpful.

Personal Information and Background

I am 5'1" and currently weigh about 120-122 pounds. I was born in 1961 and turned 56 as I was working on this book. I graduated from Penn State in 1983 with a B.S. degree in Nutrition Science and attended Denver Seminary from 1988-90. I never got married nor had children.

I did very well powerlifting way back in 1978-1985, competing in first the 114-pound weight class then the 123-pound class. For the latter, my training weight would be about 128 pounds.

But due to health problems, I had to stop competing and by the late 1980s, to stop lifting weights altogether. Over the next decade or so, all I did to stay in shape was casual walking. As a result, I gradually became increasingly lax about my diet. But I never gained weight. I fact, I lost it due to losing muscle, finally leveling off at about 112 pounds.

Then my health worsened in the 1990s. As part of my quest to find a solution to my health problems, I began becoming more meticulous about my diet, doing much research in that regard. I also began walking more intensely and later riding a bicycle, and I began working out with Nautilus strength training equipment. In addition, I began to look for treatments to help with the health problems.

Creationist Diet

The first issue I considered was allergies. I always had a problem with hay fever, so I went to an allergist (immunologist). He performed a series of skin stretch tests, and sure enough, not only was I allergic to pollen, dust, and the like, but I was also allergic to many foods. In fact, I tested positive for half of the items he tested me for. The immunologist told me I was "a very allergenic person."

He recommended I eliminate the foods I tested positive for. But then he said to reintroduce them one at a time, eating lots of that food, and to look for symptoms. If I noticed any, stop that food and wait until the symptoms cleared, then try again. If the symptoms occurred again, then I would know for sure I was allergic to that food. Then of course I should repeat that process for each of the other positively tested foods. For the environmental allergies, he recommended an allergy medication and allergy shots. These steps would have been the logical way to proceed.

However, very unfortunately, at that time (early 2000), I had begun to listen to an alternative doctor on the radio. He promoted his "natural" healing methods, which included a treatment for allergies, including food allergies. I thus decided to go to him rather than to continue with the immunologist. That was probably the biggest mistake of my life, as I now realize the alternative doctor was a quack.

That quack encouraged me to follow a vegan diet and began performing a series of his alterative allergy treatments on me. With doing both, initially I seemed to be doing better. It was at that time the First Edition of this book was published. I also switched from working out with Nautilus equipment to using free weights in the spring of 2001 for the first time since the '80s, while continuing with the cardio. With doing so, my weight rose back up to about 119 pounds.

But shortly thereafter my health became much worse, and I dropped to an adult low of 107 pounds. I was eventually diagnosed by real doctors first with fibromyalgia (chronic pain plus chronic fatigue), then with stiff person syndrome (a very rare autoimmune disorder), and finally with multiple chemical sensitivities (severe allergies). It was also around this time that I was diagnosed with low testosterone levels.

It was then that I revisited my research on diet and came across the connection between diet and testosterone levels discussed in this book, with a vegan diet being just about the worst kind of diet for such. As such, I abandoned the vegan diet and began eating animal foods again.

I also began noticing that the ill-advised allergy treatments, though they might have cured some food allergies that I was treated for, had left me sensitive to many other foods and especially to artificial food ingredients. I therefore became meticulous about consuming only all natural foods.

Then I realized the pesticide residues on commercial produce was problematic and began to consume only organic fruits and vegetables. Then the same with the antibiotic and hormone residues in factory farm animal foods, so I began consuming only old-fashioned meats, dairy, and eggs. GMO foods also seemed to be problematic, so I began looking for the "Non-GMO" label on plant foods other than produce.

My health was up and down over the next several years, but I managed to get my weight back up to about 117 pounds. It was then that I started powerlifting again, entering my first full powerlifting contest in 22 years on April 12, 2003.

I entered the 114-pound weight class, which at first meant only cutting a couple of pounds. But as I continued to lift and gain weight, I hit a high of 123 pounds, so I needed to lose up to nine pounds the week before a contest. I do so by eating only low fat animal protein and low calorie vegetables, along with water and sodium manipulation.

I mention this here as when I cut weight, I do not feel famished, nor do I get junk food cravings, like I did when I did the "detox" diet described in Chapter Three. The difference most obviously is due to consuming protein along with the vegetables. That confirms what was said in the previous chapter that protein provides satiety, along with foods high in fiber and water. All three are needed for full satisfaction.

To be clear, this is not a long-term weight loss solution. Weigh-ins are the day before a contest. And immediately after weigh-ins, I get my weight back up by downing lots of water for rehydration, eating loads of carbs to replenish glycogen, heaps of salt to replenish sodium, plus some red meat to re-elevate testosterone that drops while cutting weight.

This is one time I drink fruit and vegetable juice, namely *Lakewood Organic Orange & Carrot Juice*. It is very high in potassium, which also needs to be replenished. I use juice as it is less filling than whole oranges and carrots, which would keep me from eating copious amounts of calories. The liquid also contributes to rehydration.

This orange & carrot juice is cold pressed, unrefined, and contains the pulp, so it does not overly spike my blood sugar and would fit with the Creationist Diet. It also tastes great, so I could drink it otherwise, but it is a bit pricy.

In any case, with this eating and rehydration pattern, I usually gain at least five pounds by the next morning. As a result, I compete at just a couple of pounds shy of my normal training weight.

I take all of my food with me for this purpose if I am staying at a hotel before a contest, so I know exactly what is in it and so as not to risk eating anything I might be allergic to. For further details on all of this, see the chapter on this subject in my book *Starting and Progressing in Powerlifting* (see Appendix One). That book also presents my training philosophy at that time and other details on powerlifting.

In any case, I continued to compete until June of 2009. But during the time from 2003 to 2009, my multiple chemical sensitivities (MCS) worsened to the point that I would have a hard time being around people as people have chemicals on their bodies, clothing, and coats (perfume, cologne, make-up, hair spray, cigarette smoke, remnants of detergent, soap, etc.). As such, I had to begin to live a mostly isolated life.

The only way I was able to continue to train was to set up a home gym, and I have a home office, which enables me to do work, like writing this book. But I would rarely leave my home. When I did, it was mostly to go to doctors, go grocery shopping, to attend family get-togethers on holidays, and to compete in a powerlifting contest once or twice a year. But doing any of that was very difficult and would leave me feeling rather terrible for days afterwards, and a few times, I have gotten a cold or flu the week after a contest.

It was also during this time that I was diagnosed with reactive hypoglycemia (low blood sugar). This means that when I eat anything with carbs, my blood sugar will spike then later crash more than the average person's blood sugar would. I had long before figured out how best to eat to keep from feeling excessively hungry an hour or two after eating. But with the diagnosis, I received a blood sugar monitor, and it showed that my diet was in fact keeping my blood sugar levels within the normal range most of the time.

In addition, I was diagnosed with low blood sodium levels. But the only recommendation my doctor made for that was to drink less water. That proved to be easier said than done.

With the vegan diet having been a disaster for me, during this time, I experimented with various other eating plans. After the vegan diet, I tried a near vegetarian diet (which was still a low-fat diet), a wheat free diet, a gluten-free diet, a Paleolithic diet, a low-carb diet, and a cyclical low-carb/ high-carb diet. None of those worked well for me.

The gluten-free diet was recommended by a different alternative doctor. He "diagnosed" me as having celiac disease, but he didn't perform any diagnostic tests. He just looked at my symptoms and based on his experience, said I was gluten intolerant. Consequently, I went through the rigors of eliminating gluten from my diet for several weeks. But my health continued to deteriorate, so I reintroduced wheat into my diet and did not noticed any change in my health. Later a real doctor performed real diagnostic tests for gluten intolerance (a blood test and colonoscopy), and both tests showed I was not gluten intolerant.

I tell this story as it relates back to Chapter Three and the fact that the vast majority of people do not have gluten intolerance, no matter what alternative quacks might want to call it and how often they might diagnose it using unscientific methods or simply out for the air with no diagnostic tests, as happened to me.

In any case, after all of the dietary experimenting, I settled on what is called in this book a Promised Land Diet, which is to say, an omnivore diet, eating all kinds of healthy plant and animal foods. That works best for me. Lots of variety of beneficial foods. I also found a moderate-fat diet works best for me, with an emphasis on monounsaturated fats, which is perfectly compatible with the Promised Land/ Creationist Diet.

In addition, at this time, I experimented with many different medical treatments and medications, all of which proved to be worthless and in many cases caused adverse side effects. I also experimented with many different supplements, most of which also proved to be worthless and caused adverse side effects. I plan on writing a book on the subject of supplements later, so I won't go into details here (see Appendix Two).

But here; one of the negative reactions I would often have to a drug or supplement was that after a few days of taking it, I began having problems sleeping. If I continued with the item, it would get to the point that I couldn't sleep at all. But once I stopped the item, after a few days, I would begin to be able to sleep again.

On several occasions, I would try the same drug or supplement again a few weeks or months later, and the same thing would happen, so I know it was that item. I also noticed the same with many foods and food ingredients. As a result, I became very cautious about trying anything new, be it a medication, supplement, or food. And all of these episodes of sleeplessness led to a worsening of my health.

At one point, I tried going to an immunologist again. But strangely, this time, I tested negative to all of the skin scratch test items. All I can figure is the alternative allergy treatments in some way altered my immune system so that I no longer tested positive, but without actually eliminating the allergies. But one thing was sure—my immune system was now really screwed up. And with me now testing negative to all the skin scratch items, the immunologist was unable to help me or to recommend anything.

Despite all of this going on, with my home office and home gym, I was still able to be productive. As long as I was meticulous about my revised eating plan, I was able to function in regard to work and working out rather well. It was during this time (2008) that I wrote my other book on nutrition and the Bible, *God-given Foods Eating Plan*. It reflected my new moderate-fat eating plan. And I truly believe it was that diet plan that enabled me to function at all, let alone as well as I was doing.

My bodyweight was hovering around 123 pounds when I started cutting weight for the powerlifting contest in June of 2009. But shortly before that contest, my health took a turn for the worse, most likely due to all of the experimenting I was doing, and that contest did not go well. Then afterwards, I kept trying to work out, but I had to cut way back on the intensity and weights used.

As a result, I lost my appetite and thus lost about eight pounds of muscular bodyweight and lots of strength over the next four years. Then in the summer of 2013, I had a particularly bad spell health-wise and was in the hospital for ten days and lost another seven pounds. Therefore, by October of 2014, my bodyweight had dropped to a new adult lifetime low of 106 pounds.

But in November of 2013, I began to make gradual improvements, and I was able to gradually increase the intensity and weights in my workouts. Consequently, my appetite began to come back, and I began to gradually eat more and to regain muscular bodyweight and strength.

To be clear, nothing changed health-wise. My MCS, fatigue, and other problems are still just as severe as ever, and I still have to live a mostly isolated life. But I changed my attitude towards my problems. I ceased all of the experimenting and efforts to try to find solutions to my problems and instead just accepted them, while trusting in the LORD to enable me to do so. I discuss this attitude change at length in my book *The LORD Has It Under Control.*

But here; I began to make gradual changes to my diet and training that enabled me to regain my lost bodyweight and strength until I reached my current weight of 120-122 pounds. As a result, I entered my first powerlifting contest in almost six years on February 28, 2015.

I have entered three additional contests since then, the most recent being while I was working on this book. I have done very well at all of them, breaking three all-time masters (50-59 age) American records and one all-time world record. I have also been able to become much more productive work-wise, having published new or revised versions of several books in the past few years. I thank the LORD for all of this.

I work out four times a week, doing cardio in the morning and lifting weights in the late afternoon. On two other days, I engage in other activities that are physical in nature but not exercise, like cleaning, shopping, or preparing food in the kitchen and refrigerating or freezing it for consumption later. Then one day a week, I rest, in accordance with the principle of the Fourth Commandment (Exod 20:8-11). For details on my attitude towards Sabbath keeping, see the chapter on this subject in my *Scripture Workbook* (see Appendix One).

On a final note, I've had many people make suggestions in regards to my health problems over the years. But before you do, please understand, I've already tried just about everything that both traditional and alternative health care have to offer. As such, if you are reading this and think you somehow know what the solution to my health problems might be, please refrain from sharing your thoughts. I know people are just trying to help, but I've probably already tried whatever you might suggest. But prayer and encouraging words are always appreciated.

Dietary Implications

I tell this story as the various details influence my diet. As indicated, the MCS forces me to consume an all-natural, organic diet. Specifically, I cannot tolerate any kind of artificial food ingredients, pesticide residues on plant foods, GMO foods, or antibiotic or hormone residues in animal foods. In other words, I have no choice but to follow the recommendations in this book to consume all-natural, organic, GMO-free plant foods and old-fashioned animal foods.

Creationist Diet

To keep my energy up so as to be able to work and to work out, I need to avoid all junk foods, sweets, and the like. Even at family gatherings, I generally do not eat any of the deserts being offered. I know from experience that if I deviate from my diet, I will feel terrible afterwards and be unable to work or work out. It is thus not worth it to eat anything unhealthy. Though I do admit I ate a few cookies and pieces of candy this past Christmas and Easter at our family get-togethers, and I split a take-out pizza on Super Sunday with my dad. But those three occasions are the only times I have deviated from my diet in the past few years.

Due to my reactive hypoglycemia, I eat six times a day, with each meal containing a balance of carbs, protein, and fat and at least one serving of fruit or vegetable. In researching the previous chapter, I came across claims that eating more often does not keep blood sugar levels on an even keel any better than eating just three times a day, but my blood sugar monitor shows otherwise. And besides, I had figured out I feel better eating five or six times a day long before I was diagnosed. I usually eat breakfast, a mid-morning snack, lunch, a mid-afternoon snack (which is my pre-workout snack on workout days), supper, and a bedtime snack.

I made one change to my diet due to the blood sugar monitor readings. For most of my life, I had been eating cold sugar for breakfast. But testing with the blood sugar monitor showed that most types of cold cereal caused my blood sugar to spike then crash too much. I therefore switched to eating oatmeal with fruit and nuts for breakfast, which causes little change in my blood sugar. That is more in accordance with the Creationist Diet anyway, as discussed in Chapter Thirteen.

In regards to the low blood sodium levels, as indicated, my doctor's only recommendation was to consume less water. He probably couldn't bring himself to make the other obvious suggestion—to increase sodium intake—given the long-standing recommendation by the medical establishment to keep sodium intake low. In fact, due to that basic recommendation, I had always consumed a low sodium diet.

But now I tried increasing my sodium intake. And that not only brought my blood sodium levels up to within the normal level, but I noticed an improvement in my fatigue, and I began sleeping better. I had been consuming about 1,300 mg of sodium per day. But I increased it to about 2,300 mg and then to my current level of about 2,800 mg.

That is above the recommended level for the general population of 2,300 mg, but it is below the average American intake of 3,440 mg.

But I should mention, my blood pressure did go up slightly. But in my case, that was a good thing, as it had usually been rather low and that might have been contributing to my health problems. Specifically, my blood pressure was usually about 100/ 60. But now it is usually just a little below the normal reading of 120/ 80. My resting heart rate is usually in the mid-40s bpm. Not bad for being in my mid-50s.

I usually consume eight eggs a week by eating a spinach omelet for breakfast using two eggs instead of the oatmeal two days a week and by eating two eggs for my afternoon snack on two of the days I do not work out and do not eat the omelet for breakfast. That is in line with Chapter Fourteen, where it was said that the greatest risk of an association of eggs with heart disease and cancer are at levels of greater than one egg a day. I eat eggs at this upper limit due to the relationship of cholesterol intake and testosterone levels discussed in this book. Having been diagnosed with low testosterone levels at one time makes me very cautious in that regard. And the eggs, along with other animal foods, especially meats, help to keep my testosterone levels elevated.

I have my blood cholesterol levels checked yearly, and my LDL ("bad") cholesterol levels are a tad high, but that is offset by my very high HDL ("good") cholesterol level, and it is the LDL/ HDL ratio that matters most. The high HDL is probably due to my powerlifting training and due to emphasizing monounsaturated fats.

Of course, the USDA has been advising for 50 years, basically my entire life, to limit cholesterol and sodium intakes. That is why I had always restricted my egg intake and had always followed a low sodium diet. But I should have realized the government was wrong in these regards given that Jesus says eggs are a "good gift" and that "salt is good" (Luke 11:12; 14:34), but I did not take those statements to their logical conclusions.

In any case, to be productive in powerlifting requires a much higher protein intake than the average person would require. That is another reason I consume more animal foods than this book would seem to recommend. But I offset that high animal food intake with a copious consumption of fruits and vegetables. Probably as a result of doing so, my most recent colon test was clean.

It is also because of this high protein need that I consume a food item that would not be in line with the basic principle of the Creationist Diet of consuming foods in the most natural form possible. To that issue I now turn.

Protein Intake

I have always believed strength training increases protein needs. I can even remember giving an oral presentation back in college on this very subject. I put forth the hypothesis that strength athletes need about 1.0 grams of protein per pound of bodyweight. That is far greater than the RDA of 0.36 grams, and at that time most authorities denied that strength athletes had higher protein requirements than others. I thought the professor would object to my hypothesis, but surprisingly, she did not, and I got an "A" on that presentation.

As part of it, I stated that it was possible to attain that level of protein without the use of protein powders, so I never used them. I remember displaying a chart ranking various high-protein foods on a cost per gram of protein basis. Protein powder was the most expensive source, while non-fat dried milk was the least expensive, eggs the second least expensive, with meat, chicken, and fish in the middle.

But that was when I was in college back in the early 1980s, when the only protein powders available were soy-derived and tasted like chalk. When I started powerlifting again in my 40s (2003), protein powders were much improved, now being made with whey, casein, or egg white, and are much better tasting, less expensive, and have a higher biological value, so I have always made use of them. And with doing so, my protein intake has ranged from 1.2 to 1.5 grams/ pound.

But there have been times when I have thought back to that college presentation and debated if I really need that much protein and thus the protein powders. I even tried Googling "protein requirements for strength athletes." I found many pages on the subject. The consensus now is that strength athletes require more protein than sedentary individuals and even more than endurance athletes. That is an improvement over when I was in college.

But the exact recommendations varied, as seen in Chapter Fifteen. The range for strength athletes was 1.2-2.0 grams of protein per kilogram of bodyweight. That works out to 0.55-0.94g/ pound.

Given this evidence, on several occasions, I experimented by substituting a cup of milk for each of my one or two daily servings of protein powder. A cup of milk contains 8 grams of protein, while one serving of protein powder contains 24 grams, so that would reduce my protein intake by 16 grams per serving and my average daily intake down to about the 1.0 grams/ pound I consumed in college.

I did the experiment three times and used a different type of milk each time. The first time I used organic, pasteurized, non-fat milk, the second the same except for low-fat, and the third organic, whole, raw milk. But regardless of the type of milk, each time I tried this experiment, I ran into problems.

I would usually start to feel very sore, like I was not recovering from my workouts; my training would stagnate, and one time I even experienced a flare-up of my stiff person syndrome (SPS) and was paralyzed for the next 48 hours. But each time, about a week after going back to the protein powders, I would no longer feel sore and would start to make progress in my training again.

These experiments could prove that I need the extra protein the powders provide, or something else could be at work. I use a 50/ 50 mixture of whey and casein. This gives me 12 grams of whey protein. Milk is composed of 20% whey and 80% casein, so one cup provides 1.6 grams of whey protein. That is a big difference, so maybe there is "something" about whey protein that helps to reduce workout soreness.

That something could be the high glutamine content of whey, as I have found that supplementing with glutamine reduces post-workout soreness. Also, glutamine has a role in SPS. In fact, I first started supplementing with glutamine when an alternative doctor suggested I do so to aid my recovery from SPS.

Another possibility could be timing. Although I might be getting sufficient protein without the protein powders by the end of the day, I might not be at the two critical times I use the powders: breakfast and pre-workout. With milk having a third of the protein of the protein powders, maybe when I substituted it for the powders, that amount of protein was not enough to break the fast in the morning or to prevent muscle breakdown during the workout and to begin the recovery process afterwards. Or it could be something else.

But whatever the case, I will stick with the protein powders. That causes my diet to have 25% of calories from protein. That percentage gives me the at least 1.2 grams/ pound that by experience I know I need. Moreover, a recent blood test showed that my liver enzymes are fine, and my blood protein levels are within normal, so my high protein intake is not adversely affecting me.

However, I will freely admit that protein powders do not really fit into the basic principle of the Creationist Diet of eating unprocessed foods, as protein powders are very processed. But I know they benefit me. That is an important point. No matter what dietary philosophy you ascribe to, don't get so legalistic about it that you refuse to eat a food that you know is beneficial to you just because it does not fit that philosophy. I thus get a bit frustrated with vegetarians who refuse to eat fish, despite the overwhelming evidence for the benefits of fish.

Incidentally, "Human and bovine milk differ substantially in the ratio of whey to casein protein ($\approx$ 60:40 in human milk and $\approx$ 20:80 in bovine milk)" (Lien). Thus in some ways, my 50:50 mixture might be more natural than cow's milk.

Moreover, I try to make my protein powders sort of fit the principles of the Creationist Diet by using *Optimum Nutrition's Natural Whey* and *Natural Casein*. They do not contain the artificial flavorings, colorings, and sweeteners that most other protein powders contain.

Fat Intake

As mentioned, I have found a moderate-fat diet works best for me. Specifically, 30-35% of my calories come from fat. I have found I need at least 30% fat to keep my testosterone levels elevated, but more than 35% provides no further benefit.

Almost half of these fat calories come from monounsaturated fats, so I consume almost as much monounsaturated fats as saturated fat and polyunsaturated fat combined. Again, this high monounsaturated fat intake is probably one reason my HDL levels are so high.

Saturated fats account for less than 10% of calories, as is generally recommended. In fact, my average in 2016 was just 7.5%. Thus overall, my fat intake follows what the research supports as being the most heart protective type of diet.

Carbohydrate Intake

With consuming 30-35% of calories from fat and 25% of calories from protein, that leaves 40-45% for carbohydrates (carbs). I have found that I need at least 40% carbs for energy levels, especially for working out, but more than 45% provides no further benefit. Moreover, more than 45% spikes and crashes my blood sugar levels excessively, even with eating six times a day and consuming mostly low glycemic carbs.

Pre-Workout Snack

Another area I deviate somewhat from the Creationist Diet is with my pre-workout snack. I discuss pre- and post-workout nutrition at length in my *Starting and Progressing in Powerlifting* book and on my fitness website, so I will not repeat all of that information here.

But in sum, a pre-workout snack or meal should contain a carb source, a protein source, and a fat source, with an emphasis on the first and little of the last. The protein source for me has always been protein powders, but when I first started powerlifting again, I was using maltodextrin for the carb source and MCT oil for the fat source.

Maltodextrin is pure carbs, derived from corn or wheat, while MCT oil is derived from coconut oil. Both are highly refined products, with nothing but the carbs and fat remaining, respectively. I would put all three ingredients into a shaker cup and add water later for a pre-workout drink. But looking for something a bit more natural, I experimented with different carb sources, like whole oat powder, and with different fat sources, like olive oil. They worked, but the oat powder was still highly processed, and the drink with the olive oil tasted awful.

It was at this time that I made the switch from eating cold cereal to oatmeal for breakfast due to cold cereal spiking my blood sugar too much. But then I realized that was exactly what I wanted with my pre-workout snack. Well actually, I don't want too much of spike, just a moderate one to get me going for the workout. But if it is too much, then my blood sugar will crash in the midst of the workout, causing me to feel hungry and to drag through the rest of it.

I experimented with several different cereals. All of them were all natural, whole grain, low sugar cereals, but some would spike and crash my blood sugar more than others. The texture and fiber content of the cereal determines the response, with airy textures like puffed cereals being highest, while denser cereals like squares and high-fiber cereals being lowest, with flakes in-between, unless high fiber.

My favorite cold cereal is Barbara's *Morning Oat Squares*. It is similar to *Quaker Oat Squares*, except it is all natural. I also really like Barbara's *Multi-Grain Spoonfuls* and *High Fiber Medley*. But there are several other cereals of other natural brands that are very good as well.

For the fat source, I add a few pecans or walnuts to the cereal. Those are of course far more natural than the refined MCT oil I used to use. And again, I use protein powders instead of milk, plus some raisins to have a serving of fruit. The mixture gives me a moderate blood sugar response, which is exactly what I want.

I put all the ingredients into a container with a lid, so I can make a couple ahead of time and have them ready to go when I am ready to work out. I just add water and eat it about an hour pre-workout, and that keeps me satiated through the workout. I use glutamine immediately afterwards, shower, then eat dinner. I do the same for contests, eating one container of the cereal mixture before warming up for each lift.

Again, the cold cereal and protein powder do not strictly fit with the Creationist Diet. But again, I know this pre-workout snack works well, and it is more natural and tastes better than the drink that I used to use. And again, this shows it is good to not be too legalistic about a dietary philosophy, though these two foods are the only ones that I eat regularly that do not fully fit with the Creationist Diet.

Summary of Diet

To summarize my diet, my macronutrient distribution is:

Fat: 30-35%
Carbs: 40-45%
Protein: 25%

I keep track of my diet regularly with the *DietPower* software program. It is an old program but works just fine now that they fixed the bugs that kept it from running quite right on Windows 10. It can be downloaded for free from: www.DietPower.com. I have all my personal foods and recipes added to it, so it only takes a few minutes each day to enter my daily intake.

Its analysis shows I hit these macronutrients levels on most days. I might fall a bit short on the carbs on my rest days. But that is planned, as without doing any physical activity, I don't need as many carbs. And I tend not to be very hungry, so I reduce calories by eating fewer carbs.

This program also shows that I consume at least 100% of the RDA for the twenty-plus vitamins, minerals, and fiber the program analyzes for. In fact, for most nutrients, I consume 200-400% of the RDA.

The average number of daily servings of the various food groups I consume are as follows, with what constitutes a serving in parentheses:

Fruits: 3-4 (1 piece of fresh fruit, ½ cup berries, cherries, grapes, or dried apricots, or ¼ cup raisins)
Vegetables: 6-8 (½ cup cooked or 1 cup raw)
Nuts, Seeds, and Peanuts: 2-3 (¼ cup of nuts or 2 tablespoons of nut butters)
Grains: 4-8 (1 slice bread, ½ bun, English muffin, bagel, tortilla, or pita bread, or ½ cup rice, quinoa, pasta, or oatmeal, or ¾ -1 cup cold cereal)
Legumes: 1 (½ cup)
Red Meat and Poultry: 1-2 (3-4 ounces)
Fish: 1-2 (2-4 ounces)
Eggs: 1 large or extra-large
Dairy: 2-3 (1 scoop protein powder, 1 cup yogurt, 1 ounce cheese)
Honey and Other Sweeteners: 1-3 teaspoons
Olive and Other Oils: 1-3 teaspoons

The fruits are all raw, either fresh, frozen, or dried. I always eat a 2-cup raw salad for dinner, plus a serving or two a week of raw broccoli and of raw cauliflower. The rest of the vegetables are cooked, usually steamed or stir-fried. The nuts and seeds are about half raw and half roasted. The grains are all whole grain and about half are sprouted.

As for calories, my average for all of 2016 was 2226 per day. But that varies widely based on how active I am. On my rest days, I consume about 2,000 calories, but on workout days, I consume about 2,500 calories. That is for maintaining my weight at 120-122 pounds, to be within striking distance of the 114-pound weight class. But I might decide to move up to 123s. In that case, I would want to increase my training weight to about 128 pounds. To do so gradually so it is mostly muscle, I would increase my calories by about 200-300 per day.

Grocery Shopping

The most helpful way for me to overview the foods I eat will be to describe my grocery shopping. This will give the reader an idea of how to go about buying God-given foods that fit within the Creationist Diet.

Food Co-op:

I purchase most of my groceries at Pittsburgh's East End Food Co-op (www.eastendfood.coop). Similar but smaller stores in my area I have shopped at are Today's Market in Oakmont, PA and DeWalt Health Foods in Butler, PA, which also has three other stores in western Pennsylvania. I am sure there would be similar food co-ops or health food stores in or near most other large cities.

Pittsburgh's Co-op is a half hour drive from my home, so I only go there once a month. But when I do, I really stock up, filling up a large grocery cart to overflowing.

Produce Aisle:

As with most grocery stores, as you enter the store and go to the right, the first thing you see is the produce. What I like about the Co-op is all of the produce is organic.

I say that as I tried going to the Whole Foods store in Pittsburgh but did not like it as much as the Co-op. One problem was Whole Foods carries both organic and non-organic produce. Thus, for instance, there was a display of loose organic apples right beside a display of loose non-organic apples. I could see how easy it would be for someone to pick up a non-organic apple, decide not to buy it, and put it down with the organic apples. It is the same situation at Giant Eagle, the largest commercial grocery store chain in the Pittsburgh area.

I also like that at the Co-op, when in-season, it carries many locally grown items. That is not the case with Whole Foods or Giant Eagle. Locally grown foods are more nutritious due to less time being spent in storage, and better for the environment, due to not wasting energy transporting the foods long distances.

Opting to buy food that is grown and produced close to home has numerous benefits.
Local food is not just **fresher** than food that travels across the globe or the country to get to your kitchen, but when you buy locally produced food you are **supporting your local community's economy.**

Plus, food grown nearby has traveled fewer miles, therefore producing **less air pollution.** Food that is shipped a shorter distance has **less of a chance to become contaminated or lose nutritional value.**

Eating locally means shopping at your neighborhood farmers' market or community supported agriculture and **buying what's in season** (Los Angeles).

In any case, at the Co-op, I start by bagging at least two different types of fruit. The exact types depend on the season, but through the course of a year, I purchase: apples, apricots, bananas, blueberries, cantaloupe, grapefruit, grapes, honeydew, kiwis, mangoes, oranges, papayas, peaches, plums, pomegranates, raspberries, strawberries, tangerines, watermelon, and my favorites, cherries and nectarines.

Then comes the dark green leafy vegetables: collard greens, kale, leaf lettuce, and romaine lettuce. Along with the lettuce, other ingredients for my dinnertime salad go into my cart: celery, cucumbers, grape tomatoes, and various kinds of radishes (red, black, and daikon, which are white), plus tomatoes for both salads and my lunchtime sandwich.

Next into my cart are vegetables for my lunchtime stir-fried vegetables: broccoli, cabbage (green and red), cauliflower, carrots, rutabagas, turnips, and yellow squash, plus garlic and onions, which I mince together and use to flavor many things in addition to the stir-fry.

I also eat the broccoli and cauliflower raw for lunch and steamed for dinner. There are also other vegetables for dinner: asparagus, acorn squash, brussels sprouts, green beans, potatoes, and sweet potatoes.

Finally, there are a variety of peppers for assorted purposes: green, red, and yellow sweet peppers and jalapeno and other hot peppers.

Another very healthy item the co-op carries are avocadoes, along with prepared guacamole. But I am allergic to avocado, so I cannot take advantage of the healthy fats they provide. I found this out a while back when I tried the guacamole. I figured it would be great to dip raw vegetables into, and it is and would be the ideal dip to serve with a veggie tray at a social gathering.

But for me, after a few days of using the guacamole, I developed a rash on the underside of my left arm. It took me a few days to connect it with the guacamole. But when I stopped using it, the rash cleared up after a couple of days.

Later, I began wondering if it might have been something else in the guacamole that caused the problem other than the avocadoes themselves, so I bought a couple of avocadoes and spread them on sandwiches like mayo. That tasted great, but the rash came back after a couple of days, but then cleared up a couple of days after stopping the avocadoes. I then tried the same experiment a few months later, and the same thing happened.

I relate this story as it shows how difficult food allergies can be to identify, as it might take a couple of days for symptoms to show after eating an allergenic food, then it might take a couple of days for the symptoms to clear after the food is stopped.

In fact, I remember a while back going to a luncheon with a female friend. She ate a piece of chocolate cake, despite knowing she was allergic to chocolate, as "it just looked so good on the desert tray." I talked to her later, and she said she was sick for the next four days. She asked if eating one serving of an allergenic food could make someone sick for that long, and I told that yes, it can take that long for the food to be fully cleared out of the system.

This is important and another reason it would be best to make gradual changes rather than a wholesale change to your diet. Not only is it very difficult make a radical change, but you might inadvertently start to consume something you are allergic to, and if you start to consume many "new" foods at the same time, it will be hard to identify which is the offending food.

In any case, by the time I leave the produce aisle, my large grocery cart is usually almost half full.

Bulk Section:

Next in the Co-op is the bulk section. I used to buy many items in the bulk section, as the items are less expensive than their packaged counterparts. But I now shy away from it due to my MCS. The smells in the Co-op do not bother me that much, which is another reason I prefer it to other groceries stores, in which the smells bother me much more. But still, I don't like the idea that those smells are getting onto the unpackaged bulk foods. Of course, the produce is mostly also unpackaged, but that I can wash off, but it is not easy to wash off items like almonds. But I do buy the dried apricots, as the only other place I can get them is much more expensive.

But for those without such concerns, bulk food items can be a way to purchase quality foods at reduced prices. I used to buy all of my nuts and seeds and many grain items in bulk, but now I get them elsewhere.

Cheese Display:

Next in the Co-op is the oval cheese display. Every kind of cheese imaginable, most of it organic, grass-fed, and from local farms, and all of it is delicious. I get Mozzarella for pita pizza as I will explain shortly, plus a couple of other kinds. My favorites are *Marble* (half Colby and half Monterey Jack) and *Pepperjack* (Monterey Jack with jalapenos), both from Middlefield Farm, a farm in nearby Ohio.

For the adventurous, the Co-op carries goat cheese. I tried some white cheddar goat cheese recently. It tasted a bit "spikier" than cow's milk cheddar, though still very good.

Canned Foods:

Next comes the aisles of packaged foods. All such items in the Co-op are all-natural, and most are organic or at least non-GMO.

First up are the canned foods. They are an option, but there is always a loss of nutrients when foods are canned. I thus only buy a few items in cans, namely, legumes and tomato products. But that is because it is so time-consuming to prepare legumes from dried beans, and in the winter, fresh tomatoes are terribly expensive. It is also far easier to buy bottled spaghetti sauce and salsa than to make it myself, though I have made homemade spaghetti sauce. But for other vegetables, it is much healthier and not much more expensive or time-consuming to buy fresh or frozen vegetables and to cook them myself

509

But the Co-op carries various canned vegetables, like corn and peas, which would be options for when fresh items are not available. That is, if you can stand the taste of peas. I say that as peas are the one vegetable I simply cannot eat. I am so averse to them that I will even take the time to pick out every single pea out of a bowl of vegetable soup or stew before eating it. But peas are the only vegetable that I dislike so strongly. Most others I can at least tolerate if not actually enjoy.

I mention this as I can relate when someone says they do not like a particular vegetable, but with such a wide selection of vegetables available, I find it hard to believe someone would be so averse to all of them so as to refuse to eat any of them.

Spices:

Next is a display for spices. I get all *Simply Organic* spices and quite a variety of them. Spices are important as they keep a healthy diet from tasting bland, especially if you are limiting salt. Below is a list of the spices I use, with examples of the foods I use each on.

All-Seasons Salt: vegetables
Bay leaf: spaghetti sauce, soups
Black Pepper: eggs, chili.
Celery Salt: vegetables
Chili Powder: chili (duh)
Cinnamon: oatmeal (until I realized I was allergic to it)
Garlic Powder: soups, chili, spaghetti sauce, chicken, pizza
Garlic Salt: soups, chili, steak, chicken, veggies (this one is great)
Italian Seasoning: spaghetti sauce, chicken
Lemon Pepper: fish (until I became allergic to lemon)
Onion Powder: soups, chili, spaghetti sauce, chicken
Paprika: fish, spaghetti sauce
Parsley: chicken
Red Pepper: vegetables, eggs, pizza.
White Pepper: steak and other red meat items (also great)

Condiments:

Next up are the condiments. These can be used to flavor foods, but most are high in salt and sugar and may even contain unhealthy refined oils. They thus should only be used sparingly, if at all. Salsa is probably the healthiest condiment available, as it is pure vegetables, with only salt added. And that I use regularly, but I cannot use other condiments due to being allergic to the vinegar. How I became so is a bit of a story.

I read on the Internet somewhere that food allergies were caused by foods not being fully digested before being absorbed into the system. It was thus recommended to take a teaspoon of vinegar or lemon juice with each meal. It was said the acid in them would aid stomach acid in digesting food. I stupidly bought into that nonsense and tried it.

After a week of using that much vinegar and lemon juice, I became allergic to both, and can no longer tolerate either. As a result, I can no longer use ketchup or other condiments, and I must read food labels carefully, as these items are found in many packaged foods.

In any case, I can use sauerkraut, as it does not contain vinegar, but it is high in sodium. But again, I now eat a diet that is moderately high in sodium, and the sauerkraut tastes great on my lunchtime sandwich.

But for those who can consume vinegar, the Co-op carries a couple of different brands of organic vinegar, which is good to put on salads with one of the next items.

Vegetable Oils:

Next are the vegetable oils. The ones I buy are *Spectrum Organic* extra virgin, cold pressed olive oil, unrefined peanut oil, and refined walnut and sunflower oils.

Olive oil was discussed previously, with it being said extra virgin, cold pressed is the best. And it is great for on salads.

Peanut oil was also mentioned previously, but here, let me say that unrefined peanut oil is far different than the refined stuff that most stores carry. Unrefined peanut oil is gold and smells and tastes like actual peanuts, while refined peanut oil is clear, odorless, and tasteless. Thus unrefined peanut oil best fits with a Creationist Diet.

The sunflower and walnut oils, however, really do not fit due to being refined. However, being refined, they have a high smoke point, so they are good for stir-frying vegetables. Then again, the peanut oil works in that regard as well, but I've found oil olive has too low of a smoke point to be used for stir-frying. The refined sunflower oil is also good for use in recipes. The olive, peanut, and walnut oils are also good in that regard, but they will add distinct flavors that might not be wanted in some recipes.

Creationist Diet

The peanut and sunflower oils are high oleic, which means they are higher in monounsaturated fats than regular peanut and sunflower oils.

The Co-op also carries extra virgin coconut oil and unrefined palm oil. Tropical oils are controversial. They contain saturated fat, but many claim it is different from the saturated fat in animal foods and thus is not unhealthy. That is debatable. It also claimed by some that extra virgin coconut oil is health promoting, and that is another claim I fell for.

Specifically, the claim was that coconut oil increases thyroid levels. Even though I had had my thyroid levels tested via a blood test, and it was normal, it was said that blood tests were not reliable in this regard. The quack doctor I had gone to had made this claim and had recommended I take his supplements. Those proved to be worthless. But now I had come across several webpages making the same claim, only they were recommending coconut oil to improve the condition.

Therefore, I began using coconut oil several times a day, and just like with the vinegar and lemon juice, after about a week, I became allergic to coconut oil. As a result, I now have one more ingredient I need to check labels for. This is rather problematic, as lots of natural foods use coconut oil. But it would be a good oil for stir frying, as it has a high smoke point.

Next in that aisle is canned fish, but I also now get that elsewhere.

Rice, Pasta, and Soup:

In the next aisle are first organic rice products of various sorts. I usually get basmati brown rice, as it is the cheapest. But the Co-op also carries sprouted brown rice. It costs about twice as much as regular brown rice, but it is a bit tastier, having chewy texture to it. It also might be a bit healthier, as sprouted grains tend to be lower glycemic and are said to be easier to digest. But I only buy it when it is on sale. The Co-op also carries various specialty rice, like red rice. It has a rather unique taste to it but is also pricy. Thus again, I only buy it when it is on sale.

The same goes for quinoa (pronounced "keen-wah"). This is an "ancient grain" used by the Aztecs. Its main claim to fame is that it is higher in protein than most other grains, and the protein is "complete," meaning it contains all eight essential amino acids, whereas the protein in most other plant foods is incomplete, lacking in one or more amino acids. It is thus a favorite grain of vegans. But the amount of protein is still far less than what you would get from animal foods. Personally, I think the main value of quinoa over brown rice is brown rice takes about 45 minutes to cook, whereas quinoa only takes about 20 minutes.

Next is pasta. Being of Italian heritage, this is a must have. The Co-op carries organic refined and whole wheat pasta and even brown rice pasta for the gluten-free fanatics. I prefer the whole wheat, as the brown rice pasta tends to fall apart when cooked. That leads to another story.

My mom used to make lasagna for the whole family on Christmas Eve. But she was in a nursing home this past Christmas and has since gone to be with the LORD (see the Introductory Page in this regard), but I kept the tradition going this past Christmas Eve by making lasagna for just my dad and me. But I made it in a heathier manner by using organic brown rice noodles rather than white noodles. I would have preferred whole wheat noodles, but again, thanks to the gluten-free fanatics, brown rice is all the Co-op had. But it held together rather well

I also used old-fashioned ground turkey rather than factory farm ground meat, organic spaghetti sauce, organic grass-fed mozzarella and ricotta cheese, and a package of organic spinach. I thought it tasted just fine, as I am used to using such ingredients for spaghetti, and my dad said he liked it. But then, he never complains. We had lots leftover. But that gave both us of a couple of more meals.

I call those who refuse to eat gluten unnecessarily "fanatics" as such self-imposed restrictions are detrimental, as proven by a 2017 study:

> For people who don't have a true gluten allergy or sensitivity, **avoiding gluten may result in reduced consumption of whole grains, which actually offer cardiovascular benefits....**
>
> After additional adjustment for intake of refined grains, estimated **gluten consumption was linked to a lower risk of coronary heart disease....** Other potential **downsides to a gluten-free diet include its lack of fiber and deficiency in vitamins** (Med Page Today).

The point here is people who eat whole grains have a lower risk of heart disease and higher nutrient and fiber intake than those who do not eat whole grains, which would include those needlessly avoiding gluten.

In any case, next in this aisle is the aforementioned organic pasta sauce. I prefer *Muir Glen Garden Vegetable*, but there are many other

513

types available. I could make own pasta sauce and have done so in the past, but it is rather time consuming.

On the other side in this aisle is a bunch of different kinds of soup. The only one I usually buy is *Pacific Natural Foods Organic Light in Sodium Tomato Soup*. I make a cup of it for lunch, dipping my sandwich into it. It is also great for post-weighs for powerlifting contests, as it helps to replenish water, sodium, and potassium as even the reduced salt variety is still rather high in salt. This brand comes in an easy-open container rather than a can, so it is convenient to use in a hotel room with a microwave. I heat it up in a large Steelers mug my parents got me for Christmas a while back.

Miscellaneous Packaged Foods Aisle:

For want of a better term, I will call the next aisle the miscellaneous packaged foods aisle. First up are various kinds of crackers. Whether crackers would fit with a Creationist Diet would depend mostly if refined or whole grains and if refined or unrefined oils are used.

The brand I get is *Nairn Organic Oat Crackers*. These are imported from Scotland. The ingredients are: Organic whole grain oats (83%), organic oat bran, organic sunflower oil, organic sustainable palm oil, sea salt, raising agent: sodium bicarbonate.

The sunflower oil is probably refined but not the palm oil. And with the main ingredients being whole grain oats and oat bran, I consider these to be just about the healthiest cracker available, though they are a bit pricy. But they taste great with peanut butter and jelly on them.

Next in this aisle are baking supplies. I used to do a god bit of baking back in the day, but not so much anymore. The best tasting item I made was whole wheat muffins using molasses instead of sugar. The molasses gives them a distinctive flavor and makes them very moist.

Molasses is the byproduct of refining sugar cane into sugar. It is rather healthy, containing significant amounts of various vitamins and minerals, especially blackstrap molasses. But it is still sugar and highly refined, so it would be borderline if it fits with a Creationist Diet or not. But the Co-op carries an organic brand thereof.

In any case, the baking supplies includes a wide variety of different flours, some whole grain and some refined. Of course, only the whole grain ones would fit with a Creationist Diet.

Then there's baking powder, soda, and yeast, all needed for various kinds of baking, plus chocolate chips and baker's chocolate, vanilla and other natural flavorings for specialty items. There are also all-natural and even organic baking mixes for those who are not adventurous enough to bake from scratch.

Next are pancake and waffle mixes. The one I use is *Arrowhead Mills, Organic Sprouted Grain Pancake & Waffle Mix*. It makes the best tasting pancakes I have ever eaten, and with containing a variety of sprouted grains, it is a bit healthier than mixes with regular whole grains.

Next are various kinds of salt. These are all-natural, unlike grocery store salt, which often contains artificial ingredients. The Co-op carries various kinds of specialty salts: *Eden Sea Salt, French Celtic Sea Salt, Himalayan Salt, Real Salt*, and many others.

If you search the web, you will find all kinds of wild claims of health benefiting effects of such salts. It is also claimed that these salts do not elevate blood pressure. The reason for these claims is that these salts are unrefined, so they contain naturally occurring minerals, in addition to NaCl. However, the amounts are so tiny they are insignificant, so don't believe any of it. And for some reason, I was sensitive to some of these.

After some experimenting, I settled on *Bob Red Mills' Sea Salt*. It did not bother me allergy-wise, but it is unrefined and less expensive than other specialty salts.

Next are sweeteners. Here is where I get my organic raw honey, from *Y.S. Organic Bee Farms*. But there is also cooked honey, both organic and non-organic.

Next is brown rice syrup. It is a relatively healthy sweetener though highly processed. It differs from most other sweeteners in consisting solely of glucose and glucose polymers.

Brown rice syrup is a sweetener derived from brown rice. They make it by exposing cooked rice to enzymes that break down the starches and turn them into smaller sugars... then all the "impurities" are filtered out. What is left is a thick, sugary syrup, which really doesn't resemble brown rice at all.

Brown rice syrup contains three sugars: Maltotriose (52%), maltose (45%) and glucose (3%).

However, don't be fooled by the names. **Maltose is basically just two glucose molecules, while maltotriose is three glucose molecules** (Authority. Brown).

The reason this is important is that glucose is effective for muscle glycogen replenishment, while the fructose that composes half of the sucrose molecule of white sugar is not. I discuss this complex issue in detail in the chapter on workout nutrition in my powerlifting book and in my other book on nutrition and the Bible, so I will not pursue it here. But there is also the following difference:

The **fructose gets turned into fat**, which either lodges in the liver (causing fatty liver and insulin resistance) or is shipped out, **raising blood triglycerides**. Without getting into the gory details, these metabolic problems can lead to all sorts of diseases. However, **glucose can be metabolized by all of the body's cells, so it shouldn't have the same negative effects on liver function** (Authority. Brown).

This difference leads to the next sweetener, agave syrup. This is a popular sweetener among health fanatics, but it is not healthy due to being pure fructose, so it is even worse than white sugar. I am also allergic to it, so I wouldn't touch it.

Next in this aisle are raisins, a truly healthy and natural sweetener. The Co-op keeps changing the brand they carry, though always organic. Currently it is *Newman's Own Organics* brand, which is as good as any.

Then are granola bars. These have a reputation as being healthy, but they are not, as a large percentage of the calories come from refined sugars and refined oils, and they are highly processed.

Next are various hot cereals, like oatmeal. These would all be healthy, as they are all pure whole grains and minimally processed, though I get my oatmeal elsewhere.

Next comes the cold cereal, a wide variety of them, some whole grain, some not, but all highly processed. I've already discussed these, so I will move onto the nut butters and fruit jellies.

Peanut, almond, and cashew butter are all available and taste great. Grinding nuts into butter is a bit of processing, but all of the nutrients are retained. The only question is what is added in addition to the nuts.

If it is refined oils and a significant amount of sugar, then that make them less than God-given. The best nut butters are just pure ground nuts, with maybe salt added, and that is what I get.

This is where it is not that important to get organic or non-GMO, as nut trees and peanut plants tend not draw up as much pesticide residues into the nuts as produce, and there are no GMO nuts at this time. I still get *Once Again* organic peanut butter, as it is not much more expensive than non-organic versions. But the almond and cashew butters are quite expensive even without being organic and excessively so when organic. I thus get the non-organic versions and then only when they are on sale.

Jelly is a processed food, but only in a way that could be done at home. I can remember my grandma canning jelly back in the day. But what I get is *Crofter's Organic Just Fruit Spread*. The difference is that with jelly, sugar is the first ingredient, but with fruit spread, fruit is. And that means organic matters, just as with whole fruits. But still, being processed, I only use it sparingly, on a PB&J sandwich I eat once a week for lunch and on the aforementioned crackers once or twice a week. It comes in many flavors, though my favorites are mango and cherry.

Next are various kinds of snack bars. Mostly, these are not much better than candy bars, highly processed, with loads of sugar of some sort, or glycerin if low-carb bars. Glycerin is a by-product of soap production and is in no sense a God-given food.

But there a couple of bars I like and would sort of fit with the Creationist Diet. The first are *Clif Kit's Organic Fruit & Nut Bars*. As the name implies, they contain just dried fruit and ground nuts, though it takes quite a bit of processing to squish together it all into a bar, and they are expensive. It is better and cheaper to put some nuts and dried fruit into a zip snack bag, and use that for a portable snack.

The other bars I like are *BoBo's Oat Bars* and *Oat Bites*. These are mostly organic oats, and all of the ingredients are non-GMO, which is good. The main sweetener is brown rice syrup, which is also good. The fat source is a "buttery spread" of palm fruit, canola oil, and olive oil, two of which would be good if unrefined. And the processing doesn't appear to be much beyond basic baking that would have been possible in Bible times. In fact, I had thought of baking something similar myself, using oats, brown rice syrup or honey, and unrefined peanut oil, so Bobo got two of the three primary ingredients right.

However, they are rather caloric dense, with one bar containing two servings of about 170 calories each. The bites are half the size, so they are only one serving. But that caloric density is why they worked well for after weigh-ins and during my most recent contest. They would also be good for those who are trying to gain weight. They are available in over a dozen different flavors.

Lastly in this aisle are various chocolate products. Chocolate is somewhat of a healthy food, being high in antioxidants. But it takes a lot of processing to convert cocoa beans into chocolate, then a good bit of sugar is added, far more for milk chocolate than for dark chocolate. Therefore, if you are going to eat chocolate with the excuse that it is healthy, it should be dark chocolate that contains at least 80% cocoa.

Examples of such chocolate include *Green & Black's Organic Dark Chocolate 85%* and *Equal Exchange Organic Extreme Dark Chocolate* (88% cacao).

Dried Meats:

My oldest nephew is a hunter. This past hunting season he got both a buck and a doe. For our Christmas gathering, he brought "deer bites" made from the meat, which were dried venison. He had two kinds: mild and spicy. Both tasted great, though I preferred the spicy. On my next trip to the Co-op, I noticed they had a couple of different brands of dried meats, so I tried them.

The first are *Nick's Sticks*, which are available as beef jerky and turkey jerky. The beef is grass fed and the turkey is free range, and both taste okay, though a bit bland. Later I tried the *Spicy Beef* and *Spicy Turkey*, which are better.

The second Are *Epic Bars*. These are available in many meats: beef, bison, lamb, chicken, turkey, venison, salmon, and wild boar. The red meats are grass-fed, the poultry is free range, and the salmon is wild caught. They just happened to be on sale, so I bought one of each, except for of course of the wild boar, which is just another word for pig.

All of the *Epic Bars* are spicier than the regular *Nick's Sticks*. The venison in particular tastes fabulous, at least I think so. But when I gave one to my dad, he didn't like it at all. He even said he had a hard time finishing it. That was my experience with the salmon bar, as it was just plain awful. But the rest of the meats all taste very good.

Dried meats make for a good portable snack. I later bought a box of the venison bars from elsewhere. But they are rather pricy, so I only eat them sparingly.

Cookies and Chips:

In the next aisle are first cookies. Don't fool yourself; just because a food is sold in a health food store does not mean it is healthy, and that is the case with most "natural" cookies. Most are still made with refined flour, refined oils, and lots of refined sugar. The only difference from commercial cookies is there are no artificial ingredients. That is good, but all of the refined ingredients are not.

But to be honest, I do on occasion eat a couple of brands of cookies. The first are *Nairn Oat Cookies*. These I eat with my morning snack, if I am still hungry after eating my normal snack of canned fish and fresh fruit. They are made by same company that makes the aforementioned oat crackers and contain the same ingredients, plus sugar and various natural flavorings, depending on the flavor. But there is not much sugar in them, only two grams per cookie, so they are healthier than most other cookies. But as with the crackers, they are a bit pricy and hard to find. The Co-op no longer carries them, but I can get then elsewhere.

The next two cookies are *Barbara's Bakery Snackimals Animal Cookies Oatmeal* and *Annie's Homegrown Bunny Grahams*. These are similar to commercial animal cookies, except the former are made with whole grain oats, with cane juice and molasses as the sweeteners, and the latter with whole grain wheat and honey, and both are all natural, so they are a bit healthier than the commercial variety. But I still only eat them rarely, as a special treat. But kids would love them anytime.

Also in his aisle are chips of various kinds. Again, don't fool yourself—potato chips are potato chips, an unhealthy, highly processed snack food, no matter if they are "natural" or not. But a bit healthier are tortilla chips, if they are made with whole grain corn. But they still contain refined oils and are highly processed, so they are another borderline Creationist Diet foods at best.

But I do eat the latter on occasion. But when I do, I eat them with a bowl of vegetables, cut up meat of some sort, and salsa, all mixed together and heated up. I then use the chips as a spoon, eating the mixture with the chip. My favorites are: *Garden of Eatin' Organic Blue Tortilla Chips* and *Garden of Eatin' Corn Tortilla Chips Red Hot Blues*.

Creationist Diet

The ingredients for the former are: "Organically grown blue corn, expeller-pressed canola oil and/or safflower oil and/or sunflower oil, sea salt." The ingredients are the same of the latter, except for also containing various spices. And those spices are hot.

Next in this aisle are taco shells. The ingredients for them are about the same as for the tortilla chips, so the same comments apply. And of course, you need salsa with the chips and tacos, and that comes next. As stated previously, salsa is the healthiest condiment, being just veggies and salt.

The Co-op keeps changing the brand of salsa it sells. That is shame as they carried for a short while what I thought was the best tasting salsa I ever had: *Cadia Mango Salsa*. But they no longer carry it, and I cannot find it elsewhere. But I am content with medium hot salsa of any brand. I also like black bean and corn salsa.

Dairy Foods:

Now we come to the coolers. First is milk. I got the aforementioned raw milk at the Co-op, but it also sells organic, grass-fed pasteurized milk, both homogenized and non-homogenized, all in whole, reduced-fat, and fat-free versions. The complex issues surrounding these different kinds of milk were discussed in Chapters Ten and Eleven. But here I will say, whatever decision you come to in regards to milk, it is possible to buy milk that fits your preference.

As for myself, I don't actually drink milk. As discussed, I tried using milk rather than protein powders, but the protein powders worked better for me, so I drink that and put that on my cereal and even use it in recipes instead of milk.

But in regards to raw milk, in addition to my experiment with drinking it instead of my protein powder, I later tried drinking a glass a day in addition to the protein powder. I did so because of the claimed benefits of raw milk. But I didn't notice any improvements in my health, and with the risks, I didn't continue with it.

Also available in this section is goat's milk. I've never tried it, but it is an option for those who cannot tolerate cow's milk.

Next in this section are cheeses in a tub. The first is the ricotta cheese I used in my Christmas Eve lasagna. I used the leftover in a large stir fry, and it tasted great. But it wasn't until I was eating it that I read the label and found out ricotta cheese contains vinegar. The small amount I ate with the lasagna didn't bother me, but this larger amount did and led to a sleepless night.

Similarly, but more strangely, is cottage cheese. Throughout the 00s, the only time I would eat cottage cheese was when I was cutting weight for a contest, as it is a low-fat protein source, and I always had problems sleeping. That was very frustrating as of all times I want to sleep well is the week of a contest. It wasn't until the I entered my first contest in the '10s that I figured out it was the cottage cheese keeping me awake. I have no idea why, as there are no ingredients in it that I am allergic to otherwise, but once I stopped using it, I was able to sleep before a contest. I relate this as a warning to other athletes. Do not eat something out of the ordinary before an important game or contest.

But for those without such problems, organic, grass-fed ricotta and cottage cheeses can be high protein sources to add to one's diet.

But the next items are pure fat, with no protein: cream cheese and butter. I never use cream cheese and only use butter sparingly, mostly on baked potatoes and in recipes.

The next item is yogurt, and it I eat regularly. My favorite is *Stonyfield Farms* organic, pasture raised, low-fat, plain yogurt. It also comes in fat-free and whole-fat, but the former doesn't taste as good, while the latter tastes too rich for me. But all three are options. However, I would not recommend the vanilla or maple flavors, as they have a large amount of added sugar.

Next are eggs. The Co-op carries many different brands. Most are organic and free range and from local farms, just the kind of eggs recommended in this book.

Meats:

The meats at the Co-op were discussed in Chapter Six. But to reiterate, most are from local farms. They carry both fresh and frozen meats. The beef is organic and grass-fed, while the poultry is organic, and free range. I get most of my meats elsewhere, but I always look over the meats to see if anything looks particularly appealing or is on sale.

At a recent trip, free range chicken quarters were on sale, so I bought a couple of packages. Then another time organic, grass-fed arm roast and sirloin steak were on sale, so I bought enough for a couple of meals. All of these meats tasted great.

Creationist Diet

When I have a contest coming up, I get a couple of packages of chip steak, cook it up the week before weigh-ins, then make sandwiches after weigh-ins for the aforementioned replenishment of glycogen and testosterone levels. The bread I use will be mentioned in a moment.

But first, I might also get some grass-fed beef hot dogs and antibiotic-free chicken sausage. Given how low in fat they are, they probably do not grind up the cover fat or skin, respectively, into the products, so they sort of fit with a Creationist Diet. But still, they are higher in fat and more processed than their whole meat counterparts, so I only eat them on rare occasions for something different.

Sprouted Grain Products:

The Co-op carries many sprouted grain products. As mentioned, these are a bit healthier than regular whole grain products, so most of the bread products I eat are sprouted grain. They are all found in the freezer section. There are various types of sprouted grain bread, along with sprouted grain bagels, English muffins, hamburger buns, pita bread, and tortillas.

I use the bread for my lunchtime and post-weigh-ins sandwiches. When I eat the spinach omelet for breakfast, I eat with it a toasted bagel or English muffin with raw honey spread on it.

The pita bread I use to make pita pizza. Just spread some spaghetti or pizza sauce on the top of the pita, then add grated mozzarella cheese and chopped green peppers, and sprinkle on garlic salt and red pepper, and put in a toaster oven for 10 minutes. With a side of stir fry vegetables, it makes for a tasty and healthy lunch.

I wrap the tortilla around cut-up beef stew meat or ground turkey, cheese, and lots of veggies, and heat it up in a toaster oven. I usually heat up the meat, cheese, and veggie mixture in a bowl in the microwave for four minutes before putting it in the tortilla, otherwise, it does not get hot enough. I use wooden toothpicks to keep the tortilla from opening up while it is cooking. I then eat it with lots of salsa.

Frozen Vegetables and Fruits:

Next up are frozen vegetables. These are great for when I run out of fresh vegetables. I also use half of a ten-ounce box of thawed-out and drained frozen spinach for my breakfast spinach omelet. The frozen vegetables are all organic. I will buy a bag or two of each kind and stock up when they are on sale, while I buy several boxes of spinach.

The Co-op carries: frozen green beans, broccoli, three-color carrots, chard (not as tasty as collard greens or kale but still edible), kale, corn, okra, peas (not edible!), winter squash, mixed vegetables (which contain peas, so a no go for me), spinach, and stir fry vegetables (a mixture of green beans, broccoli, green peppers, onions, and mushrooms).

On the last item, I have to pick out the mushrooms, as I am allergic to them, and I don't actually use it for my stir-fried vegetables. For that, I use fresh vegetables. But the stir fry mixture works great in chicken catchatore. Just put skinned chicken pieces in an oven pan, add a large can of diced tomatoes, a couple of bags of the stir fry vegetables, and garlic salt to taste, and put in the oven for 90 minutes at 375 degrees. Serve over brown rice or quinoa. A simple but very tasty and healthy meal. As an alternative, can use beef stew meat instead of chicken for beef catchatore.

Next are frozen fruits, again, all organic: strawberries, blueberries, blackberries, raspberries, cherries, mango pieces, and peach slices are all available. These are a rather expensive, so I only use them in my morning oatmeal. I put a cup of the frozen fruit in a small dish the day before in the fridge, then in the morning I have not only thawed fruit but the juice in the dish to mix into my oatmeal. Add a small handful of nuts and some salt, and it is a very tasty breakfast. No sugar is needed.

I cut down on the cost by stocking up when the frozen fruits are on sale. My favorite fruit is cherries, but organic fresh cherries are terribly expensive, and non-organic cherries are one of the most pesticide contaminated fruits or vegetables there is, so I really stock up when the frozen organic cherries are on sale.

Also, the packages are usually 10 ounces, but the Co-op recently started to carry 32 ounce packages of the blueberries and strawberries. They are much less expensive on a per ounce basis, so I get them in-between sales. Instead of these frozen fruits, I will use a banana at times in my oatmeal, which also tastes great.

Prepared Frozen Foods:

The Co-op also carries many types of frozen prepared foods. Most are vegetarian: pizza, lasagna, ravioli, burritos, waffles, and the like. But these are only as healthy as the ingredients, and that usually includes refined flour, refined oils, and soy of some sort. Since I am allergic to soy and prefer not to eat refined grains and oils, I generally don't bother with them. But they do carry *PJ Organic Chicken Burritos* that tastes pretty good and makes for a quick meal in a pinch.

The Co-op also carries organic ice cream and frozen yogurt. I tried the ice cream once. It was way too high in fat for me, even fattier than *Haagan Daz* ice cream, so I didn't like it at all. While the frozen yogurt is way too high in sugar. Thus these natural alternatives are no better than their commercial counter parts and are best avoided.

That is it for the Co-op. On to another brick and mortar store I get groceries from.

Pounds' Turkey Farm:

Pounds' Turkey Farm (www.poundsturkeyfarm.com) was mentioned in Chapter Six. It is a small local farm that sells not just turkey products, but also beef products and whole chickens. They also carry eggs and other specialty items. Most of the meats are frozen, though they offer whole fresh turkeys that can be pre-ordered for Thanksgiving and Christmas.

As described in Chapter Six, Pounds' meats are not fully old-fashioned. However, they are not factory farm either, but somewhat in-between. That means their prices also are in-between that of fully old-fashioned meats and factory farm meats. That is why I get most of my meats here, and I am very thankful for it, as I couldn't afford to eat the amount of meats that I do if I had to get it all fully old-fashioned. Pounds' meats do not bother me allergy-wise, and they are much better than factory farm meats, so they work well.

Pounds' is also about half an hour drive from my home. But with a standalone freezer, I can stock up on frozen meats. Thus a quarterly trip to Pounds' suffices. And let me say, if you do not have a standalone freezer, I would highly recommend getting one. Not only can you stock up on meats, but you can stock up on all kinds of frozen foods when they are on sale, so the freezer will pay for itself over time. You can also prepare and freeze foods ahead of time, saving time later.

In any case, at Pound's, in poultry, I purchase: turkey breasts, turkey thighs, ground turkey, and whole chickens. In beef, I buy roasts, steaks of various sorts, beef stew meat, chip steak, ground meat, and maybe a soup bone.

I will cook up a turkey breast or a couple of packages of the turkey thighs (two in a package), cut it up, and freeze single serving potions for quick meals later. I cook the turkey breast, thighs, and whole chickens in a *Reynolds Oven Bag*, adding a couple of cups of water to it. That keeps the birds very moist and gives me broth to use on the poultry instead of gravy. I freeze the leftover broth and use it for soup later. Pounds' also sells turkey broth.

I cook up the ground turkey and beef stew meat and freeze it in a freezer bag. When I freeze it, I am careful to lay it out so the meat pieces don't freeze together. I then use that meat for my lunchtime sandwiches, cutting up the beef stew meat into slices.

The steaks are baked or grilled. One steak is enough for a couple of meals. The roast is cooked with vegetables and potatoes and makes enough for several meals with freezing the leftover meat. The ground meat is made into hamburgers and cooked on a *George Foreman Grill*. The ground meat is also used to make meat sauce for spaghetti, along with for chili, tacos, and stuffed peppers and cabbage.

The chip steak pieces are actually too big for sandwiches. That is why I get chip steak at the Co-op for sandwiches. That chip steak comes in very small pieces that are a bit of a pain to cook up, hence why I only use it for contests. But Pounds' chip steak works for eating like a steak.

The soup bone is used to make beef vegetable soup, using the beef stew meat and the aforementioned stir-fry vegetables.

I might also get turkey hot dogs, turkey kielbasa, and turkey sausage. Like the similar products at Co-op, these do not have the skin ground up in them, so they are low in fat as compared to their commercial counterparts. But again, I only eat them on rare occasions for something different.

Pounds is located in Leechburg, PA, but I am sure similar family farms can be found throughout the USA. You just need to look around to find one near your home. Again, a list of farms that grass feed their cattle can be found on Eat Wild's website (www.eatwild.com).

Giant Eagle:

I already mentioned about Giant Eagle and that it carries some organic foods, but the quantity and variety is not near as great as at the Co-op, especially in regards to produce. That is why I travel to the Co-op, despite Giant Eagle being much closer to my home. But I do get some items from Giant Eagle in-between Co-op trips, so I am glad it is nearby. The most important item is wild caught salmon, along with cod, flounder, and other fish.

Giant Eagle also carries both cut-up and whole chickens. They are marked as being antibiotic-free, hormone-free, and cage-free. But they are probably not fully old-fashioned like the chicken at the Co-op, though probably in line with Pounds' chicken and definitely better than fully factory farmed chicken, so I also get chicken here.

CVS Pharmacy:

Despite being a pharmacy, in a CVS store are usually several aisles of foods. Most of these are processed junk foods, like cookies, candy, and chips, but a few items are worthwhile. Foremost among these are peanuts and nuts. I get my peanuts here, as for some reason the Co-op doesn't carry them. What I like about CVS is they occasionally have BOGO sales, which is to say, "buy one get one" for half price. That is when I stock up on peanuts. They carry both salted oil-roasted and unsalted dry-roasted peanuts.

CVS also carries oil-roasted cashews and mixed nuts (salted and unsalted), roasted salted pistachios, and raw unsalted almonds, pecans, and walnuts. But none are organic nor even non-GMO. But as discussed in this book, with nuts, it is not that important to get organic, and there are not yet GMO nuts, so these are not major issues, and I can eat them without problem. As such, I get some nuts here when I can get them on a BOGO.

CVS also carries dried fruits, and some of these are organic, so they are worth getting, especially when on a BOGO.

Online Shopping:

I order some packaged foods online. Many of these are the same as the items I can get at the Co-op. But I will order them online in-between trips to the Co-op and when I can get them cheaper online. I also can find some items online that the Co-op doesn't carry.

'The first website I order from is iHerb (www.iherb.com). On my fitness website is a section titled, "iHerb Natural Foods Reviews" - www.fitnessforoneandall.com/info/merchants/iherb.htm.

On that section are reviews and direct links to various items available at iHerb. I won't repeat all of that here. But all of the items are all-natural, most are organic, and the reviews indicate which are healthy and which are not. Use referral code HOP815 to receive up to $10.00 off your first order.

But I will say, the most important items I can get at iHerb are *Now Foods* nuts and seeds. Available nuts are: almonds, brazil nuts, cashews, macadamia nuts, pecans, pine nuts, pistachio nuts, and walnuts. Available seeds are: chia seeds, hemp seeds, flax seed meal, pumpkin seeds, sesame seeds, and sunflower seeds.

Many of these nuts and seeds are available in both organic and non-organic versions, but even the non-organic nuts are non-GMO. Seeds, however, I have found I need to get organic, or they cause me problems allergy-wise.

Some of the nuts and seeds are available in both unsalted raw and salted roasted versions. There are even a few flavored varieties, but be careful with these as the extra ingredients might not be so healthy. But otherwise, all such nuts and seeds are very healthy and an integral part of a Creationist Diet, and most of the nuts and seeds I use are *Now* brand.

Many think cashews are legumes, but they are nuts:

A member of the Anacardiaceae family, **the cashew is a nut** and is botanically related to mangoes, pistachios and poison ivy (SF Gate. Are Cashews Nuts or Legumes?).

And note on the flax seed meal:

Flaxseeds are filled with omega-3 fats, fibre and lignans (antioxidants), which all benefit heart health. But **whole flaxseeds may pass through the intestines undigested**, which means you'll miss out on the health benefits inside the seed. **Buy ground flax seeds instead, or put them in a coffee or spice grinder** (Sydney).

Note also that the flax seed meal is available in both regular and golden. These are identical in nutrition and taste, except the golden variety looks a bit nicer. There are also regular and Marcona almonds. I've never tried the later, so I cannot comment.

I mix a tablespoon of the flax seed meal into my morning oatmeal and used a cup if it the last time I made a large batch of pancakes, using a whole bag of the aforementioned sprouted grain pancake mix. It gives both the oatmeal and pancakes a nutty flavor and texture. It would do the same for baked goods like bread and muffins.

I can also get the aforementioned *Nairn Oat Cookies* and *Crackers* at iHerb, which carries several different flavors of them.

A similar online store is Vitacost (www.vitacost.com). It also carries the preceding *NOW* nuts and seeds and many other similar items as iHerb. Some items are cheaper at iHerb and some at Vitacost, so I compare prices before ordering. I can usually get a coupon for Vitacost via their email and mail promotions or at: www.RetailMeNot.com.

One item I get at Vitacost that I cannot get elsewhere is *Edward & Sons Organic Breadcrumbs, Lightly Salted*. They work great for breading chicken and fish. I used to use *Kellogg's Corn Flake Crumbs*, but they are not organic and are not even non-GMO. As such, they most certainly use GMO corn, so I no longer use them. But the breadcrumbs work just as well and taste just as good.

I also order a few items from Amazon (www.Amazon.com). Unlike the preceding two stores, Amazon generally does not sell individual food items, but only boxes or cases. But for items that I use regularly, a case works well, as it is less expensive than buying the items separately. Using Amazon's "Subscribe and save" service saves even more.

I use that service to get the canned fish items I eat for my morning snack: tuna fish, salmon, mackerel, and sardines. I also get my oatmeal that way, *Bob's Red Mill Organic Quick Cooking Rolled Oats* to be exact, along with *Epic Venison Bars* and *Omega Nutrition Flax Seed Oil*, which I use on my dinner salad, alternating it with olive oil.

It is important to put oil on your salad for the following reason:

Vegetables contain fat-soluble vitamins A, E and K, and a host of antioxidants that require fat to be absorbed. If you skip the oil and vinegar, you miss out on key nutrients from the salad. Serve your greens with oil-based dressing, nuts, seeds or avocado to dramatically boost your body's ability to soak up the veggies' beneficial nutrients (Sydney).

Lastly, I order the aforementioned *Optimum Nutrition's Natural Whey* and *Natural Casein* at: www.Bodybuilding.com.

Dad's Organic Garden and Apples Trees:

I would be remiss if I did not mention one last source for food—my dad's all-organic garden and apple trees. I never got into gardening myself, but my dad has kept a garden for as long as I can remember, and I am more than willing to eat the fruits thereof!

Nothing is better than freshly picked produce. My dad often brags about picking lettuce and tomatoes in the morning then using them in a salad that day, "Can't get any fresher than that!"

Through the course of the summer, he gives me: broccoli, cabbage, carrots, cauliflower, collard greens, corn on the cob, cucumbers, green beans, green peppers, kale, leaf and romaine lettuce, grape tomatoes, onions, potatoes, and tomatoes. It all tastes great and is much appreciated, and it saves me money at the Co-op.

This is another reason having a standalone freezer is a good idea. I freeze many of these items for use later in the year. The green peppers, for instance, I chop up, bag, and freeze for use on my pita pizza. Just a few peppers give me enough for on my pizzas for the rest of the year. And I was still eating corn on the cob the following Easter this year.

But one item he grows that I cannot eat is zucchini, as I am allergic to it. That is a shame, as he always ends up with lots of it. Last year, he was giving it away to all of his neighbors. But this year I bought a couple packages of organic yellow squash seeds at the Co-op and gave them to him to plant, as that I can eat, and it is similar to zucchini.

Then in the fall, my dad's apple trees come to fruition. This past year he had such a bountiful harvest, I couldn't keep up with all of the apples he was giving me. And he made several apples pies, while also giving many apples away to his neighbors.

Keeping a garden and fruit trees is a great way to attain fresh-as-can-be, healthy, inexpensive produce. Just use natural fertilizer (i.e. manure) not chemical fertilizers on it. The latter would ruin the whole point of a garden. But of course, a garden can be time-consuming. And that leads to the final section of this book.

Time and Money

If you switch from a processed food diet to a Creationist Diet, there is no doubt you will spend more time in the kitchen preparing meals. Nothing you can make at home will be as quick or as simple as ordering in a pizza. Time must be spent purchasing then preparing the food. But that is why I have given some tips in this regard in this chapter.

As mentioned, I spend time in the kitchen preparing foods for later on two of the days I do not work out. I cut up produce, cook, cut up, and freeze meats, bake and freeze baked goods, such as the aforementioned batch of pancakes, which I separate with wax paper and freeze in freezer bags. That saves time for meals later.

Then there are the financial costs. As mentioned in the previous chapter, there is no doubt that a whole foods diet is more expensive than a junk food diet. To put it another way, your food budget will go up if you switch from a processed foods diet to a Creationist Diet. But I have mentioned a few tips on saving money that I hope are helpful.

But still, there will be extra time and money spent on food that could be spent otherwise, and only the reader can decide for yourself if it is worth it. But as for this writer, the answer is a responding "YES."

Having suffered with many health problems in my life, I know how time-consuming and expensive they can be. Consequently, in the long run, you will not be saving time nor money by eating processed foods. Eventually, all of that junk will lead to health problems that will sap all of your time and savings, and even before then, you will not have as much energy for daily activities.

As an old car repair shop advertisement said, "Pay me now, or pay me later." If you don't keep up with the upkeep on your car, eventually you will end up stranded somewhere, need to pay for a tow truck, and then expensive car repair bills. And the same goes for your health.

Your energy levels, sense of well-being, ability to enjoy life and to serve the LORD will be far less if you live on junk food than if you spend the time and money to consume a healthy diet.

Then health problems will leave you debilitated, alone in a nursing home, unable to take care of yourself but instead a burden to others. And you will die young, never seeing your children or grandchildren grow up, let alone your great-grandchildren being born, and you will have less time to serve the LORD and others.

As a result, when you die, you will not hear Jesus say, "Well done, good and faithful bondservant" (Matt 25:20).

The choice is yours.

Bibliography:

Authority Nutrition. Brown Rice Syrup: Good or Bad?
https://authoritynutrition.com/brown-rice-syrup-good-or-bad/

Lien, Eric. *American Journal of Clinical Nutrition*. Infant formulas with increased concentrations of α-lactalbumin1,2,3,4
http://ajcn.nutrition.org/content/77/6/1555S.full

Los Angeles Daily News. Nutrition: Ways to help the Earth with your choices of what to eat.
http://www.dailynews.com/lifestyle/20170417/nutrition-ways-to-help-the-earth-with-your-choices-of-what-to-eat

Med Page Today. Gluten-Free Diet Doesn't Protect Against Heart Disease. https://www.medpagetoday.com/cardiology/prevention/64981

SF Gate. Are Cashews Nuts or Legumes?
http://healthyeating.sfgate.com/cashews-nuts-legumes-3647.html

Sydney Morning Herald. Ten nutrition mistakes even really healthy people make.
http://www.smh.com.au/lifestyle/health-and-wellbeing/nutrition/ten-nutrition-mistakes-even-really-healthy-people-make-20170314-guy7y9.html

Creationist Diet

Appendixes

<u>Creationist Diet</u>

Appendix One
Current Books by the Author

The author of this book (Gary F. Zeolla) is also the author of many additional books and the translator of the *Analytical-Literal Translation of the Bible* (ALT). These books are all available in paperback and various ebook formats. Some are also available in hardback format.

The hardcopy and Acrobat Reader versions are available from Author House (www.AuthorHouse.com ~ 1-888-280-7715) or at Lulu Publishing (www.lulu.com). Most of these books are also available from online bookstores like Amazon in both hardcopy and ebook formats (like the Amazon Kindle®).

Ordering and further details on all of these books can be found on the translator's personal website: www.Zeolla.org.

Christian Books

Analytical-Literal Translation

The *Analytical-Literal Translation of the Bible* consists of four sections, with the first section containing four volumes, and each of the other sections containing one volume. They are:

Section One – The Old Testament
    Volume One – The Torah
    Volume Two – The Historical Books
    Volume Three – The Poetic Books
    Volume Four – The Prophetic Books
Section Two – Volume Five: The Apocryphal/ Deuterocanonical Books
Section Three – Volume Six: The New Testament
Section Four – Volume Seven: The Apostolic Fathers

Following is a short description of each volume:

535

Volume One - The Old Testament Torah:

This first volume contains the Torah (Genesis, Exodus, Leviticus, Numbers, Deuteronomy). These five books are foundational to the rest of the Bible, the Jewish and Christian faiths, and God's plan of redemption.

Volume Two - The Old Testament Historical Books:

This second volume contains the Historical Books (Joshua, Judges, Ruth, 1Samuel, 2Samuel, 1Kings, 2Kings, 1Chronicles, 2Chronicles, Ezra, Nehemiah, Esther). These books present the LORD's providence in the history of the ancient Israelite nation.

Volume Three - The Old Testament Poetic Books:

This third volume contains the Poetic Books (Job, Psalms, Proverbs, Ecclesiastes, Song of Solomon). These books contain praises to the LORD, honest expressions of personal struggles, wisdom sayings, and a romantic story.

Volume Four - The Old Testament Prophetic Books:

This fourth volume contains the Prophetic Books (Isaiah, Jeremiah, Lamentations, Ezekiel, Daniel, Hosea, Joel, Amos, Obadiah, Jonah, Micah, Nahum, Habakkuk, Zephaniah, Haggai, Zechariah, Malachi).

In these books, the LORD, speaking through His prophets, denounces Israel, Judah, and surrounding nations for their sins. These warnings are applicable to us today, as the USA and other nations are now engaging in similar sins. But there is also much uplifting material in these books, with the prophets expressing strong faith in the LORD in the face of hardships.

Volume Five - The Apocryphal/ Deuterocanonical Books:

This fifth volume of the ALT contains the "extra" books found in Roman Catholic and Eastern Orthodox Bibles as compared to Jewish and Protestant Bibles. There is much debate on whether these books are inspired by God or not. Only by reading them in a literal translation can you make a decision on this controversial issue. These books were written from 200 BC to 50 AD, so whether inspired or not, they provide insight into Jewish history and thought shortly before and during the time of New Testament events and thus provide important background to the New Testament.

Volume Six – The New Testament:

The ALT: NT (ALT3) is the only New Testament that is a literal translation of the second edition of the Byzantine Majority Greek Text, brings out nuances of the Greek text, and includes study aids within the text. It promotes understanding of what the New Testament writers originally wrote. No other English translation gets as close to the original text as the ALT. It is truly the ideal version for the serious student of the Bible.

Volume Seven – The Apostolic Fathers:

These are the writings of Church leaders of the late first to early second centuries (c. 80-150 AD). Some of these books were seriously considered for inclusion in the canon of the NT. They were ultimately rejected for the canon, but all of these APF books were popular in the early centuries of the Church. They provide insight into the mindset of the early Church immediately after the apostles and give background to the NT

Additional ALT Books

Analytical-Literal Translation of the New Testament: Devotional Version (ALTD):

The main difference between ALTD and ALT3 is that in ALTD the "analytical" information is footnoted, while in ALT3 such information is included within brackets within the text. The latter makes the information readily available, but it makes the text awkward to read and to quote from. By putting this information in footnotes, ALTD is a much easier to read and to quote from version.

Companion Volume to the ALT:

This volume provides aids in understanding the translations seen in the Analytical-Literal Translation of the New Testament (ALT). It includes a glossary for important words in the ALT, an-eight part

"Grammatical Renderings" section to explain the unique translations in the ALT, along with other background information to the ALT.

Concordance to the ALT:

This volume indexes every occurrence of most words in the Analytical-Literal Translation of the New Testament. Only minor words are omitted, like: the, a, etc. Sufficient context is provided for the reader to recognize the verse or to get the gist of it.

Why Are These Books in the Bible and Not Others?

Volume One – A Translator's Perspective on the Canon of the Old Testament:

This first volume looks at the 39 books in the Old Testament (OT) and discusses why they were included in the OT. It then considers books that could have been included and that some think should be included in the OT but were not.

Volume Two – A Translator's Perspective on the Canon of the New Testament:

This second volume covers the 27 books in New Testament and discusses why they were included in the NT.

Volume Three – The Apostolic Fathers and the New Testament Apocrypha:

This third and final volume first addresses the writings of the Apostolic Fathers, some of which were considered for inclusion in the NT. It then considers books that could have been included in the NT and that some think should be included but were not.

Bible Study

The LORD Has It Under Control: What the Bible Teaches About the Sovereignty of God:

This book is for the person struggling in life and for the person struggling with how God sovereignly works in people's lives. It goes through the Bible more or less in order. Along the way, I relate examples of how I believe the sovereignty of God has been operating in my life, in hopes that my experiences will help the reader to apply the principles to your life. It also addresses the question of the relationship of God's sovereignty to the human will or volition.

God's Sex Plan: Volume One - What the Old Testament Teaches About Human Sexuality:

God's Sex Plan: Volume Two - What the New Testament Teaches About Human Sexuality:

Does God have a sex plan? By that is meant, did God design the human race to function best by following a specific plan for how human beings are to interact sexually and to reproduce? What happens when this plan is followed, and when it is not followed? Are different varieties of sexual behaviors just as legitimate as God's original sex plan? This two-volume set explores these controversial questions.

Many issues are discussed that are related to sex, including but not limited to: monogamy, marital sex, polygamy, incest, homosexuality, premarital sex (fornication), extramarital sex (adultery), celibacy, transsexualism, reproduction, infertility, contraception, abortion, sexual harassment and assault, masturbation, pornography, gender roles, and school and other mass shootings (yes, those are related to this topic).

The Bible and Sexual Relationships Issues:

This book looks at what the Bible has to say on sexual types of relationships and related issues. By this is meant: dating, pre-marital sex, marriage, divorce, re-marriage, marital sex, extra-marital sex, homosexuality, polygamy, incest, abortion, and birth control.

Note: This book is an earlier version of the preceding two volumes.

Scripture Workbook: Second Edition; For Personal Bible Study and Teaching the Bible:

This book contains forty individual "Scripture Studies." It is divided into two major parts.

Part I covers the essential doctrines of the Christian faith. It is these doctrines that separate the true Christian faith from cultic and other deviations. Included here are twenty studies on such essential doctrines as the authority and reliability of the Scriptures, the attributes of God, the Trinity, and forgiveness and salvation.

Part II of this book covers controversial theologies, cultic and aberrant doctrines, and ethics and the Christian life. Included are twenty studies on Calvinism vs. Arminianism, Catholicism vs. Protestantism, Baptism, Spiritual Gifts, Mormonism, Sexual Relationships Issues, and much more.

Scripture Workbook: First Edition; For Personal Bible Study and Teaching the Bible:

This first edition of this book has been superseded by the preceding second edition, but it is still available. It contains twenty-two individual "Scripture Studies." Each study focuses on one general area of study. These studies enable individuals to do in-depth, topical studies of the Bible. They are also invaluable to the Bible study teacher preparing lessons for Sunday School or a home Bible study.

Scripture Workbook: Edition 1.1; For Personal Bible Study and Teaching the Bible:

This is a slimly updated edition of the previous book.

Bible Versions

Differences Between Bible Versions: Third Edition:

Why do Bible versions differ? Why does the same verse read differently in different versions? Why do some versions contain words, phrases, and even entire verses that other versions omit? Which Bible versions are the most reliable? These and many other questions are answered in this book. Forty versions of the Bible are compared and evaluated.

New World Translation: A Reliable Bible Version?

The NWT is the Bible of Jehovah's Witnesses. This review evaluates the NWT by looking at select passages from Paul's Epistle to the Ephesians. The standards I use are the same standards that I use in my book *Differences Between Bible Versions*. Simply put, does the translation faithfully and accurately render the Greek text into English?

Health and Fitness Books

God-given Foods Eating Plan:
For Lifelong Health, Optimization of Hormones, Improved Athletic Performance:

The approach of this book is to study different foods and food groups, with a chapter devoted to each major classification of foods. First the Biblical evidence is considered, then the modern-day scientific research is reviewed. Foods are then classified as "God-given foods" and "non-God-given foods." The main point will be a healthy eating plan is composed of a variety of God-given foods and avoids non-God-given foods. Much other dietary information is also presented.

Creationist Diet: Second Edition; A Comprehensive Guide to Bible and Science Based Nutrition:

What did God give to human beings for food? What does the Bible teach about diet and nutrition? How do the Biblical teachings on foods compare to scientific research on nutrition and degenerative disease like heart disease, cancer, and stroke? These and other questions are addressed in this book.

This Second Edition is 2½ times as long as the First Edition. It also presents a different perspective on diet. The First Edition mostly advocated a vegan diet, while this Second Edition advocates for a diet that includes animal foods. But, and this is very important, those animal foods are to be what are called "old-fashioned" meats, dairy, and eggs, not the "factory farm" products that most people eat. What is meant by these two terms and the incredible difference between them is explained in this book. This book also covers a wide range of diet related topics to

541

help the reader to understand how to live a healthier lifestyle according to God's design.

It should be noted, there is very little redundant material between the preceding two books, so to get the author's full perspective on diet and nutrition, it is best to read both books, though both advocate similar eating plans.

Starting and Progressing in Powerlifting:
A Comprehensive Guide to the World's Strongest Sport:

This 350-page book is geared towards the beginner to intermediate powerlifter, along with the person just thinking about getting into the sport. This book presents sound training, competition, dietary, and supplement advice to aid the reader in starting and progressing in the sport of powerlifting. It will also help the reader to wade through the maze of federations, divisions, and supportive gear now found in powerlifting.

Overcoming Back Pain:
A Mind-body Solution (Second Edition):

I powerlifted in college, but back pain forced me to stop lifting. Eventually, the back pain worsened to the point where I was crippled by it for six years. I tried various traditional and alternative treatments, but all to no avail. But then by utilizing mind-body techniques I was able to completely overcome the back pain, so much so that I was able to start powerlifting again.

Appendix Two
Proposed Books by the Author

Note: This appendix was updated a year after this book was first published.

On November 23, 2016, I finished my three-volume set *Why Are These Books in the Bible and Not Others?* and my translation of the Apostolic Fathers (see Appendix One). After finishing that massive project, I started work on a few smaller projects before starting my next major one. The first of these was to be an article for the next issue of my *FitTips for One and All* newsletter (see Appendix Four).

The article was to be on supplements and why I consider most of them to be a waste of money. But once I started it, it expanded into a two-part article, then a three-part article, with still much more I wanted to say. It was then that I realized that to fully cover the subject I needed to expand it into a full book. That book will be my next new book and will be titled, *Supplements: Most Are Worthless. A Few Are Worthwhile.*

But once I got to a good stopping point, I put that book on hold and started working on something I had been wanting to do. I started going over all of my previously published books, except for the seven volumes of my *Analytical-Literal Translation of the Bible* (ALT).

I am proofreading each book. As I do, I am correcting typos, updating the formatting, updating the appendixes, and making other minor changes. But these are not full new editions for most of the books. More like Edition 1.1 or 2.1. I am also updating the Scripture quotes to the most recent renderings from my ALT and adjusting the prices as needed. But a couple of these books required a full update.

One full update was the Second Edition of my *Creationist Diet* book. It greatly expanded the First Edition, so it is subtitled *A Comprehensive Guide to Bible and Science Based Nutrition.* It took me four months to finish this book.

The second full update is my two-volume set *God's Sex Plan.* The subtitles are: *Volume One: What the Old Testament Teaches About Human Sexuality* and *Volume Two: What the New Testament Teaches About Human Sexuality.*

543

Creationist Diet

These books are an update of my previous book on this subject, *The Bible and Sexual Relationships Issues*. It took me over ten months to finish these books, and they are also far longer and more detailed than the first book.

Now that that project is done, I will continue to update additional books. That will probably take me a year or so. I will then go back to working on the book on supplements. It will probably take a few months to finish and publish.

I will then update each volume of the ALT. However, these will be full updates, so they will be the Fourth Edition of the New Testament volume and the Second Edition of each of the other volumes.

If the LORD wills and all goes according to plan, as each volume is finished, I will publish the updated editions. But I will expand the title to *Analytical-Literal Translation of the Complete Bible*, with the new abbreviation of ALTC. The word "Complete" refers to the ALTC containing all books which were ever seriously considered for inclusion in the Bible or which provide background to the canonical books.

One update will be to add headings to each Bible book based on the information in this *Why These Books?* set. This set thus supplements the ALTC, providing background information and discussions of the canonicity (authoritative nature) of all the books included in the ALTC.

I will also update my *Companion Volume to the Analytical-Literal Translation*. It was written before I translated the OT, so it only addresses the NT. Most of it is still relevant to the OT, but I want to update it to specifically being so. The updated edition will also explain all of the changes for the ALTC. I will give it the new tile of *Companion Volume to the Analytical-Literal Translation of the Complete Bible*.

I will also change the format for the hardcopy versions of the seven volumes of the ALTC and for the *Companion Volume*. They are currently printed on 8-1/2" x 11" pages in double-columns. I used that format as I figured the cost would be less. And it is, for the paperback versions, but not for the hardback versions, which is what most people purchase. Meanwhile, I've had many comments that this larger size is too awkward to handle, and the double-columns difficult to read.

As such, for the new editions, they will be printed the same as this book in hardcopy format, on 6" x 9" pages in single columns. However, the print size will be smaller. Times New Roman 11 is used in this book, while the ALTC will be in Times 10. That will lessen the number of pages and thus the cost somewhat. But the *Companion Volume* and the following books will utilize Times 11, along with being in 6" x 9" size. Of course, this change will not affect the various ebook formats.

In addition, I will rearrange how the Biblical books are combined into volumes, so that there will only be four rather than seven volumes.

Once I complete updating all of these volumes of the ALTC and the *Companion Volume*, God-willing, my next major project will be to write further volumes in my *What the Bible Teaches* series.

The first volume was *The LORD Has It Under Control: What the Bible Teaches About the Sovereignty of God*. It was an expansion of "Scripture Study #21" in my *Scripture Workbook: Second Edition*. This *God's Sex Plan* two-volume set is the second installment in this series, hence the subtitles *What the Old Testament Teaches About Human Sexuality* and *What the New Testament Teaches About Human Sexuality*. They are an expansion of "Scripture Studies #35 and #36 from the *Workbook*.

The rest of the books in the series will be expansions of other Scripture Studies in my *Workbook*. But for the rest of the books, it will be best to go more or less in the order of the "Scripture Studies" as they appear in the *Workbook*, as they are in the order they are as there is a logical progression from one to the next.

I already took the time to tentatively decide how to group the studies into books and what the titles will be, checking Amazon first to be sure there were no books with those titles. In most cases, each book will be an expansion of more than one Scripture Study. Each book will have in its subtitle the phrase "What the Bible Teaches About ..."

The next volume in this series will be a book on the general dependability of the Bible. It will be titled *The Authority, Reliability, and Consistency of the Scriptures: What the Bible Teaches About Its Own Dependability*. The subtitle does not indicate circular reasoning but that there will be copious Bible quotes demonstrating its claims in these regards, which will then be critically analyzed. This volume will elaborate on the remaining Scripture Studies in Section One of my *Scripture Workbook*, namely studies #1,3,4,5,6. I will then work on additional books in the *Bible Teaches* series.

I will also include in this series a full update of my *God-given Foods Eating Plan* book, but I will expand it to include other areas of health.

Therefore, I will change the subtitle to *What the Bible Teaches About Nutrition, Exercise, and a Healthy Lifestyle*.

As I currently have the books planned out, there will be 17 books in this series. The exact number could change as I work on this project and find out how best to group the Scripture Studies together. But whatever the exact number of books, this will be a very long term project.

Another book I hope to write is *Original Language Texts and Translations of the Scriptures: How Reliable Are They?* This book will be similar to my *Differences Between Bible Versions* book, but it will address the relevant issues in a different manner.

In all of these books, the Bible quotes will be from my newly updated ALTC. As I use the ALTC for all of these purposes, I will be making any additional needed corrections or changes to the text. Eventually, God-willing, I hope to come out with a One Volume ALTC containing the Old Testament (Greek Septuagint), the Apocryphal/ Deuterocanonical Books, the New Testament (Majority Text), and the Apostolic Fathers. But this one volume *ALT Complete Bible* will be a long way off, as it will be working on all of these books while quoting from the ALTC that will enable me to notice any needed changes.

Moreover, due to page limitations with my current publisher, a one volume ALTC is not an option. That is why the current ALT is published in seven volumes and the new ALTC will be in four volumes. Consequently, I will need to find a whole new way to publish the ALTC, and it will probably be a method for which I will not be able to make any additional changes to the text. Therefore, I do not want to publish the one volume ALTC until I am sure I have made all the necessary changes and corrections to it. As such, if the reader reads the individual updated volumes of the ALTC and notices anything you think needs changed, please contact me (see Appendix Three).

Along the way, I also hope to update my *Starting and Progressing in Powerlifting* book, while writing a new book on powerlifting. It will be titled *Powerlifting to a T: Training Plans for Powerlifters and Other Strength Athletes*. The title refers to the book presenting various training plans, all beginning with the letter "T," which I have designed and used at one point or another in my own training.

I might also write a book on *Recipes and Meal Plans for Creationist Diet and God-given Foods Eating Plan*, as a companion to those books, along with a book or two on politics.

On the following pages are the proposed books, with their tentative titles. The books in the *Bible Teaches* series are divided by which part of my *Scripture Workbook: Second Edition* the studies are taken from, and in parentheses is the Scripture Studies (SS#) from the *Workbook* that the proposed book will be an expansion of.

Analytical Literal Translation

Analytical-Literal Translation of the Complete Bible (new editions of all seven volumes but now to be four volumes).

Companion Volume to the Analytical-Literal Translation of the Complete Bible: Fourth Edition.

Analytical-Literal Translation of the Complete Bible (One Volume Edition): Old Testament (Septuagint), Apocryphal/ Deuterocanonical Books, New Testament (Majority Text), The Apostolic Fathers.

Bible Teaches Series

From Part I:

1. Authority, Reliability, and Consistency of the Scriptures: What the Bible Teaches About Its Own Dependability (SS# 1,3,4,5,6).

2. God is God, and You are Not: What the Bible Teaches About the Attributes of God (SS#7,8).

3. God's Three-in-Oneness: What the Bible Teaches About the Doctrine of the Trinity (SS#9-11).

4. The Only Lord and Savior: What the Bible Teaches About Jesus and Salvation (SS#12-15, plus the first 2 questions in SS#40).

5. The Spiritual World: What the Bible Teaches About the Afterlife and Eternity and Angels and Demons (SS#16-19).

6. Christian Apologetics: What the Bible Teaches About Teaching and Defending "The Faith" (SS#20).

From Part II:

7. God-given Foods Eating Plan: What the Bible Teaches About Nutrition, Exercise, and a Healthy Lifestyle.

8. The LORD Has It Under Control: What the Bible Teaches About the Sovereignty of God (SS#21) – Started October 30, 2014. Finished April 26, 2015.

9. Divine Election: What the Bible Teaches About the Five Points of Calvinism (SS#22,23).

10. Catholicism vs. Protestantism: What the Bible Teaches About Unique Catholic Doctrines (SS#24-26).

11. The Charismata: What the Bible Teaches About Spiritual Gifts (SS#27,28).

12. End-Time Prophecy: Differing Viewpoints on What the Bible Teaches About the End-times (SS#30).

13. The Nature of Human Beings: What the Bible Teaches About Who We Are (SS#31).

14. Cultic Doctrines and Practices: What the Bible Teaches About Unique Teachings of Jehovah's Witnesses, Mormons, and Other Aberrant Groups (SS#32-34).

15a. God's Sex Plan: Volume One: What the Old Testament Teaches About Human Sexuality (SS#35,36). Started June 8, 2017. Finished March 15, 2018.

15b. God's Sex Plan: Volume Two: What the New Testament Teaches About Human Sexuality (SS#35,36). Started June 8, 2017. Finished April 15, 2018.

16. Christians and the Government: What the Bible Teaches About the Role of Government and Economics (SS#37,38).

17. Living the Christian Life: What the Bible Teaches About Church Issues and Spiritual Growth (SS#39, plus questions from SS#40).

Additional Christian Book

Original Language Texts and Translations of the Bible: How Reliable Are They?

Health Books

Creationist Diet: Second Edition: A Comprehensive Guide to Bible and Science Based Nutrition. Started January 2, 2017. Finished May 2017.

Supplements: Most Are Worthless. A Few Are Worthwhile - Started November 24, 2016. Paused December 3, 2016.

Recipes and Meal Plans for Creationist Diet and God-given Foods Eating Plan.

Powerlifting Books

Starting and Progressing in Powerlifting: A Compressive Guide to the World's Strongest Sport: Second Edition.

Powerlifting to a T: Training Plans for Powerlifters and Other Strength Athletes.

Conclusion

This is an ambitious list of books and could possibly keep me busy for the rest of my life. I had recently turned 57 years old when I finished my two-volume set *God's Sex Plan*. With doing so, I have now written 32 books in the past 18 years. My dad is 82 and still going strong, so it is feasible I could finish all 30 of these proposed books if the LORD so wills before He takes me home.

Here is trusting the LORD that He continues to give me the strength and ability to write these books to His glory and for the benefit of His people.

It will take me a very long time to finish all of these books. As such, if you are interested in a currently available book, go ahead and order the current version, as it could be many years before the new edition comes out.

Appendix Three
The Author's Websites, Newsletters, and Social Sites

This appendix provides details on my websites, newsletters, and social sites.

Zeolla.org
www.Zeolla.org

Zeolla.org is the personal website of Gary F. Zeolla. He is the author of Christian, fitness, and politics books, websites, and newsletters. He has a B.S. in Nutrition Science (Penn State; 1983) and attended Denver Seminary (1988-90). He is also a powerlifter, ranked in the Top 20 on the All-time open (all ages) ranking lists and has broken All-time masters (50-59 age) American and world records, plus dozens of federation records.

This site provides links to all of my writings, along with information about my Christian faith, powerlifting, and other personal details. A detailed autobiography is also available on the site.

Darkness to Light
www.Zeolla.org/Christian

Darkness to Light ministry is dedicated to explaining and defending the Christian faith. Currently available on the website are over 1,000 webpages, over twenty books and eBooks, and a free email newsletter. In these materials, a wide range of topics are covered, including: theology, apologetics, cults, ethics, Bible versions, and much more, so you are sure to find something of interest.

The name for the ministry is taken from the following verse:

"...to open their eyes [in order] to turn [them] back from **darkness to light** and [from] the authority of Satan to God, [in order for] them to receive forgiveness of sins and an inheritance among the ones having been sanctified by faith in Me" (Acts 26:18).

The words "darkness" and "light" have a wide range of meanings when used metaphorically in Scripture, but basically, "darkness" refers to falsehood and unrighteousness while "light" refers to truth and righteousness. People turn from darkness to light when they come to believe the teachings of the Bible and live in accordance with them.

Fitness for One and All
www.Zeolla.org/Fitness

I have a B.S. in Nutrition Science (Penn State; 1983). I competed very successfully in powerlifting in my late teens to early twenties (1978-85) and again in my 40s (2003-09), but health problems forced me to stop competing each time. But since 2015 and now in my mid-50s, I am once again competing successfully in powerlifting.

With all I have been through, dealt with, and accomplished, it is now my passion to help others achieve their health, fitness, and performance goals. To that end, I set up Fitness for One and All website.

Currently available on the website are over 500 webpages, hundreds of weightlifting videos, five books and eBooks, and a free email newsletter. These materials are directed towards a wide range of people, including beginning fitness enthusiasts, athletes, powerlifters, and those dealing with health problems. The name "Fitness for One and All" reflects this diversity of covered topics.

Biblical and Constitutional Politics
www.Zeolla.org/Politics

This website presents political articles and commentary from a conservative Christian and politically conservative perspective.

"Conservative Christian" includes the belief that the Bible is God-breathed and fully reliable in all that it teaches, including about politics. "Politically conservative" refers to the belief in limited government, separation of powers, traditional values, personal and national security, capitalism, freedom and liberty, and most of all, an adherence to the Constitution of the United States, following an originalist interpretation thereof.

Social Sites

Facebook: www.Facebook.com/GZeolla

Twitter: www.Twitter/com/GZeolla

Contacting the Author

The translator can be contacted by using the email link on any of his four websites. Click on the "Contact Information" link near the bottom of any page of any site.

Reviews

It would be appreciated if the reader would write a review of this book on Amazon and/ or wherever you purchased it. Such reviews are a help to others who might be thinking of purchasing this book, and it is a help to me to know what readers like and do not like about this book.

Creationist Diet

Printed in Great Britain
by Amazon

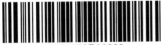

62062658R00329